Anesthesiology and Perioperative Medicine

nova
Medicine & Health
New York

Anesthesiology and Perioperative Medicine

Noninvasive Mechanical Ventilation in Anesthesiology and Perioperative Medicine
Antonio M. Esquinas, MD, PhD, FCCP, FAARC (Editor)
Peter John Papadakos, MD (Editor)
Jahan Porhomayon, MD (Editor)
Domenico Luca Grieco, MD (Editor)
Edoardo Piervincenzi, MD (Editor)
Loran Mounir, M.D. (Editor)
2022. ISBN: 978-1-68507-693-1 (Hardcover)
2022. ISBN: 978-1-68507-844-7 (eBook)

Ambulatory Multidisciplinary Management of Postoperative Pain
Irene Zapata Martínez, MD, PhD (Editor)
Jaime Ruiz-Tovar, MD, PhD (Editor)
2022. ISBN: 978-1-68507-621-4 (Hardcover)
2022. ISBN: 978-1-68507-749-5 (eBook)

Advances in PACU (Post Anesthesia Care Unit)
Ahmet Şen, MD (Editor)
2022. ISBN: 978-1-68507-506-4 (Hardcover)
2022. ISBN: 978-1-68507-543-9 (eBook)

Management of Postoperative Pain within Eras Protocols in Surgery
Jaime Ruiz-Tovar, MD, PhD (Editor)
2021. ISBN: 978-1-53619-918-5 (Hardcover)
2021. ISBN: 978-1-53619-970-3 (eBook)

More information about this series can be found at
https://novapublishers.com/?s=Noninvasive+Mechanical+Ventilation+in+Anesthesiology+and++Perioperative+Medicine&post_type=product

Ahmet Şen
and Basar Erdivanli
Editors

Organ Failure and Anesthesia Practices

nova
Medicine & Health
New York

https://doi.org/10.52305/KQRY4800

Library of Congress Cataloging-in-Publication Data

ISBN: 979-8-89113-486-7

Published by Nova Science Publishers, Inc. † New York

Contents

Preface		**vii**
Chapter 1	**Anesthetic Drugs, Fluid, Electrolyte, and Blood Replacement in Organ Failures** Seyhan Sümeyra Aşcı, Coşkun Aşcı and Ahmet Akyol	**1**
Chapter 2	**Neuraxial and Peripheral Blocks in Organ Failure Patients** Bengü Gülhan Köksal and Gamze Küçükosman	**41**
Chapter 3	**Oncological Patients, Chemotherapeutics and Anesthesia** Sinan Yılmaz and Kazim Karaaslan	**69**
Chapter 4	**Anesthesia in Cardiovascular Failures** Leman Gökçenur Aydın and Remzi İşçimen	**97**
Chapter 5	**Respiratory Insufficiencies and Anesthesia** Başar Erdivanlı and Özlem Çelebi Erdivanlı	**119**
Chapter 6	**Anesthesia Considerations in Liver Failure** Süheyla Karadağ Erkoç and Neslihan Alkış	**147**
Chapter 7	**Anesthesia During Renal Failure** Lerzan Doğan, Bülent Güçyetmez and Fevzi Toraman	**167**
Chapter 8	**Anesthesia for Endocrine Diseases** Selin Erel and Ömer Kurtipek	**187**
Chapter 9	**Neurological Insufficiencies and Anesthesia** Sadık Özmen and Yasin Tire	**225**

Chapter 10 **Postoperative Critical Care and Organ Failure in Critical Care** **261**
Cihangir Doğu and Sema Turan

Index **297**

Preface

Organ failure frequently accompanies the clinical presentations of elderly and adult patients in anesthesia practice. Today, despite the technologically advanced follow-up methods and techniques, organ failures affect the clinical picture of the patient and complicate the follow-up. Perioperative complications increase in anesthesia applications of patients with organ failure. It is important to know the physiological changes and clinical effects of organ failures and to be cautious in order to ensure that the patient is discharged as soon as possible with the least postoperative pain and side effects. Literature information about organ failure, which is very common and important in anesthesia practice, was compiled. In this book, a specific topic was chosen and it was aimed to be useful to practitioners.

Chapter 1 - Considering the patient profile in today's anesthesia practices, patients with organ failure are frequently encountered. Furthermore, the survival rates of such patients increase with the development of technology and medical practices. This will increase the number of patients with organ failure who will receive anesthesia in the future. Therefore, it is essential for us in the anesthetic approach to administer the optimum dose of anesthetic drugs to patients, regulate patient fluid and electrolyte treatments, and perform the appropriate replacement of blood products.

In this section, the authors discuss anesthetic approaches, especially in patients with renal, hepatic, heart, respiratory, and neurologic failure. If there is a contraindication to anesthetic drugs related to failure, it is important to avoid using these anesthetic drugs, and appropriate drugs should be administered by adjusting their doses and titrating. Fluid and electrolyte disorders often occur in kidney, heart, and liver failure. Necessary replacements and interventions should be performed to keep electrolytes at normal plasma levels, and in case of high plasma levels, appropriate treatment protocols should be mastered. Therefore, it is necessary to know the content and applications of crystalloid-colloid solutions. The use of blood and blood products is also of vital importance. Invasive and non-invasive methods of monitoring and biochemical tests should guide us while applying all of these treatments.

Chapter 2 - Patients with organ failure are at high risk of perioperative complications related to surgery and anesthesia. Neuraxial and peripheral nerve blocks (PNB) are believed to be beneficial for patients. However, it is important to understand the pathophysiology of the underlying disease and the physiological changes caused by the regional anesthesia techniques used so that the anesthesia technique used can provide maximum benefit to the patient and reduce the risk of complications. In the following section, neuraxial block and PNB applications in patients with organ failure will be discussed.

Chapter 3 - Today, despite the advances in diagnosis and treatment methods, cancer is increasingly ranked second worldwide as the leading cause of morbidity and mortality after cardiovascular diseases and is becoming a health problem with increasing importance day by day. According to the World Health Organization 2020 report, approximately 20 million people are diagnosed with cancer and 10 million die from cancer or related complications. Every year, 3-4 out of 1000 people are diagnosed with new cancer and it causes death in 1-2 of them. Although lung, prostate, colorectal, and breast cancers are more common, obesity and smoking are important risk factors for cancer development. Distant metastases can occur even at the diagnosis stage of cancer patients. Metastases are essential to determine the prognosis according to the type of primary tumor, the characteristics of the tissue or organ in which metastasis is detected, and the location and number of metastases. Anesthesia applications are increasing in patients receiving cancer treatment. While some of these applications are for cancer treatment, some include noncancer surgeries, diagnostic and therapeutic interventions, and imaging. Multiple anesthesia applications are increasing, especially in pediatric and disabled patient groups. In these groups of patients, changes can develop in organ and system functions that may affect the anesthesia plan and application for many different reasons.

Chapter 4 - In simple terms, heart failure means a mismatch between filling the ventricle with blood and its injection. Basically, it is defined as heart failure with low ejection fraction (HFrEF), heart failure with preserved ejection fraction (HFpEF), and HF with mildly reduced EF (HFmrEF). Heart failure patients must be well evaluated in the preoperative period and operated under hemodynamically optimal conditions. These patients must be meticulously followed during the perioperative and postoperative periods. Individuals with peripheral vascular disease represent a group with important characteristics for anesthesiologists due to the additional comorbidities that occur as a result of the primary disease or have.

Chapter 5 - This chapter discusses ways to adapt anesthetic techniques to the patient suffering from respiratory insufficiency. Traditionally, the word "respiratory" is associated with the lungs. However, the lungs are only as important as the bellows of an anesthesia workstation. The respiratory system is a complex consisting of several organs organized according to the metabolic needs of the body.

Therefore, this chapter starts with a concise review of respiratory physiology. Subsequently, pathologies related to both organs and control mechanisms are discussed. To avoid repeating things, acute pathologies are discussed first, so that comorbidities introduced due to long-standing diseases do not complicate the discussion. Pathologies are ordered from extrinsic to intrinsic as much as possible. With so many pathologies, it is difficult to summarize the text, let alone highlight the highlights. One thing to bring home though is that in many cases the treatment comes before the diagnosis. Once the patient is prevented from imminent death, treatment continues with a history and physical examination.

Anesthesia itself may cause respiratory failure. Therefore, a short section is dedicated to the mechanism, prevention, and management of crises in intraoperative and postoperative respiratory failure. Finally, some topics are suggested for future research.

Chapter 6 - Chronic liver disease (CLD) is a progressive deterioration of liver functions for more than 6 months, including protein synthesis, detoxification of harmful metabolic products, and excretion of bile. The most common causes of chronic liver diseases are chronic viral hepatitis, alcoholic liver disease, and nonalcoholic steatohepatitis. CLD causes portal hypertension that can cause complications such as ascites, gastrointestinal bleeding, encephalopathy, hepatorenal syndrome, hepatopulmonary syndrome, portopulmonary syndrome, cardiomyopathy, and coagulopathy. The reported mortality rates in patients with cirrhosis undergoing various surgical procedures range from 8.3% to 25%. This wide range of mortality rates depends on severity of liver disease, type of surgery, comorbidities, expertise of the surgical, anesthesia, and intensive care unit team. Predictors of perioperative mortality are the severity of hepatic dysfunction, the degree of portal hypertension, the urgency of surgery, and the severity of complications. The Child-Turcotte-Pugh (CTP) and end-stage liver disease model (MELD) can be used to assess the severity of liver disease and determine the risk of perioperative morbidity and mortality. The main course of anesthetic evaluation is optimizing the patient prior to surgery. Perioperative management in patients with chronic liver disease should be individualized by assessing the severity of cirrhosis and the presence of accompanying complications.

Chapter 7 - Patients with renal failure undergoing surgery pose significant challenges, given their increased vulnerability to increased morbidity and mortality. Their pre-existing medical condition and the planned surgical procedure require special consideration. Electrolyte imbalances, fluid overload, and acid-base abnormalities are among the potential medical problems these patients may face, all of which can interfere with their reactions to anesthesia and perioperative stress. Given that many anesthetics depend to some extent on renal excretion, patients with renal failure are at increased risk of experiencing adverse events due to physiologic changes associated with their condition, including reduced metabolism and elimination. Consequently, some anesthetics must be administered with caution or entirely avoided, as they can accumulate in the body or exacerbate kidney injury. Anesthetics are mainly metabolized and eliminated by the liver, so it may be preferred since the liver is able to clear them even with a low glomerular filtration rate. Therefore, it is of paramount importance to implement controlled fluid management, maintain normovolemia, optimize renal blood flow and renal perfusion, avoid hypotension, and abstain from nephrotoxic substances to prevent further renal injury. Maintenance of residual renal function should be the main goal during anesthesia, rather than the selection of anesthetic agents and techniques.

Chapter 8 - Dysfunctional endocrine organs can cause several anesthetic problems. The management of patients undergoing surgery who have primary or concomitant disease in one or more endocrine organs is discussed in this chapter. Pancreas-diabetes mellitus is the most common endocrine cause of main and secondary organ dysfunctions that affect anesthetic care. Adrenocortical hormone levels that are excessive or insufficient might lead to adrenal cortex dysfunction. Although phaeochromocytoma is uncommon, it may pose challenges during anesthesia. In the operating room, anesthesiologists may also encounter pathologies of the pituitary gland and disorders of the thyroid and parathyroid glands.

Chapter 9 - This chapter aims to provide information on the clinical features, etiology, and impact of common neurological disorders and deficiencies for anesthesia in adults, as well as the impact that these disorders have on the management of anesthesia. The topic areas in this chapter are ordered based on a combination of prevalence statistics and typical referral questions in general anesthesia clinics. This is done even though the types of neurological disorders seen in practice vary from many different variables (clinician specialty area, age range of the patients, systemic and regional issues, type, and practice affiliation). Dementia, epilepsy, multiple sclerosis, Parkinson's disease, stroke, and traumatic brain injury are some of the diseases covered in this chapter. Anesthesiologists, despite the fact that each of these disorders is unique, are frequently required to think flexibly about the characteristics of anesthesia management.

Chapter 10 - More than 300 million patients are admitted to the operation each year. This number has been shown to continue to increase the morality of noncomplication surgery is less than 1%. Postoperative complications result in a five-time increase in mortality. In surgical patients, the risk of death in the first 30 days after surgery is 1000 times higher than the surgery itself. This indicates that postoperative maintenance is as important as the operation itself. Perioperative organ damage can result in neurological complications, myocardial ischemia, acute kidney damage, respiratory failure, intestinal dysfunction, and liver failure. Acute kidney damage (AKI) is a common complication in patients admitted to the intensive care unit (ICU). More than 50% of ICU patients are AKI enhanced and 13.5% will be treated with renal replacement therapy (RRT). Perioperative myocardial injury occurs during surgery or after the administration of anesthesia and/or analgesia. 90% of patients do not show typical symptoms and the clinical diagnosis may be missed. Perioperative pulmonary complication is seen 7.9%, respiratory failure is the most common complication with 3.1%. Delirium is the most common postoperative neurological failure.

Chapter 1

Anesthetic Drugs, Fluid, Electrolyte, and Blood Replacement in Organ Failures

Seyhan Sümeyra Aşcı[1,*], MD
Coşkun Aşcı[2], MD
and Ahmet Akyol[3], MD
[1,3]Department of Anesthesiology and Reanimation, Health Sciences University, Kanuni Training and Research Hospital, Trabzon, Turkiye
[2]Department of Anesthesiology and Reanimation, Akçaabat Haçkalı Baba State Hospital, Trabzon, Turkiye

Abstract

Considering the patient profile in today's anesthesia practices, patients with organ failure are frequently encountered. Furthermore, the survival rates of such patients increase with the development of technology and medical practices. This will increase the number of patients with organ failure who will receive anesthesia in the future. Therefore, it is essential for us in the anesthetic approach to administer the optimum dose of anesthetic drugs to patients, regulate patient fluid and electrolyte treatments, and perform the appropriate replacement of blood products.

In this section, we discuss anesthetic approaches, especially in patients with renal, hepatic, heart, respiratory, and neurologic failure. If there is a contraindication to anesthetic drugs related to failure, it is important to avoid using these anesthetic drugs, and appropriate drugs should be administered by adjusting their doses and titrating. Fluid and electrolyte disorders often occur in kidney, heart, and liver failure. Necessary replacements and interventions should be performed to keep

* Corresponding Author's Email: drseyhanaydin@gmail.com.

In: Organ Failure and Anesthesia Practices
Editors: Ahmet Şen and Basar Erdivanli
ISBN: 979-8-89113-486-7

electrolytes at normal plasma levels, and in case of high plasma levels, appropriate treatment protocols should be mastered. Therefore, it is necessary to know the content and applications of crystalloid-colloid solutions. The use of blood and blood products is also of vital importance. Invasive and non-invasive methods of monitoring and biochemical tests should guide us while applying all of these treatments.

Keywords: inhalation anesthetics, intravenous anesthetics, hyponatremia, hyperkalemia, colloids

Introduction

It is crucial to choose the appropriate drug, dose, and treatment for organ failures to avoid undesirable effects and ensure optimal treatment. In this section, we review the important points to be considered in using anesthetic drugs, fluid and electrolyte irregularities, and replacement of blood and blood products in patients with organ failure.

Anesthetic Drugs in Organ Failures

Inhalation Anesthetics

As a general rule, the degree of hepatic metabolism of anesthetic agents is associated with the possibility of toxic reactions. Of the haloalkanes used in practice, halothane (available outside the United States) has been associated with the highest risk of hepatotoxicity, including acute, severe hepatitis and "halothane hepatitis." Other inhalation anesthetics currently used inhalation anesthetics (i.e., isoflurane, sevoflurane, and desflurane) can reduce hepatic blood flow but are not associated with hepatic toxicity.

Trifluoroacetyl chloride (TFA), which plays a role in the hepatic toxicity of halothane, is released less in the use of isoflurane and desflurane compared to halothane (metabolic rate: 20% for halothane, 0.2% for isoflurane, and 0.02 percent for desflurane) (Njoku et al., 1997). Liver injury is extremely rare, if any, with isoflurane and desflurane. Sevoflurane is not metabolized to TFA and has not been associated with immune-mediated liver injury.

Nitrous Oxide (N_2O)

Although N_2O is not known to cause liver injury, it can reduce liver blood flow, mainly through sympathetic stimulation. Methionine synthase can be inhibited by N_2O even after short-term exposure, but the clinical importance of impacts in healthy patients is unclear. Patients with vitamin B12 deficiency may have an increased risk of neurotoxicity when exposed to N_2O, as some patients with cirrhosis.

In some cases, total intravenous anesthesia (TIVA) may be preferred to inhalation anesthetics, which is an acceptable alternative. For example, TIVA is practical in patients with large bullous emphysema to prevent hypoxemia that may occur due to intervention in hypoxic pulmonary vasoconstriction caused by volatile agents. In such cases, it is necessary to avoid N_2O because it can cause enlargement and rupture of the bullae (Conacher, 1997). Additionally, N_2O is not recommended in patients with pulmonary hypertension (PH) due to potential increases in pulmonary vascular resistance (PVR).

Isoflurane

All inhalation anesthetics reduce hepatic blood flow (HBF) to a certain degree. Isoflurane and sevoflurane cause a small reduction in hepatic blood flow at one minimum alveolar concentration (MAC) (Schindler et al., 1996).

All inhalation agents are biodegradable to a particular degree. However, isoflurane is the agent most commonly used for the maintenance of anesthesia in liver transplants because of its low metabolic level and safe cardiovascular profile. Isoflurane is only 0.17% biodegradable. Although minimal, the hepatic metabolism of sevoflurane and desflurane leads to the release of fluoride ions. However, no reports of fluoride nephrotoxicity have been made in humans with these agents (Mcclain et al., 2015).

Desflurane

The liver does not metabolize desflurane. Therefore, it can be preferred to other inhalation anesthetic agents with respect to hepatotoxicity (Amarapurkar, 2011). Desflurane can reduce HBF by 30% at 1 MAC (Schindler et al., 1996).

It is recommended to avoid using desflurane in patients with COPD because it can increase secretions and cause cough, laryngospasm, and/or bronchospasm in smokers during induction, particularly due to its pungent odor, and it can increase airway resistance (Dikmen et al., 2003).

Sevoflurane

The theoretical renal toxicity of sevoflurane is considered due to its inorganic fluoride ion metabolite. Inhalation anesthetics (sevoflurane in particular) have previously been associated with nephrotoxicity due to the production of compound A by carbon dioxide absorbents in inhalation anesthetics. However, compound A has only been demonstrated to be nephrotoxic in rats (Anders, 2005). On the contrary, the results of the study by Bito et al., showed that compound A production during sevoflurane anesthesia did not significantly affect kidney function (Bito et al., 1997).

In patients with pre-existing renal problems, fluorinated anesthetics, particularly sevoflurane and enflurane, did not have negative impacts on postoperative renal function. None of the patients required dialysis or had a persistent worsening of renal failure (Conzen et al., 1995). Furthermore, both animal and human research has indicated that neither systemic fluoride exposure time nor fluoride peak values correspond to anesthetic nephrotoxicity (Fukazawa & Lee, 2014). In fact, there was no clinically significant renal disease or dysfunction as a result of the metabolism of enflurane to inorganic fluoride during and after surgery (Cousins et al., 1976).

The inflammatory reaction that occurs due to ischemia/reperfusion injury is the main cause of the incidence of acute kidney injury (AKI). Modern inhalation anesthetics, such as sevoflurane and isoflurane, have immunomodulatory renoprotective impacts through the activation of regulatory T lymphocytes, which stimulate the production of anti-inflammatory mediators. The study results reveal that processing inhalation anesthetics in patients with the risk of developing AKI is justified (Miklić Bublić et al., 2016). Therefore, it is possible to use sevoflurane safely in patients with stable chronic kidney disease and those undergoing dialysis.

Sevoflurane has been revealed to significantly exceed isoflurane in terms of its protective and antioxidant effects during the early phases of organ reperfusion (Dal Molin et al., 2014). Recent research demonstrated that sevoflurane preconditioning significantly decreased postoperative increase in transaminase levels in liver resection patients (Beck-Schimmer et al., 2012).

During liver transplantation, ischemic reperfusion injury occurs after blood flow is restored in the cells of the transplanted liver, which is referred to as the reperfusion phase of the liver transplant operation. Reperfusion has been considered to activate an inflammatory response. A recent randomized controlled trial argued that one of the more recent inhalation anesthetics, sevoflurane, presents greater protection against reperfusion injury (Beck-Schimmer et al., 2012). Furthermore, a short period of sevoflurane preconditioning has been shown to significantly reduce both the release of the myocardial contractile dysfunction marker and plasma cystatin C concentration levels in patients with coronary artery bypass graft surgery (Julier et al., 2003).

Sevoflurane leads to improvements in renal and cardiac functions after a major operation. Furthermore, recent research indicated that the estimated glomerular filtration rate (GFR) was better in inhalation anesthesia compared to propofol infusion in the early postoperative period after kidney transplantation (Lee et al., 2013).

Despite renal excretion of the drug, the incidence of acute renal failure was not higher with sevoflurane use among transplant recipients. Sevoflurane in liver transplant anesthesia has been argued to be as safe for renal and hepatic functions as propofol (Alonso Menarguez et al., 2012).

In case an inhalation induction technique is preferred in patients with COPD, sevoflurane is commonly preferred due to its most pronounced bronchodilator properties among the agents available (Yamakage et al., 2008). Similarly to patients with asthma, we choose a potent volatile inhalation agent (sevoflurane) with bronchodilator properties as the primary agent to maintain general anesthesia and supplement it with small doses of an opioid (fentanyl) to intensify anesthesia or suppress the cough reflex (Yamakage et al., 2008). When treating status asthmaticus, which is resistant to medical treatment, sevoflurane and isoflurane are occasionally used (Shankar et al., 2006).

Exposure to sevoflurane before, during or after hypoxic-ischemic brain injury has neuroprotective advances. Although the full mechanism is still not fully understood yet, various key processes are likely to explain this impact, and the activation of antiapoptotic gene expression, the inhibition of apoptotic cellular pathways, and changes in neuronal potassium channels are believed to provide this impact (Pasternak & Lanier, 2015).

Intravenous Anesthetics

When IV anesthetics (e.g., propofol, etomidate, and midazolam) are used for the induction of anesthesia or short procedures, they appear to not impact liver function as long as cardiac output (CO) and blood pressure (BP) are maintained.

Depending on how severe the liver disease is, different drugs require different dosage adjustments. It is usually possible to treat patients with mild liver disease with drug options similar to those of healthy ones. Susceptibility to side effects increases with worsening of liver function due to changes in pharmacokinetic and hemodynamic changes. It is necessary to consider modifications (e.g., dose reduction, titration for effect) for patients who develop cirrhosis due to advanced chronic liver disease, have portal hypertension (esophageal varices, ascites or portal gastropathy/collopathy) or renal failure.

Barbiturates

Thiopental is still among the most widely used intravenous anesthetics worldwide. It is classified as an ultrashort-acting barbiturate agent. The short duration of action following a single injection originates from the redistribution of the drug from the central circulation to the tissue of fat and muscle, rather than its metabolism. Thiopental is considerably metabolized in the liver after the redistribution described (Mcclain et al., 2015).

When the impact of cirrhosis on thiopental pharmacokinetics and binding to plasma proteins was investigated, it was demonstrated that the half-life of terminal elimination in cirrhotic patients did not change, despite the increase in the free plasma fraction secondary to low albumin levels. The researchers found that there was a small risk of long-term side effects after thiopental administration to cirrhotic patients. In contrast, considering the increased free fraction of the drug, patients were found to be more susceptible to acute poisoning (Mcclain et al., 2015). Thiopental, an intravenous anesthetic, should be administered at a lower dose, and propofol should be the preferred intravenous anesthetic agent in advanced cases of cirrhosis (Abbas et al., 2017).

When barbiturates are used alone, they can induce contraction of smooth muscles of the airways (Pizov et al., 1995). Therefore, these drugs must be avoided in patients with asthma or COPD.

Pentobarbital and thiopental infusions can be used to treat high ICP resistant to other treatments. The said agents decrease cerebral metabolism, cerebral blood flow, and cerebral blood volume. Although placing a patient in a barbiturate coma is effective for the control of ICP, it has not been indicated to increase outcomes following traumatic brain injury (TBI) (Rao & Avitsian, 2020).

Benzodiazepines

Benzodiazepines are sedative drugs that act by increasing the amount of GABA, which acts as a neurotransmitter in the nervous system. These drugs activate GABA, which suppresses neuronal function, reduces anxiety, provides muscle relaxation, and promotes sleep (Platt et al., 2016). Due to these properties, they are frequently used in anesthesia practice.

It is reasonable to use benzodiazepines as sedatives in patients with preoperative anxiety and mild asthma. Oral benzodiazepines can be administered safely in pediatric patients with asthma (Kil et al., 2003). However, the use of sedatives during asthma attacks has also been associated with some death (Bousquet et al., 2007).

Benzodiazepines are drugs with low extraction ratios. Most narcotics and benzodiazepines must be avoided, as their half-lives can be extended in cirrhosis and can worsen encephalopathy (Lewis & Stine, 2013).

Benzodiazepines are usually the first line of treatment for epilepsy and status epilepticus. Seizures should be controlled with antiepileptic drugs such as phenytoin, valproic acid, and/or levetiracetam. If seizures do not stop, benzodiazepine infusion or barbiturate coma may be necessary (Rao & Avitsian, 2020).

Ketamine

Ketamine is a crucial drug in emergency medicine and pain management all over the world due to its safety, short duration, and distinctive mode of action. It is increasingly used to treat a variety of new indications, such as pain syndromes, drug addiction, and psychiatric disorders. The main pharmacological action of ketamine is the blockade of N-methyl-d-aspartate (NMDA) receptors, ion channels primarily concerned with excitatory glutamatergic neurotransmission (Kohtala, 2021).

Administration of ketamine generally leads to significant increases in BP, heart rate (HR) and plasma epinephrine levels due to stimulation of the centrally mediated sympathetic nervous system. The impacts mentioned above are generally well tolerated, even in patients with heart failure. However, the tachycardic impact of ketamine is usually an undesirable condition in patients with ischemic heart disease. Some clinicians select a combination of 30 to 60 mg of ketamine and 20 to 30 mg of low-dose propofol with induction agents in patients with ischemic heart disease and left ventricular systolic dysfunction. In particular, the stimulating effect of ketamine depends on the presence of an adequate sympathetic reserve. Ketamine may lower blood pressure due to its mild direct myocardial depressant effect in patients who have maximally activated their sympathetic response (e.g., bleeding or cardiogenic shock).

Ketamine has bronchodilator effects and is suitable for intubation in patients with asthma (Pradal et al., 1995).

Patients with acute TBI have frequently been advised against using ketamine. Although ketamine may further increase ICP, it can be used in appropriate doses, based on the hemodynamic status of the patient, according to the physician's preference (Rao & Avitsian, 2020).

Etomidate

Etomidate is a hypnotic agent that is used to induce anesthesia. By acting as a positive allosteric modulator on the γ-aminobutyric acid (GABA) type A receptor, it produces its effect. Etomidate draws attention among other anesthetic agents because it has a stable cardiorespiratory profile that does not cause cardiovascular or respiratory depression. However, etomidate controls the adrenocortical axis by inhibiting the 11β-hydroxylase enzyme. The impact mentioned above does not make the drug suitable for long-term infusion administration (Valk & Struys, 2021).

Etomidate is beneficial in patients with HF with hemodynamic instability due to its minimal hemodynamic side effects (Das et al., 2010).

Etomidate increases airway resistance and has been associated with adrenal gland dysfunction, making it less desirable for patients with COPD to initiate IV anesthesia with it (Bruder et al., 2015).

Propofol

An intravenous hypnotic medication known as propofol is used to induce and maintain sedation and general anesthesia. Due to its potentiation of the inhibitory neurotransmitter GABA type A receptor and its acceptable drug effect profile, it has gained widespread use. Disorders in cardiopulmonary physiology are its main side effects. Propofol should only be administered by physicians trained in general anesthesia due to its small therapeutic window (Sahinovic et al., 2018).

Most propofol research has focused on its nonanesthetic effects, including its antioxidant, immunomodulatory, analgesic, and neuroprotective properties (Dogan et al., 2010). Propofol has been shown to have protective effects against ischemia-reperfusion injury in multiple organs, involving the heart, kidneys, liver, and intestines (Motayagheni et al., 2017).

The impacts of anesthetics and sedatives on recovery time and mental state of patients with cirrhosis at endoscopy and after surgery are a common source of clinical concern. The use of propofol for endoscopy has been studied with precision and has been found to not cause hypoxic encephalopathy. For cirrhosis, it seems to be quite safe to use due to its short half-life and rapid-acting effect. Propofol is preferred to the use of benzodiazepines, which can result in prolonged somnolence and encephalopathy, particularly in decompensated cirrhosis (Bamji & Cohen, 2010; Amaros et al., 2009).

If propofol is used for induction in patients with congestive heart failure (CHF), slower and lower doses (e.g., 1 to 2 mg/kg) must be used for bolus injections (Bovill, 2006). Higher bolus doses of propofol can cause profound hypotension by reducing systemic vascular resistance (SVR) due to inhibition of sympathetic vasoconstriction, reduced preload, and direct depression of myocardial contractility.

A meta-analysis comparing the impacts of propofol and volatile anesthesia in patients undergoing elective craniotomy examined intracranial pressure (ICP) and cerebral perfusion pressure (CPP). Compared to volatile anesthesia, propofol-maintained anesthesia was lower baseline mean ICP values and higher baseline mean CPP values. However, this ICP-lowering effect was not related to a reduction in brain swelling or improved operating conditions after dural dehiscence. Both techniques had similar brain relaxation scores (Chui et al., 2014).

Dexmedetomidine

Dexmedetomidine represents an α2-adrenoceptor agonist with protective effects of sedative, anxiolytic, sympatholytic, and analgesic and minimally suppressing respiratory function. Hemodynamic impacts, involving transient hypertension, bradycardia, and hypotension, are caused by the peripheral vasoconstrictive and sympatholytic properties of the drug (Weerink et al., 2017).

Dexmedetomidine is primarily metabolized in the liver. As a result, its clearance decreases and the elimination half-life can be prolonged in patients with severe liver disease. Dose titration is limited to bradycardia. Although dexmedetomidine may be related to reduced delirium and mechanical ventilation time, it has not been extensively studied in patients with liver disease (Riker et al., 2009).

Due to its short half-life, minimal respiratory depression, analgesic effects, and minimal impact on neurophysiological monitoring modalities such as evoked potential (EP) monitoring, dexmedetomidine represents a 2 adrenergic agonist that is frequently used in neuroanesthesia. In addition to the fact that it does not suppress epileptiform discharges, dexmedetomidine has recently been shown to be helpful during intraoperative seizure focus mapping (Pasternak & Lanier, 2015).

Analgesic Agents

Opioids

Opioids are still the most commonly used class of analgesics in various clinics despite the development of new analgesic agents for pain treatment. Opioids are strong, highly effective medications that have traditionally been prescribed to treat both acute and chronic pain conditions. However, the use of opioids is often associated with the development of side effects or medical problems (Mercadante et al., 2019).

These medications typically through hepatic oxidation and glucuronidation during their metabolism. Opioids are removed from the body based on their ability to bind to plasma proteins, hepatic blood flow, and hepatic enzyme activity. Oxidative enzyme pathways and opioid clearance decrease in cirrhosis, which can result in the accumulation of toxic metabolites (Tegeder et al., 1999; Chandok & Watt, 2010).

Morphine is metabolized in the liver by rapid glucuronidation. Numerous studies have shown that morphine clearance is delayed by 35 to 60% in patients with cirrhosis, despite the fact that glucuronidation is typically maintained despite decreased liver function. Furthermore, morphine has increased oral bioavailability in patients with advanced chronic liver disease or cirrhosis secondary to reduced first-pass metabolism through the liver (Tegeder et al., 1999). As a result, long-acting opioids, e.g., morphine, oxycodone, and hydromorphone, must be used in reduced doses and longer administration intervals (by reducing dose and frequency by 50%) in patients with advanced chronic liver disease or cirrhosis to prevent their accumulation and avoid side effects (seizure activity, respiratory depression, hepatic encephalopathy, etc.).

Fentanyl represents a synthetic oil-soluble opioid that is almost 80 to 100 times more potent than morphine. It is converted to inactive and nontoxic metabolites through hydroxylation and dealkylation in the liver (Haberer et al., 1982). It has a short redistribution phase and a patient-controlled fentanyl analgesia regimen can be used to control pain in the immediate postoperative period in patients with end-stage renal disease (ESRD). Elimination of the bolus dose of fentanyl does not change significantly in patients with cirrhosis, but long-term impacts can occur with repeated administration or infusion (Tegeder et al., 1999). According to the guidelines for intravenous hypnotic regimens (IHR) in patients with liver disease, opioids have been used successfully in patients with liver disease. Fentanyl is preferred the most in patients without problems with liver oxygenation and blood flow (Soleimanpour et al., 2015).

Remifentanil is rapidly hydrolyzed by esterases of blood and tissue. The clearance and elimination time of remifentanil do not change in patients with severe liver disease. It is possible to use remifentanil with the objective of facilitating laryngoscopy in patients who do not require rapid serial intubation. For the mentioned technique, 1 to 2 mg / kg propofol is administered, followed by a relatively high dose of the ultrashort-acting opioid remifentanil (e.g., 2-3 mcg/kg), which results in good intubation conditions in approximately 2 minutes. We administer 10 mg of ephedrine with propofol and remifentanil doses to minimize the deep bradycardia and hypotension that can result from the combination of high doses of both agents, particularly in a patient with ESRD.

Meperidine is an opioid used to treat postoperative tremor and analgesia. It is considerably metabolized to normeperidine by the enzymes CYP2B6 and CYP3A4. Normeperidine can cause severe central nervous system toxicity (such as neuroexcitatory effects, myoclonic activity, or seizures) in case of concomitant renal dysfunction. It is necessary to avoid the use of meperidine in patients with hepatic dysfunction due to increased bioavailability (intensive serum protein binding) and prolonged half-life of its toxic metabolite (Smith, 2009; Chandok & Watt, 2010).

The impact of tramadol on peripheral pain pathways occurs through the partial inhibition of serotonin reuptake. It causes less sedation and less respiratory depression due to its low affinity for opioid receptors. Hence, it is an additional opioid that is occasionally used in low doses in patients with cirrhosis (Kotb et al., 2008). It can be safe to use tramadol in patients with advanced liver disease or cirrhosis, but the experience is limited and therefore we do not recommend its use in patients with decompensated cirrhosis.

It is difficult to predict the impacts of codeine, and therefore alternatives should be considered. Chronic administration of any opioid requires an increase in dose in patients due to developing tolerance, which may result in an increased risk of hepatic encephalopathy.

Table 1. Metabolic changes and usage recommendations of narcotic and other analgesics in patients with cirrhosis

Drug	Potency[1]	Resulting active metabolite	Bioavailability in cirrhosis	Dose adjustment
Morphine	x1	Yes	Increases by 100%	Reduce the dose and frequency by half
Fentanyl	x75-125	No	Does not change (A or B in Child-pugh)	Usually none for a single dose[2]
Sufentanil	x500-1000	?	Does not change	Normal Dose
Remifentanil	x250	?	Does not change	Normal Dose
Meperidine	x0.1	Yes	Increases up to 80%	Avoid use in general (or reduce the dose and avoid chronic use)[3]
Codeine	x0.1	Yes	Decreases	Has a weak analgesic effect, and the drug should be avoided
Oxycodone	x1	Yes	Increases by 50-95%	Reduce the dose to avoid drug accumulation
Tramadol	x0.2	Yes	Increases by 2-3 times	Try alternative agents[4]

[1]Compared to parenteral morphine (potency = 1).

[2]It may depend on hepatic blood flow.

[3]Accumulation can cause seizures from the norpethidine metabolite.

[4]It may lower seizure thresholds in epilepsy; it is associated with serotonin syndrome when combined with SSRIs, TCAs, anticonvulsants, or morphine (Lewis & Stine, 2013).

Despite the use of gabapentinoids in some multimodal pain protocols, patients with ESRD are particularly vulnerable to the adverse effects (e.g., sedation and respiratory depression) of gabapentinoids.

In patients undergoing brain tumor resection, intraoperative remifentanil was found to be associated with a reduction in hospital mortality when patients receiving remifentanil intraoperatively were compared with patients receiving fentanyl (Uchida et al., 2012).

The prevalence and probability of renal dysfunction are high in patients with cirrhosis. Therefore, the majority opioids require a dose adjustment based on GFR. Although glucuronidation significantly alters the way morphine is metabolized, the resulting metabolite is toxic to the central nervous system and poorly excreted in cases of renal failure. Therefore, it would be prudent to decrease the dose of morphine or avoid morphine in patients with cirrhosis. Hydromorphone and fentanyl appear to be opioids the least affected by renal dysfunction and, unlike other opioids, produce less hemodynamic instability due to the absence of histamine release (Jacobi et al., 2002).

Sedation, constipation (risk of causing encephalopathy), and early indications of encephalopathy must be carefully monitored. The opioid must be stopped in the event of any manifestation of these complications. Due to the increased risk of cross-addiction, healthcare professionals must exercise caution when administering potentially addictive medications, such as opioids, to cirrhosis patients with a history of alcoholism (DiMartini et al., 2006).

Table 1 contains metabolic changes and recommendations for the use of narcotics and other analgesics in patients with cirrhosis.

Nonsteroidal Anti-inflammatory Agents (NSAIDs)

Due to their ability to effectively reduce pain and inflammation, nonsteroidal anti-inflammatory drugs (NSAIDs) are among the most widely used analgesics. In addition to their anti-inflammatory, analgesic,and antipyretic activities, NSAIDs have also been evidenced to protect against various critical disorders, including cancer and heart attacks. Furthermore, data from multiple placebo-controlled and meta-analysis research dramatically demonstrate the adverse impacts of NSAIDs on cardiovascular, gastrointestinal, renal, hepatic, cerebral, and pulmonary complications (Bindu et al., 2020). The primary effect of NSAIDs is to disrupt the final conversion of arachidonic acid to prostaglandins, prostacyclin, and thromboxanes by inhibiting cyclooxygenase (prostaglandin synthase). The form of acute renal failure induced by NSAIDs is associated with this direct decrease in prostaglandin synthesis induced by NSAIDs (Bindu et al., 2020).

Chronic use of NSAIDs in patients with ESRD can conceivably increase the risk of gastrointestinal bleeding in some patients at high risk. However, the risk of bleeding must be assessed individually because the short-term use of NSAIDs in the perioperative period has not been thoroughly studied (Karambelkar et al., 2015).

Acetaminophen is a common non-prescription drug used for analgesic and antipyretic purposes. It is the leading cause of acute liver failure in the United States. The single hepatotoxic dose of acetaminophen in healthy adults varies between 7.5-10 mg and is 150 mg/kg for children. In patients with liver disease, alcohol and malnutrition (even with therapeutic doses of acetaminophen) can increase this toxicity (Aminoshariae & Khan, 2015).

Postoperative pain control strategy in patients with liver failure usually includes a multimodal opioid-saving approach, which can include acetaminophen, antidepressants, and anticonvulsants. 2 g/day doses of acetaminophen (provided that pateints do not consume alcohol) are usually considered safe in patients with liver disease, while nonsteroidal anti-inflammatory drugs (NSAIDs) are considered less safe due to their renal toxicities and bleeding risks (Klinge et al., 2018; Rossi et al., 2008; Lewis & Stine, 2013).

Aspirin alone or in combination with other NSAIDs has been associated with variceal bleeding. In a case-control study, patients with variceal bleeding were 2.8 times more likely to use NSAIDs in the week before bleeding than patients with cirrhosis with nonbleeding esophageal varices (De Lédinghen et al., 1999).

Neuromuscular Blocking Agents (NMBAs)

Liver disease can influence the onset of action, metabolism, and duration of action of NMBAs. NMBAs should be titrated to effect and administered by being monitored with a peripheral nerve stimulator.

Patients with myasthenia gravis (MG) show an abnormal reaction to NMBAs due to the small number of acetylcholine receptors (AChR). In the case of treating patients with cholinesterase inhibitors, plasma cholinesterases are also inhibited, meaning that succinylcholine inactivation takes longer and patients are at risk of long-term blockade. Succinylcholine is relatively ineffective in depolarizing patients who do not take cholinesterase inhibitors because there is not sufficient normal AChR. In contrast, susceptibility to non-depolarizing NMBAs increases as a result of the decreased number of receptors. Because acetylcholinesterase is already maximally inhibited by the current use of pyridostigmine, attempts to invert residual block in patients treated with pyridostigmine may fail at the end of the procedure (Blichfeldt-Lauridsen & Hansen, 2012). It is necessary to avoid using neuromuscular blockers in these patients as much as possible.

Depolarizing Muscle Relaxants

Only one depolarizing NMBA, succinylcholine, also known as suxamethonium, exists. Two ACh molecules are joined together by an acetate methyl group. The postsynaptic nicotinic AChR binds to two ACh molecules, causing sharp depolarization followed by hyperpolarization and flaccid paralysis. Sufficient plasma cholinesterase activity and back diffusion of the drug from the neuromuscular junction determine the duration for which succinylcholine remains active (Zafirova & Dalton, 2018).

For patients with a potassium concentration <5.5 mEq/L, succinylcholine (SCh) can typically be selected with the aim of facilitating laryngoscopy in patients who require rapid serial intubation due to the risk of aspiration. It is possible to safely use SCh in dialysis patients if the potassium concentration is <5.5 mEq/L and there is no change in electrocardiographic (ECG) (Thapa & Brull, 2000). However, we avoid using SCh if the potassium level is ≥5.5 mEq/L or if any ECG changes are evident.

Similarly to healthy patients, a temporary increase in potassium of 0.5 to 1 mEq/L is observed after SCh administration. Nevertheless, this hyperkalemic response is not exaggerated in patients with ESRD. In particular, patients with ESRD have reduced levels of plasma cholinesterase, the enzyme that metabolizes SCh. Hence, the neuromuscular block caused by SCh may be prolonged (Ryan, 1977). During depolarization, the flow of potassium from intracellular stores causes a temporary increase in potassium levels. Due to the up-regulation of acetylcholine receptors in situations such as burns, trauma, and various neuromuscular disorders, there may be an exaggerated elevation of serum potassium (Martin & Richtsfeld, 2006).

Succinylcholine is metabolized by plasma cholinesterase, an enzyme that can decrease in patients with advanced liver disease. The period of action of succinylcholine may be prolonged in such patients, but this rarely has clinical significance.

Non-Depolarizing Muscle Relaxants

Nondepolarizing NMBAs are competitive ACh antagonists that bind specifically to the nicotinic AChR alpha subunits of the postsynaptic membrane. Nondepolarizing agents can be in the form of steroids (e.g., rocuronium, vecuronium) or benzylisoquinolinium (e.g., atracurium, cisatracurium) (Zafirova & Dalton, 2018).

For patients with a potassium concentration ≥5.5 mEq/L, we use rocuronium at a relatively high dose (1 mg/kg) when rapid serial intubation is required. Although rocuronium is basically eliminated by direct hepatic involvement and biliary excretion, part of it is excreted by the kidneys. Therefore, neuromuscular blockade can be significantly prolonged.

The liver metabolizes both rocuronium and vecuronium. The elimination time of neuromuscular blockade is prolonged in patients with advanced liver disease.

Atracurium and cisatracurium undergo organ-independent (Hofmann) elimination, and their elimination half-life and duration of action are not affected by liver disease (De Wolf et al., 1996). However, these agents are not ideal for rapid serial intubation due to their slow onset (3-4 min for atracurium and 5-7 min for cisatracurium).

Mivacurium is possible in patients with ESRD undergoing moderate surgical procedures (one or more hours) surgical procedures. Like SCh, mivacurium is hydrolyzed by plasma cholinesterase and does not have active metabolites. Its normal duration of action varies between 15 and 20 minutes, but recovery may be slower in patients with ESRD due to reduced plasma cholinesterase activity. The reversal (antagonism) of mivacurium with neostigmine or edrophonium is faster compared to spontaneous recovery.

NMBAs, such as vecuronium, rocuronium, and pancuronium, can be used safely in patients with COPD due to their higher affinity for the muscarinic-3 receptor. Atracurium and mivacurium demonstrate dose-dependent histamine-releasing results and can cause bronchoconstriction (Naguib et al., 1995).

Non-depolarizing NMBAs may cause residual postoperative curarization (Debaene et al., 2003; Kim et al., 2002). When administered perioperatively to patients with asthma or COPD, NMBAs must be carefully selected to minimize postoperative residual curarization.

Patients with Guillain-Barré syndrome (GBS) are extremely sensitive to non-depolarizing neuromuscular blocking agents. Autonomic dysfunction occurs in most patients with acute GBS and can lead to hemodynamic instability, orthostatic hypotension, and arrhythmias (Goudsouzian, 2001).

Cholinesterase Inhibitors and NMBA Antagonists

Conventional treatment to reverse neuromuscular block is via acetylcholinesterase inhibitors. The drugs in the class mentioned above prevent acetylcholine from being broken down, allowing it to develop at the neuromuscular junction and replace NMBs. Neostigmine represents the most commonly used acetylcholinesterase inhibitor in anesthesia practice (Zafirova & Dalton, 2018).

Anticholinesterase drugs (neostigmine or physostigmine) that inhibit NMBAs also increase airway secretions and cause bronchospasm. Therefore, some professionals suggest against using these medications in people with obstructive airway disease. (Hazizaj & Hatija, 2006). These drugs can be used safely in COPD patients when atropine is added (Bourgain et al., 1993).

The pharmacokinetics of the typical single dose administration of the anticholinesterase agent, neostigmine, at the end of surgery in patients with impaired renal function does not differ from patients with normal renal function.

Sugammadex is a modified gamma-cyclodextrin that consists of a ring with a central core. A molecule of sugammadex is connected to a steroidal NMB in a 1:1 ratio. A concentration gradient forms when sugammadex binds to NMBs, causing the other diffusion of NMB away from the neuromuscular junction (Zafirova & Dalton, 2018).

Patients with severe airway hypersensitivity can use sugammadex without risk because it has no anticholinesterase activity. In case high doses of rocuronium are used in a patient with ESRD and reversed with sugammadex, the sugammadex-rocuronium complexes are retained in the body longer than in healthy patients and are finally excreted by the kidneys. The clinical significance of this delay is unclear. Moreover, the sugammadex-rocuronium complex can be removed by dialysis.

Sugammadex is normally excreted without modification with the urine. Nevertheless, there are concerns about the possible recurrence of neuromuscular blockade in patients with end-stage renal disease, which may accompany severe liver disease. However, 158 surgical patients with end-stage renal disease who had their condition reversed with sugammadex were the subject of a multicenter retrospective review that found no instances of recurrence related to neuromuscular blockade (Adams et al., 2020).

Fluid and Electrolyte Balance in Organ Failures

Hyponatremia

The most common electrolyte abnormality found in hospitalized patients is hyponatremia. It is described to have a serum sodium level below 136 mmol/L. 10% of patients with HF usually have mild to moderate hyponatremia. Diuretics are among the most common causes of drug-induced hyponatremia. Although thiazide diuretics are most commonly blamed, non-thiazide agents such as spironolactone, furosemide, and indapamide have also been associated with hyponatremia. Some clinical research has shown that hyponatremia is related to a negative prognosis and decreased survival in HF (Urso et al., 2015).

It is not easy to treat apparent hyponatremia in heart failure. Conventional treatments, including fluid restriction, hypertonic saline infusion, and traditional diuretic therapies, are generally ineffective. Vasopressin receptor antagonists have been shown to increase aquaresis (removal of free water without electrolytes) and correct hyponatremia. However, the long-term beneficial impacts of such treatments on chronic heart failure have not yet been confirmed (Chatterjee, 2009).

The MELD score in liver failure is a formula-based scale computed from the patient's serum bilirubin, creatinine, and INR (higher values indicate more severe liver disease). Numerous studies have evaluated the use of the MELD score to expect postoperative morbidity and mortality in patients with cirrhosis. In general, a MELD score varying between 10 and 15 increases perioperative risk, and patients with a MELD score >15 should not undergo elective surgery.

In 2016, the MELD score was changed to include serum sodium concentration and identify hyponatremia as an independent prognostic factor not involved in the original MELD score. Patient selection based on the MELD-Na score has been indicated to successfully advance transplant waiting list results and require significant benefits to hyponatremic patients (Nagai et al., 2018).

Hypervolemic hyponatremia due to the action of an upregulated renin-angiotensin-aldosterone system (RAAS) is the most common sodium disorder in advanced liver disease. More than 20% of cirrhotic patients have serum sodium concentrations below 130 mmol/L, and about 50% have levels below 135 mmol/L. Hyponatremia is a powerful indicator of a poor prognosis, particularly in the case of a low MELD score. Sodium and fluid restriction and the use of diuretics are the recommended treatments for hypervolemic hyponatremia. Rapid resolution of hyponatremia with hypertonic saline can result in permanent neurological damage and osmotic demyelination syndrome, also known as central pontine myelinolysis (Bonavia & Singbartl, 2018).

Arginine vasopressin receptor antagonists (vaptans) act on the renal collecting ducts by blocking the selective V2 receptor. Vaptans increase the volume of urine in a dose-dependent way, causing a reduction in urine osmolarity and an increase in the excretion of free water. They have been shown to induce aquaresis and increase serum Na concentration in CHF patients. Satavaptan, a V2 receptor blocker, has been shown to be effective in the treatment of hyponatremia in patients with cirrhosis under diuretic therapy (Ginès et al., 2008).

Hyponatremia is commonly observed in patients with high ICP, particularly in association with subarachnoid hemorrhage (Rao & Avitsian, 2020).

Hypernatremia

Hypernatremia is described as the serum sodium (Na^+) concentration >145 mmol/L and is one of the most frequently observed electrolyte disorders in critically ill patients. The main cause of hypernatremia is water loss due to reduced intake or increased excretion of electrolytes. Hence, hypernatremia is usually considered a hypovolemic electrolyte disorder. According to clinical practice experience, its most common cause is loss of urine. Furthermore, it should be known that patients with severe sepsis undergoing 0.9% saline fluid resuscitation are prone to hypernatremia in the early period (Zhi et al., 2021).

Furthermore, the use of diuretics, particularly loop diuretics, which is common in patients with acute kidney injury, results in a loss of hypertonicity in the renal medulla, leading to a significant loss of free water. Extrarenal water losses related to fever, which are frequently seen in patients with sepsis, may also contribute to the development of hypernatremia (Ni et al., 2016). Additionally, hydrocortisone used to treat sepsis also contributes to hypernatremia (Chang et al., 2020).

Hyperkalemia

Hyperkalemia represents an electrolyte abnormality with life-threatening consequences, described as a serum potassium concentration (K^+) greater than 5.0 or 5.5 mEq/L (mmol/L). Individuals with chronic kidney disease (CKD), diabetes and CHF or taking RAAS inhibitors are at increased risk of developing hyperkalemia (Palmer et al., 2021).

In case the serum potassium concentration is <5.5 mEq/L and there is no change in ECG, emergency dialysis is generally not required before surgery, especially in a patient with chronic hyperkalemia. Chronic elevations in intracellular and total body potassium are present in dialysis patients. Therefore, the absence of ECG changes due to hyperkalemia must be considered until potassium is >6 to 6.5 mEq/L.

Hyperkalemia is a potential indication for consultation with a nephrologist to assess the need for preoperative dialysis, although there are no regulations indicating the maximum safe potassium level prior to induction of anesthesia.

The following is used in the treatment of hyperkalemia:

- Intravenous calcium (to antagonize membrane movements),
- Intravenous insulin (with intravenous glucose to prevent hypoglycemia),
- Sodium bicarbonate (primarily in metabolic acidosis),
- Beta-2 adrenergic agonist (to direct extracellular potassium into cells),
- Loop or thiazide diuretics if kidney function is not severely impaired,
- A gastrointestinal cation exchanger (Kayexalate),
- Dialysis (preferably hemodialysis) if kidney function is severely impaired (Sterns et al., 2016).

Hyperkalemia is not common in liver failure and most likely depends on the use of potassium-sparing diuretics (spironolactone, amiloride, or eplerenone), commonly used to treat ascites in cirrhotic patients (Bonavia & Singbartl 2018).

Hypokalemia

Hypokalemia is frequently seen in patients with CHF and is a powerful independent indicator of mortality. Hypokalemia is a serum potassium value below 3.5 mEq/L. Patients with advanced CHF who receive diuretic therapy typically exhibit hypokalemia more clearly. It is widely accepted that low potassium levels are associated with an increased risk of ventricular arrhythmias. Furthermore, hypokalemia can enhance arrhythmias related to CHF therapy (e.g., digoxin) and adversely affect the myocardium, decreasing the efficacy of antiarrhythmic drugs. The frequency of ventricular ectopic beats and sudden death is associated with both serum and total body potassium levels (Urso et al., 2015).

Mild hypokalemia must be corrected using aldosterone receptor antagonists, such as spironolactone or eplerenone, whereas more severe hypokalemia should preferably be corrected by potassium supplementation. Hypokalemia and metabolic alkalosis may occur in liver disease and trigger or exacerbate hepatic encephalopathy. Hypokalemia must be corrected preoperatively and ventilation should be managed to obtain normal end-tidal CO_2. Hypokalemia is observed more frequently compared to hyperkalemia in patients with end-stage liver disease (Bonavia & Singbartl, 2018).

Hypo-Hypercalcemia

Hypocalcemia (total serum calcium concentration <8.6 mg/dL or ionized calcium concentration <1.1 mmol/L) is a less-researched9 electrolyte problem in patients with HF. The clinical picture of hypocalcemia involves hypoparathyroidism, end-stage renal disease, and respiratory alkalosis (Urso et al., 2015).

It is essential to treat hypermagnesemia in order to treat hypocalcemia because elevated serum magnesium levels may result in decreased PTH production and secretion. Additionally, congestive heart failure may rarely occur during prolonged hypocalcemia. Several cases of hypocalcemia-caused cardiomyopathy have been reported that improved after serum calcium levels were normalized (Pepe et al., 2020).

Hypercalcemia may develop in patients with acute renal failure associated with rhabdomyolysis. Hypercalcemia is probably associated with hyperparathyroidism secondary to acute renal failure. The use of calcium, calcitriol, or vitamin D analogs in patients with end-stage renal disease or undergoing dialysis may cause hypercalcemia. In this case, hypercalcemia can also occur in relation to tertiary hyperparathyroidism. Finally, an increase in serum calcium levels can also be observed after a kidney transplant (Minisola et al., 2015).

Hypo-Hyperphosphatemia

Hypophosphatemia (serum phosphorus concentration <2.7 mg/dL) is a less studied electrolyte problem in patients with HF. Hypophosphatemia in CHF patients is usually due to phosphate loss that is attributed to respiratory alkalosis, hypomagnesemia, and the phosphaturic impacts of diuretics. Furthermore, reversible cardiomyopathy has also been associated with phosphorus deficiency (Urso et al., 2015).

In patients with heart failure (especially congestive heart failure), decreased cardiac output and effective circulating volume trigger the sympathetic nervous system to maintain hemostasis and perfusion to vital organs. Therefore, in patients with congestive heart failure, elevated levels of epinephrine and norepinephrine are observed, which has an effect on many electrolyte abnormalities. Hypophosphatemia caused by hypercatecholamine is recognized as a net shift of phosphate from the extracellular to the intracellular compartments through beta-adrenergic receptor-mediated stimulation of phosphate uptake (Christopoulou et al., 2017).

Hyperphosphatemia occurs most frequently in patients with heart failure as a result of decreased renal phosphate excretion caused by acute or chronic renal failure. It usually begins once the glomerular filtration rate drops below 40 ml/min/1.73 m^2. Additionally, elevated serum phosphate levels have been associated with the development of secondary hyperparathyroidism, induction of cardiac hypertrophy, and heart failure (Christopoulou et al., 2017).

Calcium and phosphate balance is impaired in patients with ESRD since phosphate elimination depends on renal excretion. Vitamin D3 (1,25-dihydroxycholecalciferol) produced in the kidneys is deficient, which can lead to hypocalcemia, hyperphosphatemia, and hyperparathyroidism. Due to aggressive dialysis and antacid therapy, patients may develop hypophosphatemia (phosphate below 1.5 mg/dl), resulting in muscle weakness, tremors, respiratory failure, osteoporosis, and hemolytic anemia (Ladjević et al., 2011).

Hypo-Hypermagnesemia

Magnesium plays a role in numerous enzymatic processes and is an essential element in mitochondrial structure and function; it controls cellular potassium permeability and affects calcium uptake and distribution. Hypomagnesemia (serum magnesium <1.5 mg/dL) can also be studied in CHF patients. However, its pathophysiology has been less investigated in comparison with other electrolyte changes. Additionally, there is evidence to indicate that early detection and correction of magnesium abnormalities can improve potentially dangerous arrhythmogenic effects. Especially magnesium deficiency in magnesium balance has been documented to cause cellular potassium depletion. Furthermore, it was assumed that the detection of electrolyte disorders such as hypokalemia, hypocalcemia, hypophosphatemia, hyponatremia, and especially refractory potassium depletion in CHF patients must draw attention to the possibility of coexisting magnesium depletion. It is believed that increased mortality in CHF patients with hypomagnesemia is associated with the development of ventricular arrhythmias rather than clinical and hemodynamic deterioration (Urso et al., 2015).

Hypomagnesemia affects CHF patients more frequently, ranging from 7% in outpatients to 52% in more advanced CHF patients receiving aggressive diuretic therapy (Ralston et al., 1990).

Hypermagnesemia is a frequent finding in patients with ESRD and is the result of inadequate dialysis or magnesium intake and antacids most commonly. It may cause weakness in the skeletal muscle and increase the impacts of muscle relaxants (Ladjević et al., 2011).

Intravenous Fluids

Intraoperative fluid therapy in CHF patients is adjusted to provide adequate preload to support cardiac output (CO) and tissue perfusion while avoiding harmful elevated filling pressures. It is particularly important to maintain euvolemia in these patients, considering the risk of perioperative worsening of renal function (Fernando et al., 2020).

In the preoperative period, patients with CHF may have intravascular volume overload due to the underlying disease or volume loss due to the administration of diuretics. Fluid shift and/or bleeding during surgery and conditions that require fluid administration can significantly reduce preload. However, care should be taken to limit volume expansion in hypotensive patients. For example, anesthesia-induced vasodilation that leads to transient hypotension should not be treated with excessive fluid administration. Instead of this, the administration of alpha receptor agonists (e.g., phenylephrine) or direct/indirect sympathomimetics (e.g., ephedrine) would be appropriate.

The fluid response (i.e., an increase in stroke volume after IV fluid administration) can be predicted using the following:

- Standard hemodynamic measurements (e.g., noninvasive BP and HR),
- Transesophageal echocardiography,
- One or more invasive monitors of dynamic hemodynamic parameters in selected cases.

Fluid replacement is important for CHF patients in comparatively short, minimally, or moderately invasive surgeries in which early postoperative ambulation is planned. We usually recommend administering a smaller fluid volume (e.g., less than 1 L) rather than the 1-2 L fluid typically administered to patients without CHF. For major invasive surgical procedures, we recommend using a restrictive and balanced approach minimizing fluid administration or a targeted approach with vasopressor/inotropic support.

The use of intravenous fluids is common in the perioperative period to maintain ventricular preload conditions and compensate for losses in hemorrhage, fluid, and third space. Patients with chronic kidney disease (CKD) develop fluid overload in the early period and have impaired ability to concentrate or dilute urine. Studies conducted in critically ill patients have shown that weight gain with organ edema formation is closely related to the development of acute kidney injury (AKI) and the progression to more severe forms of AKI. Nevertheless, it is not recommended to use intraoperative diuretics to prevent AKI, except for the management of severe fluid overload (Meersch et al., 2016).

Crystalloid Solutions

For hemodialysis patients undergoing elective surgery, hemodialysis treatment is generally carried out practically the day before or the day of the procedure. If hemodialysis is provided on the day of surgery, it is necessary to take precautions for long-term anticoagulation. Providing intensive hemodialysis therapy to patients has not been demonstrated to improve results.

Therefore, we do not recommend additional hemodialysis therapy before surgery.

Patients on peritoneal dialysis should be in their dry weight before surgery, similar to those on hemodialysis. After the peritoneal dialysate is removed from the abdomen, the patients must undergo surgery. In order to treat vasodilation and negative inotropy caused by the induction and maintenance of anesthetic agents, as well as surgical bleeding, fluid replacement is typically necessary during the intraoperative period.

During the preoperative period, intravascular volume overload and pulmonary edema may be exacerbated by intraoperative fluid infusion or transfusion, which may require immediate postoperative dialysis and/or a period of non-invasive positive pressure ventilation or controlled mechanical ventilation.

If there is no hyperkalemia in a patient, we usually select a balanced electrolyte solution. In such cases, we choose normal saline. However, the administration of large volumes of normal saline can cause hyperchloremic metabolic acidosis compared to the administration of balanced electrolyte solutions (Potura et al., 2015). A recently published meta-analysis that included 6253 patients and 21 studies reconfirmed that AKI, metabolic acidosis, and hyperchloremia occurred at higher rates in fluids with high chloride content (Krajewski et al., 2015).

High ICP can be treated with a class of hypertonic solutions that cannot cross the blood-brain barrier. For the treatment of intracranial hypertension, hypertonic solutions of mannitol or sodium chloride are frequently chosen. Some studies have reported higher lactic acid levels in patients taking mannitol compared to those taking hypertonic saline. The above-mentioned findings suggest that, compared to hypertonic saline, mannitol leads to a possibly more significant decrease in intravascular volume, which can cause tissue hypoperfusion (Pasternak, 2019).

Free water (including 5% dextrose, 0.45% saline, and enteral free water) should be avoided, and only isotonic or slightly hypertonic fluids should be infused in patients with increased ICP (Rao & Avitsian, 2020).

Colloid Solutions

Colloids are administered in rare cases in which immediate and significant volume expansion is required when transfusion of packed red blood cells (RBCs) is not available or not indicated in a patient with ESRD.

Albumin is recommended in place of crystalloid for perioperative volume expansion to minimize postoperative edema in liver disease patients with ascites or hypoalbuminemia. Specific indications for albumin are as follows:

- in the presence of spontaneous bacterial peritonitis to prevent worsening of kidney failure,
- together with splanchnic vasoconstrictors for type 1 hepatorenal syndrome,
- for intravascular volume expansion after large volume (4 to 5 L) paracentesis (Bernardi et al., 2014; Runyon, 2009; Terg et al., 2009).

The detrimental effect of hydroxyethyl starch (HES) on kidney function has been known since the publication of studies comparing HES and crystalloids in critically ill patients (Perner et al., 2012; Myburgh et al., 2012).

When hemorrhagic shock is not present, the guidelines suggest using isotonic crystalloids rather than colloids and avoiding the use of diuretics and other nephrotoxic agents.

Blood Replacement in Organ Failures

Erythrocyte Suspensions

Anemia in patients with ESRD is more commonly of normochromic normocytic type, with hematocrits varying between 25% and 28%. It is mainly caused by impaired erythropoiesis (due to reduced erythropoietin synthesis and release), followed by shorter half-life of the RBC, hemolysis and bleeding activation, recurrent blood losses during hemodialysis, suppression of bone marrow due to uremia, aluminum toxicity, and vitamin deficiencies (iron, folate, vitamin B6 and B12). Preoperative transfusion is not shown in patients with stable chronic anemia and hematocrit values greater than 25%. The unnecessary transfusion increases the risk of infection and edema. If necessary, it must be administered during dialysis with the objective of maintaining fluid balance, potassium level, and blood pH (Ladjević et al., 2011).

Anemia and iron deficiency (ID) are two significant comorbidities that are frequently observed in patients with CHF and are related to poor clinical status and worse results (Anand & Gupta, 2018).

Although the exact cause of anemia in HF is unknown, some evidence points to renal dysfunction, neurohormonal and proinflammatory cytokine activation, and chronic disease anemia as contributing factors. Although packaged red blood cell transfusion can be used as a short-term therapy, transfusions are dangerous and have only transient benefits. Packaged red blood cell transfusion is considered not necessarily beneficial in patients with HF and anemia and may even be associated with worse outcomes. Hence, routine blood transfusion cannot be recommended in asymptomatic patients, especially those with nonacute anemia. Since the hemoglobin threshold for packaged RBC transfusions varies according to clinical practice procedures, it can be recommended to carefully consider individual factors when determining clinical indications for transfusion in patients with HF, involving age, comorbidities and the need for surgical intervention (Anand & Gupta, 2018).

Perioperative blood transfusion is avoided as much as possible in patients with ESRD. However, if hemoglobin <7 g / dL, a transfusion of RBC is frequently required, particularly in ongoing surgical bleeding. It is necessary to check potassium on a regular basis during transfusions because hyperkalemia can develop in an anuric patient.

RBCs are utilized to compensate for intraoperative blood loss in the event that a transfusion threshold exceeds. Erythrocyte transfusion is appropriate for patients with HF with borderline hemoglobin levels (<8 g/dL), ongoing bleeding, coagulopathy, or evidence of inadequate perfusion of vital organs. When infusions of significant volumes of blood or other fluids are required, the risk of excess volume is managed by adjusting the infusion rate and using diuretics when needed. Erythrocyte suspensions are more advantageous than whole blood because anemia patients with heart failure cannot tolerate an excessive volume increase.

In general, very few patients with a Hb value of 10 g/dL or above need transfusion. Most patients with a Hb value of 7g/dL or less require transfusion. The patient's age, other comorbidities, duration of anemia, the possibility of peroperative blood loss, and the type and duration of the operation should be taken into account in addition to the Hb value when deciding on blood transfusion.

A study examining the outcomes of nonhepatic surgery in patients with liver cirrhosis showed that perioperative mortality was high, particularly in emergencies. Furthermore, the mortality rate was reported to be very high in patients with poor liver function (CHILD/MELD) and/or in need of blood transfusion (Neeff et al., 2011).

Fresh Frozen Plasma

Viscoelastic tests, thromboelastography (TEG), and rotational thromboelastometry (ROTEM) are increasingly used in algorithms to diagnose and treat bleeding in high-risk patients (Ganter & Spahn, 2010).

Fresh frozen plasma is not routinely recommended for the purpose of correcting INR in patients with liver failure. Viscoelastic tests (thromboelastography [TEG] or thromboelastometry) can be beneficial in guiding the preoperative correction of hemostatic abnormalities in patients with liver disease. In a small study, 60 patients with cirrhosis and significant coagulopathy were randomly divided into two groups. In anticipation of invasive procedures, one group received fresh frozen plasma and/or platelet transfusion under TEG guidance, while the other under standard laboratory guidelines. TEG guidance resulted in reduced blood product transfusion without an increase in bleeding complications (De Pietri et al., 2016).

For patients undergoing closed-cavity surgery (e.g., craniotomy), perioperative hemostatic management must be individualized and more aggressive efforts may be required to correct INR with cryoprecipitate or fresh frozen plasma.

Fibrinogen plays a central role in clot stabilization. Procedures for the treatment of patients with severe perioperative bleeding and patients with severe liver disease undergoing surgery recommend maintaining a fibrinogen level between 150 and 200 mg/dL (Kozek-Langenecker et al., 2017; Rossaint et al., 2016; Nadim et al., 2016; Spahn et al., 2013). These recommendations for higher fibrinogen levels are compatible with the fibrinogen levels required for optimal clot formation in the viscoelastic test (Spahn et al., 2013). It is recommended to use cryoprecipitate instead of fresh frozen plasm for fibrinogen administration.

Platelets

Platelet transfusion is a common practice used to prevent or treat bleeding in thrombocytopenic patients. Patients with oncohemological diseases and/or those undergoing hematopoietic stem cell transplantation receive more than 50% of the platelets they need. To help physicians make the best choices regarding platelet transfusion, some guidelines have been developed based on the most recent scientific research.

Table 2. Thresholds for prophylactic platelet transfusion according to different guidelines

Indication/Procedure	AAAB	ASCO	BSH
Major Surgery	<50,000/µL (WR)	<40,000–50,000/µL (WR)	<50,000/µL(WR)
CNS or ophthalmic surgery	NR	NR	<100,000/µL (WR)
Central venous catheter placement	<20,000/µL (WR)	NR	<20,000/µL (SR)
Lumbar puncture	<50,000/µL (WR)	NR	<40,000/µL (WR)
Epidural or spinal anesthesia	NR	NR	<80,000/µL (WR)
Bone marrow aspiration or biopsy	NR	NR	Platelet transfusion not indicated (SR)
Percutaneous liver biopsy	NR	NR	<50,000/µL (MR)
Hypoproliferative thrombocytopenia after chemotherapy or allogeneic BMT	<10,000/µL (SR)	<10,000/µL (SR)	<10,000/µL (SR)
Hypoproliferative thrombocytopenia after autologous BMT	NR	Platelet transfusion not indicated (MR)	Platelet transfusion not indicated (MR)
Chronic bone marrow failure (including patients receiving low-dose oral chemotherapy or azacitidine)	NR	NR	Platelet transfusion not indicated (SR)
Chronic bone marrow failure in patients receiving intensive chemotherapy	NR	NR	<10,000/µL (SR)

Abbreviations: AABB, American Association of Blood Banks (former name); ASCO, American Society of Clinical Oncology; BSH, British Society of Hematology; BMT, bone marrow transplantation; CNS, central nervous system; NR, no recommendations presented; MR, moderate recommendation; SR, strong recommendation; WR, weak recommendation (Yuan & Otrock, 2021).

Nevertheless, there are some debated points and the available scientific evidence is still insufficient for their resolution. The clinical risk of bleeding is high in thrombocytopenic patients, particularly those with a platelet count ≤5000/μL (Solves Alcaina, 2020).

We suggest platelet transfusion to increase platelet count to ≥50,000/μL and cryoprecipitate replacement to maintain fibrinogen levels at ≥200 mg/dL both preoperatively and intraoperatively in patients with microvascular bleeding in CL failure or at risk of bleeding due to percutaneous procedures. We keep the platelet count as N>100,000/μL in patients with active bleeding and undergoing craniotomy (Table 2).

ESRD patients may tend to bleed during and/or after surgery. A patient with suspected uremia-induced platelet dysfunction can be administered IV desmopressin or, in the event of actively bleeding, platelets (one apheresis unit or six units of pooled platelets), even if there is no thrombocytopenia. In particular, platelet therapy will be only a temporary treatment for uremic platelet dysfunction because transfused platelets become dysfunctional by the uremic milieu at a variable rate.

Conclusion

In conclusion, patients with organ failure are more frequently encountered in medical practice nowadays. The use of anesthetic drugs, the balance of fluid-electrolyte and the replacement of blood-blood products in these patients vary according to the failure status and the patient. Hence, we must individualize the appropriate treatment methods on a patient basis as anesthesiologists. If a drug is contraindicated, the use of that drug and the treatment regimen should be avoided, the dose should be adjusted, and it is recommended to administer it by titration. Attention must be paid to optimizing all medical treatments and practices because this patient group is at higher risk in terms of mortality and morbidity.

References

Abbas, N., Makker, J., Abbas, H., & Balar, B. (2017). Perioperative Care of Patients With Liver Cirrhosis: A Review. *Health services insights*, 10, 1178632917691270. https://doi.org/10.1177/1178632917691270.

Adams, D. R., Tollinche, L. E., Yeoh, C. B., Artman, J., Mehta, M., Phillips, D., Fischer, G. W., Quinlan, J. J., & Sakai, T. (2020). Short-term safety and effectiveness of sugammadex for surgical patients with end-stage renal disease: a two-centre retrospective study. *Anaesthesia,* 75(3), 348–352. https://doi.org/10.1111/anae.14914.

Alonso Menárguez, B., Gajate Martín, L., García Suárez, J., Martín Martín, A., Moreno Ballesteros, R., Arribas Pérez, P., & García Fernández, J. (2012). Estudio retrospectivo comparativo entre sevoflurano y propofol en el mantenimiento de la anestesia durante el trasplante hepático. Efectos sobre la función renal y hepática [Retrospective comparative study between sevoflurane and propofol in maintaining anaesthesia during liver transplant: Effects on kidney and liver function]. *Revista espanola de anestesiologia y reanimacion,* 59(5), 237–243. https://doi.org/10.1016/j.redar.2012.03.021.

Amarapurkar D. N. (2011). Prescribing medications in patients with decompensated liver cirrhosis. *International journal of hepatology,* 2011, 519526. https://doi.org/10.4061/2011/519526.

Aminoshariae, A., & Khan, A. (2015). Acetaminophen: old drug, new issues. *Journal of endodontics,* 41(5), 588–593. https://doi.org/10.1016/j.joen.2015.01.024.

Amorós, A., Aparicio, J. R., Garmendia, M., Casellas, J. A., Martínez, J., & Jover, R. (2009). Deep sedation with propofol does not precipitate hepatic encephalopathy during elective upper endoscopy. *Gastrointestinal endoscopy,* 70(2), 262–268. https://doi.org/10.1016/j.gie.2008.10.038.

Anand, I. S., & Gupta, P. (2018). Anemia and Iron Deficiency in Heart Failure: Current Concepts and Emerging Therapies. *Circulation,* 138(1), 80–98. https://doi.org/10.1161/CIRCULATIONAHA.118.030099.

Anders M. W. (2005). Formation and toxicity of anesthetic degradation products. *Annual review of pharmacology and toxicology,* 45, 147–176. https://doi.org/10.1146/annurev.pharmtox.45.120403.095847.

Bamji, N., & Cohen, L. B. (2010). Endoscopic sedation of patients with chronic liver disease. *Clinics in liver disease,* 14(2), 185–194. https://doi.org/10.1016/j.cld.2010.03.003.

Beck-Schimmer, B., Breitenstein, S., Bonvini, J. M., Lesurtel, M., Ganter, M., Weber, A., Puhan, M. A., & Clavien, P. A. (2012). Protection of pharmacological postconditioning in liver surgery: results of a prospective randomized controlled trial. *Annals of surgery,* 256(5), 837–845. https://doi.org/10.1097/SLA.0b013e318272df7c.

Bernardi, M., Ricci, C. S., & Zaccherini, G. (2014). Role of human albumin in the management of complications of liver cirrhosis. *Journal of clinical and experimental hepatology,* 4(4), 302–311. https://doi.org/10.1016/j.jceh.2014.08.007.

Bindu, S., Mazumder, S., & Bandyopadhyay, U. (2020). Non-steroidal anti-inflammatory drugs (NSAIDs) and organ damage: A current perspective. *Biochemical pharmacology,* 180, 114147. https://doi.org/10.1016/j.bcp.2020.114147.

Bito, H., Ikeuchi, Y., & Ikeda, K. (1997). Effects of low-flow sevoflurane anesthesia on renal function: comparison with high-flow sevoflurane anesthesia and low-flow isoflurane anesthesia. *Anesthesiology,* 86(6), 1231–1237. https://doi.org/10.1097/00000542-199706000-00003.

Blichfeldt-Lauridsen, L., & Hansen, B. D. (2012). Anesthesia and myasthenia gravis. *Acta anaesthesiologica Scandinavica,* 56(1), 17–22. https://doi.org/10.1111/j.1399-6576.2011.02558.x.

Bonavia, A., & Singbartl, K. (2018). Kidney Injury and Electrolyte Abnormalities in Liver Failure. *Seminars in respiratory and critical care medicine,* 39(5), 556–565. https://doi.org/10.1055/s-0038-1673616.

Bourgain, J. L., Debaene, B., Meistelman, C., & Donati, F. (1993). Respiratory mechanics in anaesthetised patients after neostigmine-atropine. A comparison between patients with and without chronic obstructive pulmonary disease. *Acta anaesthesiologica Scandinavica,* 37(4), 365–369. https://doi.org/10.1111/j.1399-6576.1993.tb03730.x.

Bousquet, J., Clark, T. J., Hurd, S., Khaltaev, N., Lenfant, C., O'byrne, P., & Sheffer, A. (2007). GINA guidelines on asthma and beyond. *Allergy,* 62(2), 102–112. https://doi.org/10.1111/j.1398-9995.2006.01305.x.

Bovill J. G. (2006). Intravenous anesthesia for the patient with left ventricular dysfunction. *Seminars in cardiothoracic and vascular anesthesia,* 10(1), 43–48. https://doi.org/10.1177/108925320601000108.

Bruder, E. A., Ball, I. M., Ridi, S., Pickett, W., & Hohl, C. (2015). Single induction dose of etomidate versus other induction agents for endotracheal intubation in critically ill patients. *The Cochrane database of systematic reviews,* 1(1), CD010225. https://doi.org/10.1002/14651858.CD010225.pub2.

Chandok, N., & Watt, K. D. (2010). Pain management in the cirrhotic patient: the clinical challenge. *Mayo Clinic proceedings,* 85(5), 451–458. https://doi.org/10.4065/mcp.2009.0534.

Chang, P., Liao, Y., Guan, J., Guo, Y., Zhao, M., Hu, J., Zhou, J., Wang, H., Cen, Z., Tang, Y., & Liu, Z. (2020). Combined Treatment With Hydrocortisone, Vitamin C, and Thiamine for Sepsis and Septic Shock: A Randomized Controlled Trial. *Chest,* 158(1), 174–182. https://doi.org/10.1016/j.chest.2020.02.065.

Chatterjee K. (2009). Hyponatremia in heart failure. *Journal of intensive care medicine,* 24(6), 347–351. https://doi.org/10.1177/0885066609344941.

Christopoulou, E. C., Filippatos, T. D., Megapanou, E., Elisaf, M. S., & Liamis, G. (2017). Phosphate imbalance in patients with heart failure. *Heart failure reviews,* 22(3), 349–356. https://doi.org/10.1007/s10741-017-9615-6.

Chui, J., Mariappan, R., Mehta, J., Manninen, P., & Venkatraghavan, L. (2014). Comparison of propofol and volatile agents for maintenance of anesthesia during elective craniotomy procedures: systematic review and meta-analysis. *Canadian journal of anaesthesia = Journal canadien d'anesthesie*, 61(4), 347–356. https://doi.org/10.1007/s12630-014-0118-9.

Conacher I. D. (1997). Anaesthesia for the surgery of emphysema. *British journal of anaesthesia*, 79(4), 530–538. https://doi.org/10.1093/bja/79.4.530.

Conzen, P. F., Nuscheler, M., Melotte, A., Verhaegen, M., Leupolt, T., Van Aken, H., & Peter, K. (1995). Renal function and serum fluoride concentrations in patients with stable renal insufficiency after anesthesia with sevoflurane or enflurane. *Anesthesia and analgesia*, 81(3), 569–575. https://doi.org/10.1097/00000539-199509000-00026.

Cousins, M. J., Greenstein, L. R., Hitt, B. A., & Mazze, R. I. (1976). Metabolism and renal effects of enflurane in man. *Anesthesiology*, 44(1), 44–53. https://doi.org/10.1097/00000542-197601000-00009.

Dal Molin, S. Z., Kruel, C. R., de Fraga, R. S., Alboim, C., de Oliveira, J. R., & Alvares-da-Silva, M. R. (2014). Differential protective effects of anaesthesia with sevoflurane or isoflurane: an animal experimental model simulating liver transplantation. *European journal of anaesthesiology*, 31(12), 695–700. https://doi.org/10.1097/EJA.0000000000000127.

Das, S., Forrest, K., & Howell, S. (2010). General anaesthesia in elderly patients with cardiovascular disorders: choice of anaesthetic agent. *Drugs & aging*, 27(4), 265–282. https://doi.org/10.2165/11534990-000000000-00000.

Debaene, B., Plaud, B., Dilly, M. P., & Donati, F. (2003). Residual paralysis in the PACU after a single intubating dose of nondepolarizing muscle relaxant with an intermediate duration of action. *Anesthesiology*, 98(5), 1042–1048. https://doi.org/10.1097/00000542-200305000-00004.

De Lédinghen, V., Heresbach, D., Fourdan, O., Bernard, P., Liebaert-Bories, M. P., Nousbaum, J. B., Gourlaouen, A., Becker, M. C., Ribard, D., Ingrand, P., Silvain, C., & Beauchant, M. (1999). Anti-inflammatory drugs and variceal bleeding: a case-control study. *Gut*, 44(2), 270–273. https://doi.org/10.1136/gut.44.2.270.

De Pietri, L., Bianchini, M., Montalti, R., De Maria, N., Di Maira, T., Begliomini, B., Gerunda, G. E., di Benedetto, F., Garcia-Tsao, G., & Villa, E. (2016). Thrombelastography-guided blood product use before invasive procedures in cirrhosis with severe coagulopathy: A randomized, controlled trial. *Hepatology*, 63(2), 566–573. https://doi.org/10.1002/hep.28148.

De Wolf, A. M., Freeman, J. A., Scott, V. L., Tullock, W., Smith, D. A., Kisor, D. F., Kerls, S., & Cook, D. R. (1996). Pharmacokinetics and pharmacodynamics of cisatracurium in patients with end-stage liver disease undergoing liver transplantation. *British journal of anaesthesia*, 76(5), 624–628. https://doi.org/10.1093/bja/76.5.624.

Dikmen, Y., Eminoglu, E., Salihoglu, Z., & Demiroluk, S. (2003). Pulmonary mechanics during isoflurane, sevoflurane and desflurane anaesthesia. *Anaesthesia*, 58(8), 745–748. https://doi.org/10.1046/j.1365-2044.2003.03285.x.

DiMartini, A., Day, N., Dew, M. A., Javed, L., Fitzgerald, M. G., Jain, A., Fung, J. J., & Fontes, P. (2006). Alcohol consumption patterns and predictors of use following liver transplantation for alcoholic liver disease. *Liver transplantation: official publication of the American Association for the Study of Liver Diseases and the International Liver Transplantation Society*, 12(5), 813–820. https://doi.org/10.1002/lt.20688.

Dogan, Z., Yuzbasioglu, M. F., Kurutas, E. B., Yildiz, H., Coskuner, I., Senoglu, N., Oksuz, H., & Bülbüloglu, E. (2010). Thiopental improves renal ischemia-reperfusion injury. *Renal failure*, 32(3), 391–395. https://doi.org/10.3109/08860221003611752.

Fernando, R. J., Marchant, B. E., Jao, G. T., & Royster, R. L. (2020). Renal Function and Heart Failure: Assessment, Goals, and Perioperative Implications. *Journal of cardiothoracic and vascular anesthesia*, 34(12), 3175–3179. https://doi.org/10.1053/j.jvca.2020.07.010.

Fukazawa, K., & Lee, H. T. (2014). Volatile anesthetics and AKI: risks, mechanisms, and a potential therapeutic window. *Journal of the American Society of Nephrology: JASN*, 25(5), 884–892. https://doi.org/10.1681/ASN.2013111215.

Ganter, M. T., & Spahn, D. R. (2010). Active, personalized, and balanced coagulation management saves lives in patients with massive bleeding. *Anesthesiology*, 113(5), 1016–1018. https://doi.org/10.1097/ALN.0b013e3181f22b7c.

Ginès, P., Wong, F., Watson, H., Milutinovic, S., del Arbol, L. R., Olteanu, D., & HypoCAT Study Investigators (2008). Effects of satavaptan, a selective vasopressin V(2) receptor antagonist, on ascites and serum sodium in cirrhosis with hyponatremia: a randomized trial. *Hepatology*, 48(1), 204–213. https://doi.org/10.1002/hep.22293.

Goudsouzian N. G. (2001). Rapacuronium and bronchospasm. *Anesthesiology*, 94(5), 727–728. https://doi.org/10.1097/00000542-200105000-00006.

Haberer, J. P., Schoeffler, P., Couderc, E., & Duvaldestin, P. (1982). Fentanyl pharmacokinetics in anaesthetized patients with cirrhosis. *British journal of anaesthesia*, 54(12), 1267–1270. https://doi.org/10.1093/bja/54.12.1267.

Hazizaj, A., & Hatija, A. (2006). Bronchospasm caused by neostigmine. *European journal of anaesthesiology*, 23(1), 85–86. https://doi.org/10.1017/S0265021505241820.

Jacobi, J., Fraser, G. L., Coursin, D. B., Riker, R. R., Fontaine, D., Wittbrodt, E. T., Chalfin, D. B., Masica, M. F., Bjerke, H. S., Coplin, W. M., Crippen, D. W., Fuchs, B. D., Kelleher, R. M., Marik, P. E., Nasraway, S. A., Jr, Murray, M. J., Peruzzi, W. T., Lumb, P. D., & Task Force of the American College of Critical Care Medicine (ACCM) of the Society of Critical Care Medicine (SCCM), American Society of Health-System Pharmacists (ASHP), American College of Chest Physicians (2002). Clinical practice guidelines for the sustained use of sedatives and analgesics in the critically ill adult. *Critical care medicine*, 30(1), 119–141. https://doi.org/10.1097/00003246-200201000-00020.

Karambelkar, A., Kasekar, R., & Palevsky, P. M. (2015). Perioperative Pharmacologic Management of Patients with End Stage Renal Disease. *Seminars in dialysis*, 28(4), 392–396. https://doi.org/10.1111/sdi.12384.

Klinge, M., Coppler, T., Liebschutz, J. M., Dugum, M., Wassan, A., DiMartini, A., & Rogal, S. (2018). The assessment and management of pain in cirrhosis. *Current hepatology reports*, 17(1), 42–51. https://doi.org/10.1007/s11901-018-0389-7.

Kil, N., Zhu, J. F., VanWagnen, C., & Abdulhamid, I. (2003). The effects of midazolam on pediatric patients with asthma. *Pediatric dentistry*, 25(2), 137–142.

Kim, K. S., Lew, S. H., Cho, H. Y., & Cheong, M. A. (2002). Residual paralysis induced by either vecuronium or rocuronium after reversal with pyridostigmine. *Anesthesia and analgesia*, 95(6). https://doi.org/10.1097/00000539-200212000-00033.

Kohtala S. (2021). Ketamine-50 years in use: from anesthesia to rapid antidepressant effects and neurobiological mechanisms. *Pharmacological reports*: PR, 73(2), 323–345. https://doi.org/10.1007/s43440-021-00232-4.

Kotb, H. I., Fouad, I. A., Fares, K. M., Mostafa, M. G., & Abd El-Rahman, A. M. (2008). Pharmacokinetics of oral tramadol in patients with liver cancer. *Journal of opioid management*, 4(2), 99–104. https://doi.org/10.5055/jom.2008.0014.

Kozek-Langenecker, S. A., Ahmed, A. B., Afshari, A., Albaladejo, P., Aldecoa, C., Barauskas, G., De Robertis, E., Faraoni, D., Filipescu, D. C., Fries, D., Haas, T., Jacob,

M., Lancé, M. D., Pitarch, J. V. L., Mallett, S., Meier, J., Molnar, Z. L., Rahe-Meyer, N., Samama, C. M., Stensballe, J., Van der Linden P. J. F., Wikkelsø A. J., Wouters P., Wyffels P., Zacharowski, K. (2017). Management of severe perioperative bleeding: guidelines from the European Society of Anaesthesiology: First update 2016. *European journal of anaesthesiology*, 34(6), 332–395. https://doi.org/10.1097/EJA.0000000000000630.

Krajewski, M. L., Raghunathan, K., Paluszkiewicz, S. M., Schermer, C. R., & Shaw, A. D. (2015). Meta-analysis of high- versus low-chloride content in perioperative and critical care fluid resuscitation. *The British journal of surgery*, 102(1), 24–36. https://doi.org/10.1002/bjs.9651.

Julier, K., da Silva, R., Garcia, C., Bestmann, L., Frascarolo, P., Zollinger, A., Chassot, P. G., Schmid, E. R., Turina, M. I., von Segesser, L. K., Pasch, T., Spahn, D. R., & Zaugg, M. (2003). Preconditioning by sevoflurane decreases biochemical markers for myocardial and renal dysfunction in coronary artery bypass graft surgery: a double-blinded, placebo-controlled, multicenter study. *Anesthesiology*, 98(6), 1315–1327. https://doi.org/10.1097/00000542-200306000-00004.

Ladjević, N., Kalezić, N., Ladjević, I. L., Vuksanović, A., Durutović, O., & Jovanović, D. (2011). Preoperative assessment of patients with end stage renal failure. *Acta chirurgica Iugoslavica*, 58(2), 131–136. https://doi.org/10.2298/aci1102131l.

Lee, J. H., Joo, D. J., Kim, J. M., Park, J. H., Kim, Y. S., & Koo, B. N. (2013). Preconditioning effects of the anesthetic administered to the donor on grafted kidney function in living donor kidney transplantation recipients. *Minerva anestesiologica*, 79(5), 504–514.

Lewis, J. H., & Stine, J. G. (2013). Review article: prescribing medications in patients with cirrhosis - a practical guide. *Alimentary pharmacology & therapeutics*, 37(12), 1132–1156. https://doi.org/10.1111/apt.12324.

Martyn, J. A., & Richtsfeld, M. (2006). Succinylcholine-induced hyperkalemia in acquired pathologic states: etiologic factors and molecular mechanisms. *Anesthesiology*, 104(1), 158–169. https://doi.org/10.1097/00000542-200601000-00022.

Meersch, M., Schmidt, C., & Zarbock, A. (2016). Patient with chronic renal failure undergoing surgery. *Current opinion in anaesthesiology*, 29(3), 413–420. https://doi.org/10.1097/ACO.0000000000000329.

Mercadante, S., Arcuri, E., & Santoni, A. (2019). Opioid-Induced Tolerance and Hyperalgesia. *CNS drugs*, 33(10), 943–955. https://doi.org/10.1007/s40263-019-00660-0.

Mcclain, R. L., Ramakrishna, H., Aniskevich, S., III, Cartwright, J. A., Phar, L. G., Pai, S. L., Rodrigues, E. S., Martin, A. K., & Shine, T. S. (2015). Anesthetic pharmacology and perioperative considerations for the end stage liver disease patient. *Current clinical pharmacology*, 10(1), 35–46. https://doi.org/10.2174/1574884709666140212110036.

Miklić Bublić, M., Tonković, D., Sakan, S., Misir, A., & Bandić Pavlović, D. (2016). Effect of Inhalational Anesthetics on Acute Kidney Injury. *Acta clinica Croatica*, 55(3), 464–468. https://doi.org/10.20471/acc.2016.55.03.16.

Minisola, S., Pepe, J., Piemonte, S., & Cipriani, C. (2015). The diagnosis and management of hypercalcaemia. *BMJ*, 350, h2723. https://doi.org/10.1136/bmj.h2723.

Motayagheni, N., Phan, S., Eshraghi, C., Nozari, A., & Atala, A. (2017). A Review of Anesthetic Effects on Renal Function: Potential Organ Protection. *American journal of nephrology*, 46(5), 380–389. https://doi.org/10.1159/000482014.

Myburgh, J. A., Finfer, S., Bellomo, R., Billot, L., Cass, A., Gattas, D., Glass, P., Lipman, J., Liu, B., McArthur, C., McGuinness, S., Rajbhandari, D., Taylor, C. B., Webb, S. A., CHEST Investigators, & Australian and New Zealand Intensive Care Society Clinical Trials Group (2012). Hydroxyethyl starch or saline for fluid resuscitation in intensive care. *The New England journal of medicine*, 367(20), 1901–1911. https://doi.org/10.1056/NEJMoa1209759.

Nadim, M. K., Durand, F., Kellum, J. A., Levitsky, J., O'Leary, J. G., Karvellas, C. J., Bajaj, J. S., Davenport, A., Jalan, R., Angeli, P., Caldwell, S. H., Fernández, J., Francoz, C., Garcia-Tsao, G., Ginès, P., Ison, M. G., Kramer, D. J., Mehta, R. L., Moreau, R., Mulligan, D., Olson J. C., Pomfret E. A., Senzolo M., Steadman R. H., Subramanian R. M., Vincent JL, Genyk, Y. S. (2016). Management of the critically ill patient with cirrhosis: A multidisciplinary perspective. *Journal of hepatology*, 64(3), 717–735. https://doi.org/10.1016/j.jhep.2015.10.019.

Nagai, S., Chau, L. C., Schilke, R. E., Safwan, M., Rizzari, M., Collins, K., Yoshida, A., Abouljoud, M. S., & Moonka, D. (2018). Effects of Allocating Livers for Transplantation Based on Model for End-Stage Liver Disease-Sodium Scores on Patient Outcomes. *Gastroenterology*, 155(5), 1451–1462.e3. https://doi.org/10.1053/j.gastro.2018.07.025.

Naguib, M., Samarkandi, A. H., Bakhamees, H. S., Magboul, M. A., & el-Bakry, A. K. (1995). Histamine-release haemodynamic changes produced by rocuronium, vecuronium, mivacurium, atracurium and tubocurarine. *British journal of anaesthesia*, 75(5), 588–592. https://doi.org/10.1093/bja/75.5.588.

Neeff, H., Mariaskin, D., Spangenberg, H. C., Hopt, U. T., & Makowiec, F. (2011). Perioperative mortality after non-hepatic general surgery in patients with liver cirrhosis: an analysis of 138 operations in the 2000s using Child and MELD scores. *Journal of gastrointestinal surgery: official journal of the Society for Surgery of the Alimentary Tract*, 15(1), 1–11. https://doi.org/10.1007/s11605-010-1366-9.

Ni, H. B., Hu, X. X., Huang, X. F., Liu, K. Q., Yu, C. B., Wang, X. M., & Ke, L. (2016). Risk Factors and Outcomes in Patients With Hypernatremia and Sepsis. *The American journal of the medical sciences*, 351(6), 601–605. https://doi.org/10.1016/j.amjms.2016.01.027.

Njoku, D., Laster, M. J., Gong, D. H., Eger, E. I., 2nd, Reed, G. F., & Martin, J. L. (1997). Biotransformation of halothane, enflurane, isoflurane, and desflurane to trifluoroacetylated liver proteins: association between protein acylation and hepatic injury. *Anesthesia and analgesia*, 84(1), 173–178. https://doi.org/10.1097/00000539-199701000-00031.

Palmer, B. F., Carrero, J. J., Clegg, D. J., Colbert, G. B., Emmett, M., Fishbane, S., Hain, D. J., Lerma, E., Onuigbo, M., Rastogi, A., Roger, S. D., Spinowitz, B. S., & Weir, M. R. (2021). Clinical Management of Hyperkalemia. *Mayo Clinic proceedings*, 96(3), 744–762. https://doi.org/10.1016/j.mayocp.2020.06.014.

Pasternak, J. J., & Lanier, W. L. (2015). Neuroanesthesiology update. *Journal of neurosurgical anesthesiology*, 27(2), 87–122. https://doi.org/10.1097/ANA.0000000000000167.

Pasternak J. J. (2019). Neuroanesthesiology Update. *Journal of neurosurgical anesthesiology*, 31(2), 178–198. https://doi.org/10.1097/ANA.0000000000000581.

Pepe, J., Colangelo, L., Biamonte, F., Sonato, C., Danese, V. C., Cecchetti, V., Occhiuto, M., Piazzolla, V., De Martino, V., Ferrone, F., Minisola, S., & Cipriani, C. (2020). Diagnosis and management of hypocalcemia. *Endocrine*, 69(3), 485–495. https://doi.org/10.1007/s12020-020-02324-2.

Perner, A., Haase, N., Guttormsen, A. B., Tenhunen, J., Klemenzson, G., Åneman, A., Madsen, K. R., Møller, M. H., Elkjær, J. M., Poulsen, L. M., Bendtsen, A., Winding, R., Steensen, M., Berezowicz, P., Søe-Jensen, P., Bestle, M., Strand, K., Wiis, J., White, J. O., Thornberg, K. J., Quist L., Nielsen J., Andersen L. H., Holst L. B., Thormar K., Kjældgaard A. L., Fabritius M. L., Mondrup F., Pott F. C., Møller T. P., Winkel P., Wetterslev J., 6S Trial Group, Scandinavian Critical Care Trials Group (2012). Hydroxyethyl starch 130/0.42 versus Ringer's acetate in severe sepsis. *The New England journal of medicine*, 367(2), 124–134. https://doi.org/10.1056/NEJMoa1204242.

Pizov, R., Brown, R. H., Weiss, Y. S., Baranov, D., Hennes, H., Baker, S., & Hirshman, C. A. (1995). Wheezing during induction of general anesthesia in patients with and without asthma. A randomized, blinded trial. *Anesthesiology*, 82(5), 1111–1116. https://doi.org/10.1097/00000542-199505000-00004.

Platt, L. M., Whitburn, A. I., Platt-Koch, A. G., & Koch, R. L. (2016). Nonpharmacological Alternatives to Benzodiazepine Drugs for the Treatment of Anxiety in Outpatient Populations: A Literature Review. *Journal of psychosocial nursing and mental health services*, 54(8), 35–42. https://doi.org/10.3928/02793695-20160725-07.

Potura, E., Lindner, G., Biesenbach, P., Funk, G. C., Reiterer, C., Kabon, B., Schwarz, C., Druml, W., & Fleischmann, E. (2015). An acetate-buffered balanced crystalloid versus 0.9% saline in patients with end-stage renal disease undergoing cadaveric renal transplantation: a prospective randomized controlled trial. *Anesthesia and analgesia*, 120(1), 123–129. https://doi.org/10.1213/ANE.0000000000000419.

Pradal, M., Vialet, R., Soula, F., Dejode, J. M., & Lagier, P. (1995). The risk of anesthesia in the asthmatic child. Pediatric pulmonology. Supplement, 11, 51–52. https://doi.org/10.1002/ppul.1950191127.

Ralston, M. A., Murnane, M. R., Unverferth, D. V., & Leier, C. V. (1990). Serum and tissue magnesium concentrations in patients with heart failure and serious ventricular arrhythmias. *Annals of internal medicine*, 113(11), 841–846. https://doi.org/10.7326/0003-4819-113-11-841.

Rao, S., & Avitsian, R. (2020). Anesthesia for Neurosurgical Emergencies. *Anesthesiology clinics*, 38(1), 67–83. https://doi.org/10.1016/j.anclin.2019.10.004.

Riker, R. R., Shehabi, Y., Bokesch, P. M., Ceraso, D., Wisemandle, W., Koura, F., Whitten, P., Margolis, B. D., Byrne, D. W., Ely, E. W., Rocha, M. G., & SEDCOM (Safety and Efficacy of Dexmedetomidine Compared With Midazolam) Study Group (2009). Dexmedetomidine vs midazolam for sedation of critically ill patients: a randomized trial. *JAMA*, 301(5), 489–499. https://doi.org/10.1001/jama.2009.56.

Rossaint, R., Bouillon, B., Cerny, V., Coats, T. J., Duranteau, J., Fernández-Mondéjar, E., Filipescu, D., Hunt, B. J., Komadina, R., Nardi, G., Neugebauer, E. A., Ozier, Y., Riddez, L., Schultz, A., Vincent, J. L., & Spahn, D. R. (2016). The European guideline on management of major bleeding and coagulopathy following trauma: fourth edition. *Critical care*, 20, 100. https://doi.org/10.1186/s13054-016-1265-x.

Rossi, S., Assis, D. N., Awsare, M., Brunner, M., Skole, K., Rai, J., Andrel, J., Herrine, S. K., Reddy, R. K., & Navarro, V. J. (2008). Use of over-the-counter analgesics in patients with chronic liver disease: physicians' recommendations. *Drug safety*, 31(3), 261–270. https://doi.org/10.2165/00002018-200831030-00007.

Runyon, B. A., & AASLD Practice Guidelines Committee (2009). Management of adult patients with ascites due to cirrhosis: an update. *Hepatology*, 49(6), 2087–2107. https://doi.org/10.1002/hep.22853.

Ryan D. W. (1977). Preoperative serum cholinesterase concentration in chronic renal failure. Clinical experience of suxamethonium in 81 patients undergoing renal transplant. *British journal of anaesthesia*, 49(9), 945–949. https://doi.org/10.1093/bja/49.9.945.

Sahinovic, M. M., Struys, M. M. R. F., & Absalom, A. R. (2018). Clinical Pharmacokinetics and Pharmacodynamics of Propofol. *Clinical pharmacokinetics*, 57(12), 1539–1558. https://doi.org/10.1007/s40262-018-0672-3.

Schindler, E., Müller, M., Zickmann, B., Kraus, H., Reuner, K. H., & Hempelmann, G. (1996). Untersuchungen zur Durchblutung der Leber beim Menschen nach 1 MAC Desfluran im Vergleich zu Isofluran und Halothan [Blood supply to the liver in the human after 1 MAC desflurane in comparison with isoflurane and halothane]. *Anasthesiologie, Intensivmedizin, Notfallmedizin, Schmerztherapie : AINS*, 31(6), 344–348. https://doi.org/10.1055/s-2007-995933.

Shankar, V., Churchwell, K. B., & Deshpande, J. K. (2006). Isoflurane therapy for severe refractory status asthmaticus in children. *Intensive care medicine*, 32(6), 927–933. https://doi.org/10.1007/s00134-006-0163-0.

Smith H. S. (2009). Opioid metabolism. *Mayo Clinic proceedings*, 84(7), 613–624. https://doi.org/10.1016/S0025-6196(11)60750-7.

Soleimanpour, H., Safari, S., Rahmani, F., Jafari Rouhi, A., & Alavian, S. M. (2015). Intravenous hypnotic regimens in patients with liver disease; a review article. Anesthesiology and pain medicine, 5(1), e23923. https://doi.org/10.5812/aapm.23923.

Solves Alcaina P. (2020). Platelet Transfusion: And Update on Challenges and Outcomes. *Journal of blood medicine*, 11, 19–26. https://doi.org/10.2147/JBM.S234374.

Spahn, D. R., Bouillon, B., Cerny, V., Coats, T. J., Duranteau, J., Fernández-Mondéjar, E., Filipescu, D., Hunt, B. J., Komadina, R., Nardi, G., Neugebauer, E., Ozier, Y., Riddez, L., Schultz, A., Vincent, J. L., & Rossaint, R. (2013). Management of bleeding and coagulopathy following major trauma: an updated European guideline. *Critical care*, 17(2), R76. https://doi.org/10.1186/cc12685.

Sterns, R. H., Grieff, M., & Bernstein, P. L. (2016). Treatment of hyperkalemia: something old, something new. *Kidney international*, 89(3), 546–554. https://doi.org/10.1016/j.kint.2015.11.018.

Tegeder, I., Lötsch, J., & Geisslinger, G. (1999). Pharmacokinetics of opioids in liver disease. *Clinical pharmacokinetics*, 37(1), 17–40. https://doi.org/10.2165/00003088-199937010-00002.

Terg, R., Gadano, A., Cartier, M., Casciato, P., Lucero, R., Muñoz, A., Romero, G., Levi, D., Terg, G., Miguez, C., & Abecasis, R. (2009). Serum creatinine and bilirubin predict renal failure and mortality in patients with spontaneous bacterial peritonitis: a retrospective study. *Liver international: official journal of the International Association for the Study of the Liver*, 29(3), 415–419. https://doi.org/10.1111/j.1478-3231.2008.01877.x.

Thapa, S., & Brull, S. J. (2000). Succinylcholine-induced hyperkalemia in patients with renal failure: an old question revisited. *Anesthesia and analgesia*, 91(1), 237–241. https://doi.org/10.1097/00000539-200007000-00044.

Uchida, K., Yasunaga, H., Miyata, H., Sumitani, M., Horiguchi, H., Matsuda, S., & Yamada, Y. (2012). Impact of remifentanil use on early postoperative outcomes following brain tumor resection or rectal cancer surgery. *Journal of anesthesia*, 26(5), 711–720. https://doi.org/10.1007/s00540-012-1397-3

Urso, C., Brucculeri, S., & Caimi, G. (2015). Acid-base and electrolyte abnormalities in heart failure: pathophysiology and implications. *Heart failure reviews*, 20(4), 493–503. https://doi.org/10.1007/s10741-015-9482-y.

Valk, B. I., & Struys, M. M. R. F. (2021). Etomidate and its Analogs: A Review of Pharmacokinetics and Pharmacodynamics. *Clinical pharmacokinetics*, 60(10), 1253–1269. https://doi.org/10.1007/s40262-021-01038-6.

Weerink, M. A. S., Struys, M. M. R. F., Hannivoort, L. N., Barends, C. R. M., Absalom, A. R., & Colin, P. (2017). Clinical Pharmacokinetics and Pharmacodynamics of Dexmedetomidine. *Clinical pharmacokinetics*, 56(8), 893–913. https://doi.org/10.1007/s40262-017-0507-7.

Yamakage, M., Iwasaki, S., & Namiki, A. (2008). Guideline-oriented perioperative management of patients with bronchial asthma and chronic obstructive pulmonary disease. *Journal of anesthesia*, 22(4), 412–428. https://doi.org/10.1007/s00540-008-0650-2.

Yuan, S., & Otrock, Z. K. (2021). Platelet Transfusion: An Update on Indications and Guidelines. *Clinics in laboratory medicine*, 41(4), 621–634. https://doi.org/10.1016/j.cll.2021.07.005.

Zafirova, Z., & Dalton, A. (2018). Neuromuscular blockers and reversal agents and their impact on anesthesia practice. Best practice & research. *Clinical anaesthesiology*, 32(2), 203–211. https://doi.org/10.1016/j.bpa.2018.06.004.

Zhi, D., Lin, J., Dong, L., Ji, X., Zhuang, H., Liu, Z., Liu, J., & Duan, M. (2021). Risk predictive role of hypernatremia for occurrence of sepsis-induced acute kidney injury. *Annals of palliative medicine*, 10(4), 4705–4715. https://doi.org/10.21037/apm-21-792.

Chapter 2

Neuraxial and Peripheral Blocks in Organ Failure Patients

Bengü Gülhan Köksal, MD
and Gamze Küçükosman*, MD
Department of Anesthesiology and Reanimation, Zonguldak Bülent Ecevit University, Zonguldak, Turkiye

Abstract

Patients with organ failure are at high risk of perioperative complications related to surgery and anesthesia. Neuraxial and peripheral nerve blocks (PNB) are believed to be beneficial for patients. However, it is important to understand the pathophysiology of the underlying disease and the physiological changes caused by the regional anesthesia techniques used so that the anesthesia technique used can provide maximum benefit to the patient and reduce the risk of complications. In the following section, neuraxial block and PNB applications in patients with organ failure will be discussed.

Keywords: organ failure, neuraxial blocks, peripheral nerve blocks

Introduction

The anesthesia method to be chosen after a detailed clinical and laboratory examination in patients who will undergo surgery should be the most comfortable for patients and least invasive. Although the safety profile of

---

* Corresponding Author's Email:gamzebeu@gmail.com.

In: Organ Failure and Anesthesia Practices
Editors: Ahmet Şen and Basar Erdivanli
ISBN: 979-8-89113-486-7

general anesthesia (GA) has improved in recent years, regional anesthesia (RA) has many advantages over GA. Regional anesthesia helps prevent hemodynamic disruptions, increased stress response, and GA-related hypercoagulability. Eliminating sedatives and intubation is necessary to make RA more physiological and allows a positive effect on postoperative mortality and morbidity (Perlas et al., 2016; Abe et al., 2020; Turan et al., 2019; Hadzic, 2017). At this point, peripheral nerve blocks (PNB) come to the fore in especially upper extremity surgeries as a better alternative to GA and other RA techniques. With the use of ultrasonography (USG) in PNB, these advantages have been more prominent and while the dosages of local anesthetics (LA) used have decreased, the chances of success of the block have increased (Kelsaka & Guldogus, 2013). Although complications encountered in USG-accompanied interventions have decreased, complications such as intraarterial-neural LA injection and pneumothorax can still be observed. In addition, unsuccessful and partial block can also be seen. The biggest disadvantage of USG is that it is a method that depends on the person who is performing it and requires specific skills (Gurkan, 2015).

The principle in anesthesia selection is to reduce the impact of anesthesia on organ functions provided that the requirements of the surgery are met. Unlike general and neuraxial anesthesia, PNB has a minimal effect on hemodynamics and leads to fewer complications, particularly in patients with high risk of cardiopulmonary dysfunction (Pu & Sun, 2019; Mei et al., 2019).

Organ failure patients are at high risk in terms of perioperative complications related to surgery and anesthesia. In general, neuraxial block and PNB are believed to be beneficial for patients. However, in order for the technique used to ensure maximum benefit for the patient and reduce the risk of complications, physiological changes, as well as pathophysiology, that occur in the neuraxial and PNB techniques must be understood and evaluated. In the following section, neuraxial block and PNB applications in patients with organ failure will be discussed.

Regional Anesthesia

Regional anesthesia is the reversible elimination of nerve transmission and pain in certain areas of the body without causing loss of consciousness (Hadzic, 2017). Regional anesthesia is divided into two groups as peripheral and neuraxial blocks. Consequently, peripheral nerve, ganglion, and plexus blocks are PNB, and spinal, combined spinal-epidural (CSE), and epidural

(EA) blocks are neuraxial blocks. When general anesthesia and neuraxial anesthesia are compared, PNB is minimally invasive and an effective perioperative analgesic method with unique advantages (Zhang et al., 2019). Peripheral nerve block is the temporary stop of nerve transmission by injecting local anesthetic around a nerve. Peripheral nerve blocks are techniques applied to nerves that usually innervate usually upper and lower extremities for the purpose of anesthesia and pain therapy. The most important advantage ofperipheral nerve blocks over both GA and other RA methods is that the block effect is limited to the area that the plexus or nerve innervates. For this reason, PNBs have become alternative methods to both GA and neuraxial blocks. Upper extremity PNBs frequently used in anesthesia practice are classified as cervical and brachial plexus block, interscalene, supraclavicular, infraclavicular and axillary nerve blocks, and thoracic and lumbar paravertebral somatic blocks and psoas compartment and intercostal nerve block (Kaya & Elmas, 2010). The technical applicability of neuraxial blocks and the provision of quality anesthesia and analgesia with a single injection have over shadowed the plexus and PNB applied to the lower extremity to some extent. However, due to the introduction of techniques that allow easy finding of peripheral nerves as a result of developing technology and complication of neuraxial hematoma that can develop as a result of venous thromboembolism prophylaxis that is frequently applied in the perioperative process, plexus and peripheral nerve blocks applied in the lower extremity have become a good option in the anesthesia management of patients with poor general condition for whom GA and neuraxial blocks are not appropriate Lower extremity PNBs are classified as sciatic, femoral, lateral, femoral cutaneous, obturator and pudendal nerve blocks (Hadzic, 2017; Kelsaka & Guldogus, 2013).

Before regional anesthesia, the intervention to be performed should be explained in full to the patient and, following the patient's permission, should be performed in an area where all the necessaryequipment for nerve block is available. As it can lead to premedication respiratory depression, hypoventilation, and hypoxia, vascular access should definitely be established for patients to whom RA will be applied, and should be monitored. The patient should be followed for at least 30 minutes under conditions that include routine ECG, pulsoxymeter, noninvasive monitoring of blood pressure and respiration rate, oxygen, emergency airway equipment, and drugs such as atropine, ephedrine, propofol, succinylcholine, and 20 > % intralipid (Hadzic, 2017; Kelsaka & Guldogus, 2013).

Systemic Toxicity of Local Anesthetic

Local anesthetics are drugs that temporarily and reversibly prevent sensory, motor, and autonomous nerve transmission (Hadzic, 2017). Although local anesthetics create local anesthesia in therapeutic concentrations, as a result of the entry of high-dose LA agent into systemic circulation through absorption during various applications or undesirable increase in plasma LA concentration related to intravascular injection, local anesthetic systemic toxicity (LAST) can develop. Furthermore, LAST development in therapeutic doses has also been reported (Wadlund, 2017; Tunney et al., 2018; Kramer et al., 2019; Digala & Lucchese, 2020). The plasma concentration of local anesthetics is determined by the balance between systemic absorption and elimination. Different ratios of the incidence of local anesthetic systemic toxicity have been reported in publications. Consequently, the incidence of LAST in epidural anesthesia applications has been reported to be 0.7-1.8/100,000 and in PNB as 2-2.8/10.000 (Macfarlane et al., 2021; Barrington & Kluger, 2013; Auroyet al., 2003). Determining the maximum safe dosage of LA specific to the patient by evaluating in detail several factors such as patient comorbid diseases, liver and renal dysfunction history, pregnancy, and age is critical to preventing the development of LAST (Neal et al., 2018).

As the metabolic rate and organ perfusion decrease in patients at advanced ages, drug clearance and elimination also decrease. Due to the weakening of ventricular contractility, these patients are more sensitive to the cardiac depressing effects of LA. Along with the decrease in muscle mass in advanced ages and slowing down of the circulation, tissue and plasma LA concentrations increase. In addition, the sensitivity of the central nervous system to LAs has increased in elderly patients. Therefore, it is recommended to reduce LA dosage by 10-20% (El-Boghdadly & Chin, 2016; Waldinger et al., 2020; Paqueron et al., 2002). The risk of developing LAST is elevated in cases of cardiac, hepatic, and renal dysfunction disorder. Patients with ventricular dysfunction, arrythmia history, transmission anomalies, myocardial ischemia, and congestive heart failure are more vulnerable to the toxic effects of LAs on the cardiovascular system. In hepatic function disorder, as the metabolization and bonding of amide-type local anesthetics to plasma protein are reduced, the risk of LAST increases. In patients with terminal stage renal failure, the presence of uremia or acidosis increases the free fraction of LA in the blood and thus the risk of LAST increases (Macfarlane et al., 2021). Protein binding is one of the major factors that affect peak plasma concentration. In diseases that lead to hypoproteinemia or in cases such as acidosis in which the bond to protein is reduced, the free drug fraction increases and therefore the risk of LAST increases as a result of increased plasma concentration (Gitman et al., 2019; Grigg et al., 2015; Calenda et al., 2014).

In truncal blocs that have started to be used in anesthesia applications along with current developments, the block is applied to the transversus abdominis, rectus sheath, quadratus lumborum, and pectoral facial planes (Tran et al., 2017). The planes to which local anesthetics are applied in truncal blocks are highly vascular, and it is necessary to apply local anesthetic in large volumes. In this regard, the risk of LAST development is high in truncal blocs (Vasques et al., 2015; Gitman & Barrington, 2018). The LAST risk related to truncal nerve blocks can be reduced by using LA at lower concentrations, adjusting the dosage according to body weight, giving additional epinephrine, and observing for at least 30-45 minutes after the block. Patients who receive liposomal bupivacaine should not be evaluated as less risk compared to patients who receive other local anesthetics and should be observed with the same attention. Although there are no extended scientific data on the relationship between liposomal bupivacaine and LAST development, LAST development has been reported (Aggarwal, 2018). The incidence of vascular punction has also been reported to decrease with the use of USG in peripheral nerve blocks (Abrahams et al., 2009). However, LAST symptoms have been reported to have developed in a 0.26/1.000 ratio despite the use of USG (Neal, 2016).

Regional Anesthesia in Liver Failure

The liver plays a role in homeostasis of many physiological systems such as drug metabolism, protein synthesis, hemostatic factors, and detoxification (Mushlin, 2011). Chronic liver disease (CLD) is a progressive disruption of liver functions. This situation is a continuous process of inflammation, destruction, and regeneration that causes fibrosis and cirrhosis in the liver parenchyma. Cirrhosis is the terminal stage of CLD, and progresses from the asymptomatic phase to the symptomatic decompensated phase with the development of acid, hemorrhage, encephalopathy with symptoms of decompensation. As soon as the patient enters the symptomatic decompensated phase, it turns into a systemic disease (Bernardi et al., 2015; Heidelbaugh & Bruderly, 2006). In patients with liver disease, the need for surgery, intraoperative complications, and postoperative morbidity and mortality risk are generally high. Although elective surgery is considered only in only CLD who are well compensated, urgent patient optimization is compulsory in urgent patients, and intravascular volume status, coagulation function, neurological condition, and infection scanning should be considered (Gropper et al., 2023).

The selection of anesthesia technique for patients with liver disease, similarly to patients without liver disease, should be based on the surgical procedure and the factors of the patient. Neuraxial anesthesia, GA, and monitored anesthesia care can be options. GA and surgery can lead to complications that might cause severe morbidity and mortality in a large portion of patients who have been well compensated or have latent cirrhosis (EndaleSimegn et al., 2022).

Critical issues for RA in patients with liver disease include LA metabolism, the effect of RA on hepatic perfusion, and potential coagulopathy related to liver function disorder (Hadzic, 2017).

Effect of Regional Anesthesia on Hemodynamics in Patients with Liver Failure

All anesthesia methods can decrease mean arterial pressure (MAP) and thus reduce hepatic blood flow. Systemic hypotension that results from sympathectomy caused by spinal or epidural blockage can lead to decreased hepatic blood flow. Hepatic blood flow does not have autoregulation (Kennedy et al., 1971). Intravenous fluids and vasopressors are usually applied to reverse this hypotension. In a study conducted, it was reported that despite maintainingnormotension through hydroxyethyl starch infusion, hepatic blood flow decreased with epidural anesthesia and this decrease was reversed by adding a dopamine infusion, while in another study, it was found that thoracic epidural anesthesia along with norepinephrine infusion led to a greater decrease in hepatic blood flow (Meierhenrich et al., 2009; Tanaka et al., 1997). On the other hand, sympathetic blockage originating from neuraxial block in the intraoperative period has been reported to be beneficial, as it leads to low central venous pressure and decreases blood loss and the need for transfusions during the hepatic procedure in patients undergoing liver resection (Gurusamy et al., 2009). As long as MAP is maintained and kept close to initial values, hepatic blood flow is also maintained; therefore, blood pressure should be monitored closely with hemodynamic monitoring during anesthesia (Zinn et al., 1985; Igarashi, 1995).

Effect of Liver Disease on Local Anesthetic Drug Administration

Local anesthetics are commonly used in clinical practice and are classified as amino ester or aminoamide compounds. While ester-type local anesthetics are hydrolyzed by cholinesterase, amide-type local anesthetics that include bupivacaine, levobupivacaine, lignocaine, and ropivacaine are metabolized in the liver. All LAs may be associated with a higher risk of adverse effects due to decreased clearance, altered protein binding, and volume of distribution in patients with liver disease. Furthermore, with a decrease in hepatic blood flow due to portacaval shunt, hemodynamic changes, or decreased hepatic entry during liver resection, the effectiveness of drug elimination can be restricted (Becker & Reed, 2012; Murphy, 2005). Amide metabolism is much slower than plasma hydrolysis, and therefore amide-type LAs are more prone to hepatic function disorder or accumulation in the presence of decreased hepatic blood flow (Peck & Harris, 2021). When high doses of LAs are used, factors that must be considered with respect to the patient include age, renal and hepatic function disorders, heart failure, pregnancy, and drug interactions. As clearance of local anesthetics (CL) decreases along with advanced age, renal, hepatic, and cardiac dysfunction, in continuous regional blocks where low doses of drug are used, the drug and its metabolites are allowed to accumulate (Rosenberg et al., 2004). Due to the wide individual differences in pharmacokinetics in patients with liver failure, a definitive dosage instruction can not be provided. It has been reported that in terminal stage liver disease, ropivacaine clearance decreases by 60% on average, but since the maximum plasma concentration after a single dose is not affected by liver disorder, a single dose can be used. If ropivacaine infusion is to be used, it is recommended to use the least effective dose for a short time and to closely monitor the patients (Jokinen et al., 2007). The clearance of drugs with a high ratio of hepatic extraction is significantly affected by hepatic flow. Lidocaine has a high ratio of hepatic extraction. Clearance depends on hepatic blood flow, and it does not change relatively with changes in hepatic enzyme activity. Current data show that both lidocaine protein bonding and its Alpha1 acid glycoprotein (α1-AGP) concentration decrease as the severity of hepatic disease increases. It has been reported that severe cirrhosis can be associated with increased fractions of free drugs in plasma, such as lidocaine, and that the probability of these patients showing symptoms of lidocaine toxicity can be higher (Barry et al., 1990). When levobupivacaine, which is metabolized by CYP3A4 and CYO1A2, whichare members of cytochrome P450 in the liver, was used in patients with liver function disorder for epidural anesthesia, the metabolism oflevobupivacaineslowed and plasma concentration was elevated (Ran et al., 2015). It has been stated that dosage adjustment would not be required in PNB where single-dose amide-type LA is applied in patients with liver disease (Hadzic, 2017). In addition to amide-type LAs, since plasma cholinesterase levels also decrease in advanced liver failure, ester-type LAs such as procaine were shown to be slowly metabolized (Reidenberg et al., 1972).

Coagulopathy and Regional Anesthesia

In particular in terminal stage CLD, both the coagulant and anticoagulant factors show changes with respect to normal level. A decrease in the levels of most procoagulant factors other than Factor VIII and Willebrand factor and anticoagulants such as antithrombin and protein C is observed (Northup et al., 2007). Thrombocytopenia and thrombocyte dysfunction are common. In alcoholic cirrhosis, dysfibrinogenemia and fibrinolysis may develop (Wiklund, 2004).

As the risk of hemorrhage is not present in each cirrhosis patient, there is a tendency to thrombosis in patients with cholestatic liver, such as primary sclerosing cholangitis (Tripodi & Mannucci, 2011). Especially when liver synthesis function is disrupted more prominently, along with D-dimer, anomalies including prolongation of prothrombin time, international normalized ratio (INR), and active partial thromboplastin time are frequently seen. These tests are very poor at predicting the risk of hemorrhage in individuals with liver disease because they only reflect changes in procoagulant factors. The prolongation of INR in cirrhosis does not indicate hypocoagulation or hypercoagulation (Northup et al., 2021). When possible, viscoelastic tests (thromboelastography, thromboelastometry, etc.) can be beneficial in terms of providing guidance for the correction of preoperative hemostatic anomalies in patients with liver disease (Bedreli et al., 2016).

Neuraxial anesthesia procedures are contraindicated in patients with severe coagulopathy and/or thrombocytopenia due to an increased risk of spinal-epidural hematoma. Intraspinal hematoma is a rare situation and can be seen as a result of neuraxial anesthesia. Its incidence is higher in thrombocytopenic patients taking anticoagulants and in those with liver disease and alcoholism. For this reason, neuraxial anesthesia is usually contraindicated in the presence of coagulopathy (Horlocker & Wedel, 1998; Hadzic, 2017). Regional anesthesia and analgesia are recommended for patients with an appropriate coagulation profile. The dose should be carefully adjusted and the patient should be followed up in terms of possible side effects (Rahimzadeh et al., 2014; Starczewska et al., 2017). Epidural anesthesia and analgesia are a vital part of the enhanced recovery after surgery program, as it often suppresses the neuroendocrine response to surgical stress and provides better postoperative pain control and faster mobilization (Van Dam et al., 2008). Epidural anesthesia is commonly used in the field of open liver surgery and provides positive results in terms of reducing pain scores (Page et al., 2008; Matot et al., 2002; Ganapathi et al., 2015). In an experimental study conducted, it was emphasized that thoracic epidural anesthesia reduced liver damage that developed in relation to acute necrotizing pancreatitis and could protect liver function in systemic inflammatory disorders (Freise et al., 2009).

Changes in coagulation profile after liver resection are common and are related to preoperative liver function and intraoperative factors such as duration of surgery, degree of hemorrhage during surgery, and especially the size and mass of liver tissue resected, and due to this coagulation disorder, that develops, the placement of the epidural catheter and its management can create potential risks (Oguro et al., 1993). Therefore, if it is considered to use an epidural catheter in a patient planned to undergo liver resection, contacting the surgery team to estimate the size of the liver resection and anticipated blood loss could be helpful in the decision to place an epidural catheter. Following placement, serial coagulation measurements should be performed in patients at risk in terms of hemostatic abnormalities, and considering deficiency before removing the catheter, fresh frozen plasma or thrombocyte application should be considered (Shontz et al., 2009). To understand the severity of epidural hematoma and reduce its incidence, the American Regional Anesthesia and Pain Medicine Association has developed guidelines for patients with hemostatic abnormalities. Although there is no specific suggestion for the treatment of neuraxial analgesia in patients who have undergone liver resection, it should be considered if the INR is >1.5 and the thrombocyte count is 100,000 mm^3 (Vaja et al., 2010; Narouze et al., 2018).

In addition to epidural anesthesia, other RA techniques, including subcostal transversus abdominis plan, erector spinae, and quadratus lumborum blocks, provide benefits without any risk of hemorrhage. These are performed in conjunction with USG, and a permanent catheter can also be placed. Studies have shown that these blocks alone ensured better pain control compared to intravenous opioids and reduced the need for postoperative opioids. Erector spinae and quadratus lumborum blocks have been defined more recently (Karanicolas et al., 2014). With these blocks, in addition to somatic analgesia, visceral analgesia can also be provided (Chin et al., 2017).

Serious sequelae may occur during PNB applications in bleeding disorders. There is no definitive guide for performing PNBs. The risks related to the application of PNB in patients with abnormal coagulation parameters are less clear. In techniques in which the needle is placed close to a large blood vessel, the risk of hemorrhage increases. Deep blocks such as anterior sciatic or lumbar plexus blocks should be applied with care in patients with coagulopathy. Furthermore, blocks around unclamped blood vessels should also be carefully evaluated (Li & Oprea, 2020; Ashken & West, 2021; Hadzic, 2017).

Renal Failure

Acute renal failure is a clinical syndrome characterized by sudden disruption of renal functions and affects many organs and systems with symptoms such as disruption in acid-base and fluid-electrolyte balance and deficiency in the clearance of nitrogenous wastes and oliguria (Li et al., 2013). Chronic renal failure (CRF) can be defined as glomerular filtration rate (GFR) being < 60 ml/min/1.73 m^2 for more than 3 months or the presence of findings of kidney damage on pathology and laboratory examinations (proteinuria, hematuria, microalbuminuria) examinations or radiological imaging (Levey et al., 2005). The incidence of CRF incidence in our country has been reported to be 15.7% (Süleymanlar et al., 2011).

Patients with renal failure constitute a challenging group of patients for anesthesia in the perioperative period, both due to complications that develop in the natural course of the disease and diseases that contribute to its etiology (Eilers et al., 2010). Considering serious comorbidities, it is not surprising that these patients have significant perioperative risks (Smith et al., 2015). In the evaluation of physical and laboratory examinations to be performed, independently of the anesthesia method to be applied and surgical interventions to be performed in these patients in order to make sure that their medical condition is optimal, special emphasis should be placed on particularly cardiac and respiratory functions. Perioperative dialysis is necessary on the day ofanesthesia application or the day before it (Gropper et al., 2023).

Renal failure is a disease that affects all systems. It is frequently accompanied by disorders in the renin-angiotensin system and systemic arterial hypertension related to sodium retention. Hypovolemia can be observed in these patients due to hydration or fluid overdrawing during dialysis (Butterworth et al., 2022; Gropper et al., 2023). The incidence of left ventricular hypertrophy, transmission anomalies, and atherosclerosis is increased. There is an increase in cardiac output, an increase in heart metabolic need related to hypertension, congestive heart failure due to anemia and sodium retention resulting from extracellular hydration, lung edema, and hypoxemia (Gradaus et al., 2001; Craig & Hunter, 2008; London, 2003). In these patients, the accumulation of uremic toxins inhibits thrombocyte function and thrombocyte-vein wall interactions (Kaw & Malhotra, 2006). In thromboelastographic studies conducted in CRF patients, all steps of the coagulation cascade (fibrine formation, fibrine-platelet interaction, etc.) have been reported to be activatedand coagulation anomalies have developed in 42.9% of patients (Pivalizza et al., 1997; Darlington et al., 2011). In patients with renal failure, the functions of the thrombocyte and leukocyte are altered. Consequently, prolonged bleeding time and increased susceptibility to infections can be observed in patients. Bleeding time values are above normal and platelet count is generally within normal limits. The decrease in ADP deposit in platelets and the decrease in thromboxane A2 levels are responsible for platelet dysfunction. Chronic anemia also increases susceptibility to bleeding. Anemia contributes to dialysis, low drug clearance, and disruption of anticoagulation hemostasis applied during dialysis (Bennett, 2013). Anemia that is observed at a 6-8 g/dL level of hemoglobin concentration is always present in uremic patients whose creatinine clearance is below 30 mL/min (Gropper et al., 2023). Peripheral and autonomic neuropathies are neurological complications seen in patients with CRF. In patients in whom autonomic neuropathy develops, gastric emptying can be delayed and susceptibility to aspiration increases. Autonomic neuropathy is frequently seen, especially in advanced stage renal failure, and this situation has a considerable effect on arterial pressure. CRF-related autonomic dysfunction is characterized by decreased baroreceptor activity, sympathetic hyperactivity, and parasympathetic dysfunction. Parasympathetic activity manifests itself with decreased heart rate variation and bradycardia that does not respond to atropine. It should be noted that due to the possibility of developing autonomic neuropathy, decreases in blood pressure in these patients cannot be tolerated as much as in a normal patient (Wagener & Brentjens, 2010). Peripheral neuropathies develop in the distal region of the low extremities and are typically sensorial (Sanya & Ogunniyi, 2004). As paresthesia symptoms can be seen in patients who developed uremic neuropathy, the place of RA is an issue of debate (Akça et al., 2016).

The Effect of Regional Anesthesia on Renal Function

Renal failure is rather common among the surgical population, and when providing anesthesia in these patients, RA techniques alone or their combination with GA are ideal options (Hadimioglu et al., 2005; Freiret al., 2012; Dhir & Fuller, 2007). In the treatment of patients who have the risk of perioperative renal function disorder, avoiding nephrotoxic agents and maintaining kidney perfusion are basic principles (Meersch et al., 2016).

As loss of renal function affects drug pharmacokinetics and dynamics, anesthesia specialists should carefully assess possible changes in drug distribution, metabolism, elimination, and protein bonding, and should take care when using LA to prevent complications. Local anesthetics do not have any nephrotoxic properties on their own, and the low bicarbonate value related to terminal stage renal failure leads to a delay in local anesthetics, while the low protein bonding effect causes a prolongation of the time of taking effect (Al-Mustafa et al., 2010). Especially in these patients who are acidotic and have hyperkalemia, the total dosa of LA used should be reduced by 25% (Tsuchiya et al., 2012). In these patients, renal clearance of lidocaine or ropivacaine metabolites decreases. As these metabolites have central nervous system toxicity, symptoms of the nervous system should be followed, especially in high doses and long-term applications. These pharmacokinetic changes can increase the possibility of LAST, so they should be applied with care (De Martin et al., 2006; Pere et al., 2003). Hemodialysis is ineffective in terms of eliminating lidocaine from plasma; therefore, it is not reliable in treating toxicity (Grossman et al.,1982). On the other hand, lipid emulsion has been successfully used to treat cardiovascular and neurological systemic toxicity in patients with renal failure (De Martin et al., 2006). Even if there are no acid-base or electrolyte disorders, plasma levels of LA after PNB have been reported to be high in CRF patients. Although the cause of this situation is not exactly known, it is believed that it can be associated with increased blood flow (withdrawal at the injection site) related to hyperdynamic circulation seen frequently in uremic patients (Mostert et al., 1970). In addition, α1-acid glycoprotein levels increase in uremia, and this situation can provide a protective effect by causing both the current free fraction for hepatic metabolism to decrease and the volume of distribution to decrease (Vasson et al., 1993).

The risk of epidural hematoma increasesin patients with renal failure due to thrombocyte dysfunction and the residual effects of heparin administered during dialysis. This situation has raised concerns related to neuraxial blockage. However, there are studies that reported theuse of EA in CRF patients at different stages (Sharrock et al., 2006; Dauri et al., 2003). A possible relationship between hemodialysis and spontaneous epidural hematoma has also been reported (Shahlaie et al., 2004). In patients with CRF, anticoagulants and antiplatelet drugs are frequently used for reasons such as comorbid atrial fibrillation, thromboembolic events, and coronary or peripheral artery disease. Since these drugs are discharged through the kidney, they accumulate in the body and can cause increased effects and hemorrhages. While heparin can be used safely in patients with CRF, heparins with low molecular weight can accumulate. Direct oral anticoagulants should be avoided in patients with severe CRF or hemodialysis. If neuraxial or deep plexus block is indicated in patients with renal failure, indications for anticoagulation and antiplatelet treatment must be ensured and careful dosage adjustment and follow-up of renal function are necessary (Narouze et al., 2015; Olcay & Akdemir, 2018; Gropper et al., 2023; Hadzic, 2017). Uremic patients are at increased risk in terms of thrombotic events (Wu et al., 2022; Boccardo et al., 2004). A case of hypoxia that developed after brachial plexus blockage in a uremic patient has been reported to later become secondary to pulmonary embolism (Rose & Ness, 2002). There is no significant difference between CRF patients and healthy patients in terms of PNB latency, duration, and quality (Pere et al., 2003; Rice et al., 1991; McEllistrem et al., 1989). It has been reported that, unlike healthy patients, spinal anesthesia quality is similar in CRF patients, but that in uremic patients, both the initial time and duration of the block were shortened (Orko et al., 1986).

Preventing especially anesthesia-induced hypotension in patients with renal failure is highly important in terms of maintaining renal perfusion. Kidneys can perform autoregulation at mean arterial pressures (MAP) of 80-100 mmHg and GFH can be maintained. Although neuraxial anesthesia and sympathectomy can decrease MAP, renal blood flow is generally maintained (Suleiman et al.,1997; Gropper et al., 2023). In a study which demonstrated that although renal blood flow was minimally affected by T10 spinal anesthesia, it was significantly decreased by T1 sensory block, it was reported that in patients with renal failure, lumbar and subthoracic neuraxial anesthesia levels were physiologically well tolerated and that significant changes did not occur until higher levels were reached (Sivarajan et al., 1975).

Heart Failure

Hemodynamic Effects of Regional Anesthesia

High levels of sympathetic block are associated with increased hypotension. Blocking of cardioaccelerator fibers (T1, T4) contributes to hypotension through increased heart rate and cardiac output. When the same dermatomal block is achieved with epidural anesthesia, a similar hypotension is observed, but the onset of hypotension could be slower (Bonica et al., 1996). The reason for the difference in hypotension incidence and risk factors has been reported in the literature to be the difference in hypotension definition and tension measurement methods. Hypovolemia, <40-50 years of age, emergency surgery, obesity, chronic alcohol consumption, and chronic hypertension are among the risk factors for hypotension observed during spinal anesthesia. Neuraxial anesthesia can also lead to bradycardia and different types of heart block (Hartmann et al., 2002; Carpenter et al., 1992).

Heart Failure and Regional Anesthesia

Heart failure (HF) patientsare at risk of acute heart failure, hypotension, hypertension, and arrythmia during surgery. Among the causes of hemodynamic instability is the response to surgery, changes in intravascular volume, and the effects of anesthetics and other agents (Mangano et al., 1991). No matter what anesthesia technique is used, after understanding the pathophysiology of HF, there are hemodynamic targets for the perioperative period, which are protecting heart output and minimizing myocardial work. If possible, local or RA should be recommended to patients who are applying minor peripheral procedures. In moderate and low-risk surgeries that include the lower extremity, perineum, and lower abdominal region, neuraxial anesthesia methods could be a good choice. There is no evidence on the advantages of RA over GA for major surgeries (Hedge et al., 2017; Pirracchio et al., 2007). As a high dose of LA application could lead to myocardial toxicity and depression, care should be taken. The use of epinephrine with local anesthetics is not recommended (Breen & Park, 2002). In neuraxial anesthesia, a decrease in vasodilatation and preload related to sympathetic blockage results in hypotension. The possibility of hypotension development is greater in patients with high sensitivity to preload and diastolic dysfunction. Although volume application that is titrated with increases of 250 ml can be helpful in regulating blood pressure, excessive hydration should be avoided to prevent postoperative complications such as pulmonary edema. Therefore, if hypotension develops, rather than rapid or significant volume loading, it is appropriate to apply an α1 receptor agonist (e.g., epinephrine) or direct/indirect sympathomimetic (e.g., ephedrine). Modified neuraxial anesthesia techniques (e.g., intrathecal opioids, or low-dose combined spinal-epidural without opioids, or very slowly titrated EA) are a reasonable choice for especially patients with HF susceptible to hypotension (e.g., recently decompensated HF) (Holte et al., 2004). In preload-dependent cardiac disorders (e.g., aorta stenosis or hypertrophic cardiomyopathy), there is the risk of a severe decrease in cardiac output and hypotension as a result of sympathectomy accompanying neuraxial anesthesia (Hadzic, 2017).

Tachycardia and hypertension that develop in relation to perioperative pain and inadequate depth of anesthesia should be treated, as they will disrupt the balance of myocardial oxygen supply / demand. Additionally, pain management is also important to reduce hypercoagulopathy. This situation can be prevented by increasing the depth of anesthesia and applying neuraxial or PNB (Schneider, 2018).

In a patient with valvular heart disease, there can be perioperative arrythmias of the cardia, such as HF or atrial fibrillation. These patients with comorbid atrial fibrillation generally use anticoagulant drugs. These patients can come to the surgery room as emergency or electively under the residual effect of anticoagulants or under alternative intravenous medications. Therefore, preoperative anesthesia evaluation of these patients should include a history of hemorrhage and blood coagulation tests (Nkomo et al., 2006; Horlocker et al., 2003). Intraoperative neuraxial anesthesia and postoperative neuraxial analgesia are contraindicated in patients with distinct anticoagulation or antiplatelet effect; treatment and anesthesia management should be planned accordingly.

Aorta stenosis leads to excessive pressure load due to output obstruction, causing left ventricle workload to increase. The duration of diastole is reduced, the ejection time is prolonged, and it leads to a shorter filling duration and subendocardial perfusion ischemia. Ventricular filling depends on the preservation of preload and sinus rhythm. The perioperative targets are to maintain contractility and afterload and to avoid bradycardia and tachycardia. The choice of anesthesia techniques for aortic stenosis depends on the requirements of surgical procedures, as well as hemodynamic goals. Neuraxial anesthesia can cause a rapid and major decrease in systemic vascular resistance due to its strong sympatholytic effect. This leads to hypotension and decreases in coronary perfusion; these changes are changes that patients with severe aortic stenosis can not compensate for (Herrera, 2012; McDonald, 2004). Although neuraxial anesthesia is contraindicated in patients with aortic stenosis, it has been reported in case reports that LAs were slowly and gradually applied and EA or CSEA wasapplied in patients with a moderate degree of aortic stenosis to minimize hemodynamic changes in appropriate surgical procedures. However, this can typicallybe avoided in patients with severe aortic stenosis, and continuous spinal anesthesia can be used as an alternative to these methods (Boso, 2008; Xia etal., 2006; López et al., 2016). However, it has been stated that PNB could be used safely and effectively in close hemodynamic monitoring in suitable surgeries on a case-by-case basis (Yamane et al., 2017; Forero et al., 2015).

Patients with hypertrophic cardiomyopathy have obstruction of the left ventricular outflow tract, and the incidence of ischemic heart disease increases with anesthesia and surgery (Spoladore et al., 2012). PNB has been reported to be safely applied with LA providing long-term analgesia such as ropivacaine (Mitra et al., 2020).

The use of neuraxial techniques in coronary artery bypass graft (CABG) for postoperative analgesia is controversial (Ho et al., 2000). Intrathecal and epidural techniques provide safe analgesia in patients who have undergone heart surgery, as they decrease the stress response and ensure thoracic cardiac sympathectomy. In CABG, high thoracic epidural analgesia (TEA) applied in addition to general anesthesiahas been reported to normalize myocardial blood flow and provided decreased oxygen requirement, regional improvement in left ventricular function, decrease in supraventricular arrythmia incidence, decrease in stress response to surgery, intraoperative hemodynamic stability and postoperative analgesia (Nygård et al., 2005). However, concerns related to hypotension that develops as a result of epidural hematoma and sympathetic blockage continue to exist in patients who require complete heparinization for CABG. In a retrospective study that included patients who had undergone peripheral vascular surgery, epidural catheterization before systemic heparinization was safe. However, it was stated that the degree of coagulation in this study was considerably lower than the degree of coagulation in patients who had undergone heart surgery (Baron et al., 1987). In a study conducted in patients who had undergone CABG and who applied and did not apply TEA and analgesia, it was reported that continuous TEA considerably increased recovery quality after CABG compared to conventional narcotic analgesia, and no neurological complications related to TEA use were developed (Scott et al., 2001).

Conclusion

Neuraxial and peripheral nerve blocks are useful and safe in patients with organ failure, as they not only reduce the patient's exposure to many anesthetic drugs, but also reduce the risks associated with GA. It is known that RA techniques, which will be selected considering the accompanying comorbidities and surgical methods, provide minimum drug use, better postoperative analgesia, and faster recovery.

References

Abe, H., Sumitani, M., Matsui, H., Aso, S., Inoue, R., Fushimi, K., Uchida, K., Yasunaga, H., & Yamada, Y. (2020). Comparing outcomes after peripheral nerve block versus general anesthesia for lower extremity amputation: a nationwide exploratory retrospective cohort study in Japan. *Regional anesthesia and pain medicine, 45*(6), 399–404. https://doi.org/10.1136/rapm-2019-101208.

Abrahams, M. S., Aziz, M. F., Fu, R. F., & Horn, J. L. (2009). Ultrasound guidance compared with electrical neurostimulation for peripheral nerve block: a systematic review and meta-analysis of randomized controlled trials. *British journal of anaesthesia*, 102(3), 408–417. https://doi.org/10.1093/bja/aen384.

Aggarwal N. (2018). Local anesthetics systemic toxicity association with exparel (bupivacaine liposome)- a pharmacovigilance evaluation. *Expert opinion on drug safety, 17*(6), 581–587. https://doi.org/10.1080/14740338.2017.1335304.

Akça, B., Yılbaş, A. A., Kanbak, M. (2016). Chronic renal disease and anesthetic management. *Journal of Anesthesia – JARSS, 24*(1): 2–7.

Al-mustafa, M. M., Massad, I., Alsmady, M., Al-qudah, A., & Alghanem, S. (2010). The effect of low serum bicarbonate values on the onset of action of local anesthesia with vertical infraclavicular brachial plexus block in patients with end-stage renal failure. *Saudi journal of kidney diseases and transplantation: an official publication of the Saudi Center for Organ Transplantation, Saudi Arabia, 21*(3), 494–500.

Ashken, T., & West, S. (2021). Regional anaesthesia in patients at risk of bleeding. *BJA education, 21*(3), 84–94. https://doi.org/10.1016/j.bjae.2020.11.004.

Auroy, Y., Benhamou, D., Bargues, L., Ecoffey, C., Falissard, B., Mercier, F. J., Bouaziz, H., & Samii, K. (2002). Major complications of regional anesthesia in France: The

SOS Regional Anesthesia Hotline Service. *Anesthesiology, 97*(5), 1274–1280. https://doi.org/10.1097/00000542-200211000-00034.

Baron, H. C., LaRaja, R. D., Rossi, G., & Atkinson, D. (1987). Continuous epidural analgesia in the heparinized vascular surgical patient: a retrospective review of 912 patients. *Journal of vascular surgery, 6*(2), 144–146. https://doi.org/10.1067/mva.1987.avs0060144.

Barrington, M. J., & Kluger, R. (2013). Ultrasound guidance reduces the risk of local anesthetic systemic toxicity following peripheral nerve blockade. *Regional anesthesia and pain medicine, 38*(4), 289–299. https://doi.org/10.1097/AAP.0b013e318292669b.

Barry, M., Keeling, P. W., Weir, D., & Feely, J. (1990). Severity of cirrhosis and the relationship of alpha 1-acid glycoprotein concentration to plasma protein binding of lidocaine. *Clinical pharmacology and therapeutics, 47*(3), 366–370. https://doi.org/10.1038/clpt.1990.41.

Becker, D. E., & Reed, K. L. (2012). Local Anesthetics: Review of Pharmacological Considerations. *Anesthesia Progress, 59*(2), 90–102. https://doi.org/10.2344/0003-3006-59.2.90.

Bedreli, S., Sowa, J. P., Malek, S., Blomeyer, S., Katsounas, A., Gerken, G., Saner, F. H., & Canbay, A. (2016). Rotational thromboelastometry can detect factor XIII deficiency and bleeding diathesis in patients with cirrhosis. *Liver International, 37*(4), 562–568. https://doi.org/10.1111/liv.13254.

Bennett, L. (2013). Patient independence in chronic kidney disease and anaemia: implications of the 2012 KDIGO guideline. *Journal of renal care, 39*(2), 108–117. https://doi.org/10.1111/j.1755-6686.2013.12010.x.

Bernardi, M., Moreau, R., Angeli, P., Schnabl, B., & Arroyo, V. (2015). Mechanisms of decompensation and organ failure in cirrhosis: From peripheral arterial vasodilation to systemic inflammation hypothesis. *Journal of Hepatology, 63*(5), 1272–1284. https://doi.org/10.1016/j.jhep.2015.07.004.

Breen, P., & Park, K. W. (2002). General anesthesia versus regional anesthesia. *International anesthesiology clinics, 40*(1), 61–71. https://doi.org/10.1097/00004311-200201000-00006.

Boccardo, P., Remuzzi, G., & Galbusera, M. (2004). Platelet dysfunction in renal failure. *Seminars in thrombosis and hemostasis, 30*(5), 579–589. https://doi.org/10.1055/s-2004-835678.

Bonica, J. J., Kennedy, W. F., Jr, Ward, R. J., & Tolas, A. G. (1966). A comparison of the effects of high subarachnoid and epidural anesthesia. Acta anaesthesiologica Scandinavica. *Supplementum, 23*, 429–437. https://doi.org/10.1111/j.1399-6576.1966.tb01043.x.

Boso E. B. (2008). A case for combined spinal-epidural anesthesia for Cesarean section in a patient with aortic stenosis. *The West Virginia medical journal, 104*(2), 20–21.

Butterworth, J. F., Mackey, D. C., Wasnick, J. D. (2022). *Morgan & Mikhail's Clinical Anesthesiology* (7th ed). McGraw Hill Medical Books.

Calenda, E., Baste, J. M., Hajjej, R., Danielou, E., & Peillon, C. (2014). Toxic plasma concentration of ropivacaine after a paravertebral block in a patient suffering from severe hypoalbuminemia. *Journal of clinical anesthesia, 26*(2), 149–151. https://doi.org/10.1016/j.jclinane.2013.11.008.

Carpenter, R. L., Caplan, R. A., Brown, D. L., Stephenson, C., & Wu, R. (1992). Incidence and risk factors for side effects of spinal anesthesia. *Anesthesiology, 76*(6), 906–916. https://doi.org/10.1097/00000542-199206000-00006.

Chin, K. J., Malhas, L., & Perlas, A. (2017). The Erector Spinae Plane Block Provides Visceral Abdominal Analgesia in Bariatric Surgery: A Report of 3 Cases. *Regional anesthesia and pain medicine, 42*(3), 372–376. https://doi.org/10.1097/AAP.0000000000000581.

Craig, R. G., & Hunter, J. M. (2008). Recent developments in the perioperative management of adult patients with chronic kidney disease. *British journal of anaesthesia, 101*(3), 296–310. https://doi.org/10.1093/bja/aen203.

Darlington, A., Ferreiro, J. L., Ueno, M., Suzuki, Y., Desai, B., Capranzano, P., Capodanno, D., Tello-Montoliu, A., Bass, T. A., Nahman, N. S., & Angiolillo, D. J. (2011). Haemostatic profiles assessed by thromboelastography in patients with end-stage renal disease. *Thrombosis and haemostasis, 106*(1), 67–74. https://doi.org/10.1160/TH10-12-0785.

Dauri, M., Costa, F., Servetti, S., Sidiropoulou, T., Fabbi, E., & Sabato, A. F. (2003). Combined general and epidural anesthesia with ropivacaine for renal transplantation. *Minerva anestesiologica, 69*(12), 873–884.

De Martin, S., Orlando, R., Bertoli, M., Pegoraro, P., & Palatini, P. (2006). Differential effect of chronic renal failure on the pharmacokinetics of lidocaine in patients receiving and not receiving hemodialysis. *Clinical pharmacology and therapeutics, 80*(6), 597–606. https://doi.org/10.1016/j.clpt.2006.08.020.

Dhir, S., & Fuller, J. (2007). Case report: pregnancy in hemodialysis-dependent end-stage renal disease: anesthetic considerations. *Canadian journal of anaesthesia = Journal canadien d'anesthesie, 54*(7), 556–560. https://doi.org/10.1007/BF03022320.

Digala, L. P., & Lucchese, S. (2020). IV Lidocaine Infusion Leading to the Toxic Levels in Serum Causing Asystole- A Case Report. *Headache, 60*(1), 269–270. https://doi.org/10.1111/head.13699.

Eilers, H., Liu, K. D., Gruber, A., & Niemann, C. U. (2010). Chronic kidney disease: implications for the perioperative period. *Minerva anestesiologica*, 76(9), 725–736.

El-Boghdadly, K., & Chin, K. J. (2016). Local anesthetic systemic toxicity: Continuing Professional Development. *Canadian journal of anaesthesia = Journal canadien d'anesthesie, 63*(3), 330–349. https://doi.org/10.1007/s12630-015-0564-z.

Endale Simegn, A., Yaregal Melesse, D., Belay Bizuneh, Y., & Mekonnen Alemu, W. (2022). Perioperative management of patients with liver disease for non-hepatic surgery: A systematic review. *Annals of Medicine and Surgery, 75*, 103397. https://doi.org/10.1016/j.amsu.2022.103397.

Forero, M., Kruisselbrink, R., & Leon, S. J. (2015). Ultrasound-guided peripheral nerve blocks for total knee arthroplasty in the context of severe aortic stenosis: avoiding the general anesthetic. *Canadian journal of anaesthesia = Journal canadien d'anesthesie, 62*(6), 665–666. https://doi.org/10.1007/s12630-015-0314-2.

Freir, N. M., Murphy, C., Mugawar, M., Linnane, A., & Cunningham, A. J. (2012). Transversus abdominis plane block for analgesia in renal transplantation: a randomized controlled trial. *Anesthesia and analgesia, 115*(4), 953–957. https://doi.org/10.1213/ANE.0b013e3182642117.

Freise, H., Lauer, S., Konietzny, E., Hinkelmann, J., Minin, E., Van Aken, H. K., Lerch, M. M., Sielenkaemper, A. W., & Fischer, L. G. (2009). Hepatic effects of thoracic epidural analgesia in experimental severe acute pancreatitis. *Anesthesiology, 111*(6), 1249–1256. https://doi.org/10.1097/ALN.0b013e3181c1494e.

Ganapathi, S., Roberts, G., Mogford, S., Bahlmann, B., Ateleanu, B., & Kumar, N. (2015). Epidural analgesia provides effective pain relief in patients undergoing open liver surgery. *British journal of pain, 9*(2), 78–85. https://doi.org/10.1177/2049463714525140.

Gitman, M., Fettiplace, M. R., Weinberg, G. L., Neal, J. M., & Barrington, M. J. (2019). Local Anesthetic Systemic Toxicity: A Narrative Literature Review and Clinical Update on Prevention, Diagnosis, and Management. *Plastic and reconstructive surgery, 144*(3), 783–795. https://doi.org/10.1097/PRS.0000000000005989.

Gitman, M., & Barrington, M. J. (2018). Local Anesthetic Systemic Toxicity: A Review of Recent Case Reports and Registries. *Regional anesthesia and pain medicine, 43*(2), 124–130. https://doi.org/10.1097/AAP.0000000000000721.

Gradaus, F., Ivens, K., Peters, A. J., Heering, P., Schoebel, F. C., Grabensee, B., & Strauer, B. E. (2001). Angiographic progression of coronary artery disease in patients with end-stage renal disease. *Nephrology, dialysis, transplantation: official publication of the European Dialysis and Transplant Association- European Renal Association, 16*(6), 1198–1202. https://doi.org/10.1093/ndt/16.6.1198.

Grigg, E., Anderson, C., Pankovich, M., Martin, L., & Flack, S. (2015). Systemic ropivacaine toxicity from a peripheral nerve infusion in a medically complex patient. *Journal of clinical anesthesia, 27*(4), 338–340. https://doi.org/10.1016/j.jclinane.2015.03.021.

Gropper, M. A., Cohen, N. H., Eriksson, L. I., Fleisher, L. A., Leslie, K., Wienner-Kronish, J. P. (2023). *Miller's Anesthesia* (9th ed.). Elsevier.

Grossman, S. H., Davis, D., Kitchell, B. B., Shand, D. G., & Routledge, P. A. (1982). Diazepam and lidocaine plasma protein binding in renal disease. *Clinical pharmacology and therapeutics, 31*(3), 350–357. https://doi.org/10.1038/clpt.1982.45.

Gurusamy, K. S., Li, J., Sharma, D., & Davidson, B. R. (2009). Cardiopulmonary interventions to decrease blood loss and blood transfusion requirements for liver resection. *The Cochrane database of systematic reviews,* (4), CD007338. https://doi.org/10.1002/14651858.CD007338.pub2.

Gurkan, Y. (2015). Ultrasound Use in Regional Anesthesia Practice. *Turkiye Klinikleri J Anest Reanim-Special Topics. 8*(3), 15-19.

Hadimioglu, N., Ertug, Z., Bigat, Z., Yilmaz, M., & Yegin, A. (2005). A randomized study comparing combined spinal epidural or general anesthesia for renal transplant surgery. *Transplantation proceedings, 37*(5), 2020–2022. https://doi.org/10.1016/j.transproceed.2005.03.034.

Hadzic, A. (2017). *Hadzic's Textbook of Regional Anesthesia and Acute Pain Management, Second Edition* (2nd ed.). McGraw Hill / Medical.

Hartmann, B., Junger, A., Klasen, J., Benson, M., Jost, A., Banzhaf, A., & Hempelmann, G. (2002). The Incidence and Risk Factors for Hypotension After Spinal Anesthesia Induction: An Analysis with Automated Data Collection. *Anesthesia &Amp; Analgesia, 94*(6), 1521–1529. https://doi.org/10.1213/00000539-200206000-00027.

Hedge, J., Balajibabu, P. R., & Sivaraman, T. (2017). The patient with ischaemic heart disease undergoing non cardiac surgery. *Indian journal of anaesthesia, 61*(9), 705–711. https://doi.org/10.4103/ija.IJA_384_17.

Heidelbaugh J. J., & Bruderly M. (2006). Cirrhosis and chronic liver failure: part I. Diagnosis and evaluation. *American Academy of Family Physicians., 74*(5), 756-62.

Herrera, A. (2012). Valvular heart disease. In: R. L. Hines & K. E. Marschall (Eds.), *Stoelting's anesthesia and co-existing disease* (pp. 40-42). PA: Philadelphia, Saunders.

Ho, A. M., Chung, D. C., & Joynt, G. M. (2000). Neuraxial blockade and hematoma in cardiac surgery: estimating the risk of a rare adverse event that has not (yet) occurred. *Chest, 117*(2), 551–555. https://doi.org/10.1378/chest.117.2.551.

Holte, K., Foss, N. B., Svensén, C., Lund, C., Madsen, J. L., & Kehlet, H. (2004). Epidural anesthesia, hypotension, and changes in intravascular volume. *Anesthesiology, 100*(2), 281–286. https://doi.org/10.1097/00000542-200402000-00016.

Horlocker, T. T., Wedel, D. J., Benzon, H., Brown, D. L., Enneking, F. K., Heit, J. A., Mulroy, M. F., Rosenquist, R. W., Rowlingson, J., Tryba, M., & Yuan, C. S. (2003). Regional anesthesia in the anticoagulated patient: defining the risks (the second ASRA Consensus Conference on Neuraxial Anesthesia and Anticoagulation). *Regional anesthesia and pain medicine, 28*(3), 172–197. https://doi.org/10.1053/rapm.2003.50046.

Horlocker, T. T., & Wedel, D. J. (1998). Anticoagulation and neuraxial block: historical perspective, anesthetic implications, and risk management. *Regional anesthesia and pain medicine, 23*(6 Suppl 2), 129–134. https://doi.org/10.1016/s1098-7339(98)90137-7.

Igarashi, M., Kawana, S., Iwasaki, H., & Namiki, A. (1995). Masui. *The Japanese journal of anesthesiology, 44*(1), 96–99.

Jokinen, M. J., Neuvonen, P. J., Lindgren, L., Höckerstedt, K., Sjövall, J., Breuer, O., Askemark, Y., Ahonen, J., & Olkkola, K. T. (2007). Pharmacokinetics of ropivacaine in patients with chronic end-stage liver disease. *Anesthesiology,* 106(1), 43–55.

Karanicolas, P., Cleary, S., McHardy, P., McCluskey, S., Sawyer, J., Ladak, S., Law, C., Wei, A., Coburn, N., Ko, R., Katz, J., Kiss, A., Khan, J., Coimbatore, S., Lam-McCulloch, J., & Clarke, H. (2014). Medial open transversus abdominis plane (MOTAP) catheters for analgesia following open liver resection: study protocol for a randomized controlled trial. *Trials, 15*, 241. https://doi.org/10.1186/1745-6215-15-241.

Kaw, D., & Malhotra, D. (2006). Platelet dysfunction and end-stage renal disease. *Seminars in dialysis, 19*(4), 317–322. https://doi.org/10.1111/j.1525-139X.2006.00179.x.

Kaya, K. & Elmas, C. (2010). Peripheral Nerve and Plexus Blocks. In: Tüzüner F. (Eds.) *Anesthesia Intensive Care Pain.* (1st Edition, pp. 561-600). Ankara: MN Medikal and Nobel Medicine Press.

Kelsaka, E. & Guldogus, F. (2013). Regional Anesthesia Room. In: Güldoğuş F, Gürkan Y. (Eds.) *Regional Anesthesia* (1st edition, pp. 11-18). Istanbul: Nobel Medicine Press.

Kennedy, W. F., Jr, Everett, G. B., Cobb, L. A., & Allen, G. D. (1971). Simultaneous systemic and hepatic hemodynamic measurements during high peridural anesthesia in normal man. *Anesthesia and analgesia, 50*(6), 1069–1077. https://doi.org/10.1213/00000539-197150060-00029.

Kramer, M. E., Holtan, E. E., Ives, A. L., & Wall, R. T. (2019). Perioperative Intravenous Lidocaine Infusion Adverse Reaction: A Case Report. *A&A practice, 13*(3), 96–98. https://doi.org/10.1213/XAA.0000000000001002.

Levey, A. S., Eckardt, K. U., Tsukamoto, Y., Levin, A., Coresh, J., Rossert, J., De Zeeuw, D., Hostetter, T. H., Lameire, N., & Eknoyan, G. (2005). Definition and classification of chronic kidney disease: a position statement from Kidney Disease: Improving Global Outcomes (KDIGO). *Kidney international, 67*(6), 2089–2100. https://doi.org/10.1111/j.1523-1755.2005.00365.x.

Li, P. K., Burdmann, E. A., & Mehta, R. L. (2013). World Kidney Day 2013: acute kidney injury-global health alert. *American journal of kidney diseases: the official journal of the National Kidney Foundation, 61*(3), 359–363. https://doi.org/10.1053/j.ajkd.2013.01.002.

Li, J., & Oprea, A. D. (2020). Periprocedural management of patients on oral anticoagulation: focus on regional anesthesia. *Polish Archives of Internal Medicine, 130*(12): 1081-1092. https://doi.org/10.20452/pamw.15416.

London, G. M. (2003). Cardiovascular disease in chronic renal failure: pathophysiologic aspects. *Seminars in dialysis, 16*(2), 85–94. https://doi.org/10.1046/j.1525-139x.2003.16023.x.

López, M. M., Guasch, E., Schiraldi, R., Maggi, G., Alonso, E., & Gilsanz, F. (2016). Raquianestesia contínua com monitoração hemodinâmica minimamente invasiva para cirurgia de reparação do quadril em dois pacientes com estenose aórtica grave [Continuous spinal anaesthesia with minimally invasive haemodynamic monitoring for surgical hip repair in two patients with severe aortic stenosis]. *Brazilian Journal of Anesthesiology, 66*(1), 82–85. https://doi.org/10.1016/j.bjan.2013.03.010.

Macfarlane, A. J. R., Gitman, M., Bornstein, K. J., El-Boghdadly, K., & Weinberg, G. (2021). Updates in our understanding of local anaesthetic systemic toxicity: a narrative review. *Anaesthesia, 76* Suppl 1, 27–39. https://doi.org/10.1111/anae.15282.

Mangano, D. T., Hollenberg, M., Fegert, G., Meyer, M. L., London, M. J., Tubau, J. F., & Krupski, W. C. (1991). Perioperative myocardial ischemia in patients undergoing noncardiac surgery--I: Incidence and severity during the 4 day perioperative period. *The Study of Perioperative Ischemia (SPI) Research Group. Journal of the American College of Cardiology, 17*(4), 843–850. https://doi.org/10.1016/0735-1097(91)90863-5.

Marhofer, P., Harrop-Griffiths, W., Kettner, S. C., & Kirchmair, L. (2010). Fifteen years of ultrasound guidance in regional anaesthesia: part 1. *British journal of anaesthesia, 104*(5), 538–546. https://doi.org/10.1093/bja/aeq069.

Matot, I., Scheinin, O., Eid, A., & Jurim, O. (2002). Epidural anesthesia and analgesia in liver resection. *Anesthesia and analgesia, 95*(5), 1179-1181. https://doi.org/10.1097/00000539-200211000-00009.

McDonald, S. B. (2004). Is neuraxial blockade contraindicated in the patient with aortic stenosis? *Regional anesthesia and pain medicine, 29*(5), 496–502. https://doi.org/10.1016/j.rapm.2004.06.010.

McEllistrem, R. F., Schell, J., O'Malley, K., O'Toole, D., & Cunningham, A. J. (1989). Interscalene brachial plexus blockade with lidocaine in chronic renal failure--a pharmacokinetic study. *Canadian journal of anaesthesia = Journal canadien d'anesthesie*, *36*(1), 59–63. https://doi.org/10.1007/BF03010889.

Meersch, M., Schmidt, C., & Zarbock, A. (2016). Patient with chronic renal failure undergoing surgery. *Current opinion in anaesthesiology*, *29*(3), 413–420. https://doi.org/10.1097/ACO.0000000000000329.

Mei, B., Lu, Y., Liu, X., Zhang, Y., Gu, E., & Chen, S. (2019). Ultrasound-guided lumbar selective nerve root block plus T12 paravertebral and sacral plexus block for hip and knee arthroplasty: Three case reports. *Medicine, 98*(22), e15887. https://doi.org/10.1097/MD.0000000000015887.

Meierhenrich, R., Wagner, F., Schütz, W., Rockemann, M., Steffen, P., Senftleben, U., & Gauss, A. (2009). The effects of thoracic epidural anesthesia on hepatic blood flow in patients under general anesthesia. *Anesthesia and analgesia, 108*(4), 1331–1337. https://doi.org/10.1213/ane.0b013e3181966e6f.

Mitra, M., Basu, M., Shailendra, K., & Jain, A. C. (2020). Use of Peripheral Nerve Blocks in Perioperative Management of Cases with Hypertrophic Cardiomyopathy Undergoing Lower Limb Orthopedic Surgeries. *Anesthesia, essays and researches, 14*(2), 277–282. https://doi.org/10.4103/aer.AER_48_20.

Mostert, J. W., Evers, J. L., Hobika, G. H., Moore, R. H., Kenny, G. M., & Murphy, G. P. (1970). The haemodynamic response to chronic renal failure as studied in the azotaemic state. *British journal of anaesthesia*, *42*(5), 397–411. https://doi.org/10.1093/bja/42.5.397.

Murphy, E. J. (2005). Acute Pain Management Pharmacology for the Patient with Concurrent Renal or Hepatic Disease. *Anaesthesia and Intensive Care, 33*(3), 311–322. https://doi.org/10.1177/0310057x0503300306.

Mushlin, P. S. & Gelman S. (2011). Anesthesia and the Liver. In: P. G. Barash, B. F. Cullen, R. K. Stoelting, M. K. Cahalan, M. C. Stock (Eds.) *Clinical Anesthesia* (pp. 121-140). Philadelphia: Lippincott Williams & Wilkins.

Narouze, S., Benzon, H. T., Provenzano, D., Buvanendran, A., De Andres, J., Deer, T., Rauck, R., & Huntoon, M. A. (2018). Interventional Spine and Pain Procedures in Patients on Antiplatelet and Anticoagulant Medications (Second Edition): Guidelines From the American Society of Regional Anesthesia and Pain Medicine, the European Society of Regional Anaesthesia and Pain Therapy, the American Academy of Pain Medicine, the International Neuromodulation Society, the North American Neuromodulation Society, and the World Institute of Pain. *Regional anesthesia and pain medicine,* *43*(3), 225–262. https://doi.org/10.1097/AAP.0000000000000700.

Narouze, S., Benzon, H. T., Provenzano, D. A., Buvanendran, A., De Andres, J., Deer, T. R., Rauck, R., & Huntoon, M. A. (2015). Interventional spine and pain procedures in patients on antiplatelet and anticoagulant medications: guidelines from the American Society of Regional Anesthesia and Pain Medicine, the European Society of Regional Anaesthesia and Pain Therapy, the American Academy of Pain Medicine, the International Neuromodulation Society, the North American Neuromodulation Society, and the World Institute of Pain. *Regional anesthesia and pain medicine, 40*(3), 182–212. https://doi.org/10.1097/AAP.0000000000000223.

Neal, J. M., Barrington, M. J., Fettiplace, M. R., Gitman, M., Memtsoudis, S. G., Mörwald, E. E., Rubin, D. S., & Weinberg, G. (2018). The Third American Society of Regional Anesthesia and Pain Medicine Practice Advisory on Local Anesthetic Systemic Toxicity: Executive Summary 2017. *Regional anesthesia and pain medicine, 43*(2), 113–123. https://doi.org/10.1097/AAP.0000000000000720.

Neal J. M. (2016). Ultrasound-Guided Regional Anesthesia and Patient Safety: Update of an Evidence-Based Analysis. *Regional anesthesia and pain medicine, 41*(2), 195–204. https://doi.org/10.1097/AAP.0000000000000295.

Nkomo, V. T., Gardin, J. M., Skelton, T. N., Gottdiener, J. S., Scott, C. G., & Enriquez-Sarano, M. (2006). Burden of valvular heart diseases: a population-based study. *Lancet (London, England), 368*(9540), 1005–1011. https://doi.org/10.1016/S0140-6736(06)69208-8.

Northup, P. G., Sundaram, V., Fallon, M. B., Reddy, K. R., Balogun, R. A., Sanyal, A. J., Anstee, Q. M., Hoffman, M. R., Ikura, Y., & Caldwell, S. H. (2007). Hypercoagulation and thrombophilia in liver disease. *Journal of Thrombosis and Haemostasis, 6*(1), 2-9. https://doi.org/10.1111/j.1538-7836.2007.02772.x.

Northup, P. G., Garcia-Pagan, J. C., Garcia-Tsao, G., Intagliata, N. M., Superina, R. A., Roberts, L. N., Lisman, T., & Valla, D. C. (2021). Vascular Liver Disorders, Portal Vein Thrombosis, and Procedural Bleeding in Patients With Liver Disease: 2020 Practice Guidance by the American Association for the Study of Liver Diseases. *Hepatology, 73*(1), 366–413. https://doi.org/10.1002/hep.31646.

Nygård, E., Kofoed, K. F., Freiberg, J., Holm, S., Aldershvile, J., Eliasen, K., & Kelbaek, H. (2005). Effects of high thoracic epidural analgesia on myocardial blood flow in patients with ischemic heart disease. *Circulation, 111*(17), 2165–2170. https://doi.org/10.1161/01.CIR.0000163551.33812.1A.

Oguro, A., Taniguchi, H., Daidoh, T., Itoh, A., Tsukuda, N., & Takahashi, T. (1993). Factors relating to coagulation, fibrinolysis and hepatic damage after liver resection. *HPB surgery: a world journal of hepatic, pancreatic and biliary surgery, 7*(1), 43–49. https://doi.org/10.1155/1993/91843.

Olcay, A. & Akdemir, B. (2018). Direct Oral Anticoagulants in Patients with Chronic Renal Failure. *Turkiye Klinikleri J Cardiol-Special Topics.11*(2),142–146.

Orko, R., Pitkänen, M., Rosenberg, P., H. (1986). Subarachnoid anaesthesia with 0.75% bupivacaine in patients with chronic renal failure. *Br J Anaesth, 58*:605–609.

Page, A., Rostad, B., Staley, C. A., Levy, J. H., Park, J., Goodman, M., Sarmiento, J. M., Galloway, J., Delman, K. A., & Kooby, D. A. (2008). Epidural analgesia in hepatic resection. *Journal of the American College of Surgeons, 206*(6), 1184–1192. https://doi.org/10.1016/j.jamcollsurg.2007.12.041.

Paqueron, X., Boccara, G., Bendahou, M., Coriat, P., & Riou, B. (2002). Brachial plexus nerve block exhibits prolonged duration in the elderly. *Anesthesiology, 97*(5), 1245–1249. https://doi.org/10.1097/00000542-200211000-00030.

Peck, T., & Harris, B. (2021). *Pharmacology for anaesthesia and intensive care.* Cambridge University Press.

Pere, P., Salonen, M., Jokinen, M., Rosenberg, P. H., Neuvonen, P. J., & Haasio, J. (2003). Pharmacokinetics of ropivacaine in uremic and nonuremic patients after axillary brachial plexus block. *Anesthesia and analgesia, 96*(2), 563-569. https://doi.org/10.1097/00000539-200302000-00048.

Perlas, A., Chan, V. W., & Beattie, S. (2016). Anesthesia Technique and Mortality after Total Hip or Knee Arthroplasty: A Retrospective, Propensity Score-matched Cohort Study. *Anesthesiology, 125*(4), 724–731. https://doi.org/10.1097/ALN.0000000000001248.

Pirracchio, R., Cholley, B., De Hert, S., Solal, A. C., & Mebazaa, A. (2007). Diastolic heart failure in anaesthesia and critical care. *British journal of anaesthesia, 98*(6), 707–721. https://doi.org/10.1093/bja/aem098.

Pivalizza, E. G., Abramson, D. C., & Harvey, A. (1997). Perioperative hypercoagulability in uremic patients: a viscoelastic study. *Journal of clinical anesthesia, 9*(6), 442–445. https://doi.org/10.1016/s0952-8180(97)00097-4.

Pu, X., & Sun, J. M. (2019). General anesthesia vs spinal anesthesia for patients undergoing total-hip arthroplasty: A meta-analysis. *Medicine, 98*(16), e14925. https://doi.org/10.1097/MD.0000000000014925.

Rahimzadeh, P., Safari, S., Faiz, S. H., & Alavian, S. M. (2014). Anesthesia for patients with liver disease. *Hepatitis monthly, 14*(7), e19881. https://doi.org/10.5812/hepatmon.19881.

Ran, J., Wang, Y., Li, F., Zhang, W., & Ma, M. (2015). Pharmacodynamics and Pharmacokinetics of Levobupivacaine Used for Epidural Anesthesia in Patients with Liver Dysfunction. *Cell biochemistry and biophysics, 73*(3), 717–721. https://doi.org/10.1007/s12013-015-0677-6.

Reidenberg, M. M., James, M., & Dring, L. G. (1972). The rate of procaine hydrolysis in serum of normal subjects and diseased patients. *Clinical pharmacology and therapeutics, 13*(2), 279–284. https://doi.org/10.1002/cpt1972132279.

Rice, A. S., Pither, C. E., & Tucker, G. T. (1991). Plasma concentrations of bupivacaine after supraclavicular brachial plexus blockade in patients with chronic renal failure. *Anaesthesia, 46*(5), 354–357. https://doi.org/10.1111/j.1365-2044.1991.tb09542.x.

Rose, M., & Ness, T. J. (2002). Hypoxia following interscalene block. *Regional anesthesia and pain medicine, 27*(1), 94–96. https://doi.org/10.1053/rapm.2002.29709.

Rosenberg, P. H, Veering, B. T., & Urmey, W. F. (2004) Maximum recommended doses of local anesthetics: a multifactorial concept. *Regional anesthesia and pain medicine. 29*(6), 564-75. https//doi.org/10.1016/j.rapm.2004.08.003. PMID: 15635516.

Sanya, E. O., & Ogunniyi, A. (2004). Cardiovascular autonomic neuropathy in non-diabetic Nigerian patients with chronic renal failure. *West African journal of medicine, 23*(1), 15–20. https://doi.org/10.4314/wajm.v23i1.28073.

Schneider, A. C. (2018). A review of aortic stenosis: an anesthetic perspective. *J Anesth Crit Care Open Access.,10*(6):262-264. https//doi.org/10.15406/jaccoa.2018.10.00401.

Scott, N. B., Turfrey, D. J., Ray, D. A., Nzewi, O., Sutcliffe, N. P., Lal, A. B., Norrie, J., Nagels, W. J., & Ramayya, G. P. (2001). A prospective randomized study of the potential benefits of thoracic epidural anesthesia and analgesia in patients undergoing coronary artery bypass grafting. *Anesthesia and analgesia, 93*(3), 528–535.

Shahlaie, K., Fox, A., Butani, L., & Boggan, J. E. (2004). Spontaneous epidural hemorrhage in chronic renal failure. A case report and review. *Pediatric nephrology (Berlin, Germany), 19*(10), 1168–1172. https://doi.org/10.1007/s00467-004-1551-8.

Sharrock, N. E., Beksac, B., Flynn, E., Go, G., & Della Valle, A. G. (2006). Hypotensive epidural anaesthesia in patients with preoperative renal dysfunction undergoing total hip replacement. *British journal of anaesthesia, 96*(2), 207–212. https://doi.org/10.1093/bja/aei308.

Shontz, R., Karuparthy, V., Temple, R., & Brennan, T. J. (2009). Prevalence and risk factors predisposing to coagulopathy in patients receiving epidural analgesia for hepatic surgery. *Regional anesthesia and pain medicine, 34*(4), 308–311. https://doi.org/10.1097/AAP.0b013e3181ac7d00.

Sivarajan, M., Amory, D. W., Lindbloom, L. E., & Schwettmann, R. S. (1975). Systemic and regional blood-flow changes during spinal anesthesia in the rhesus monkey. *Anesthesiology, 43*(1), 78–88. https://doi.org/10.1097/00000542-197507000-00017.

Smith, M. C., Boylan, M. R., Tam, S. F., Lee, R., Alfonso, A. E., & Sugiyama, G. (2015). End-stage renal disease increases the risk of mortality after appendectomy. *Surgery, 158*(3), 722–727. https://doi.org/10.1016/j.surg.2015.03.064.

Spoladore, R., Maron, M. S., D'Amato, R., Camici, P. G., & Olivotto, I. (2012). Pharmacological treatment options for hypertrophic cardiomyopathy: high time for evidence. *European heart journal, 33*(14), 1724–1733. https://doi.org/10.1093/eurheartj/ehs150.

Starczewska, M. H., Mon, W., & Shirley, P. (2017). Anaesthesia in patients with liver disease. *Current Opinion in Anaesthesiology, 30*(3), 392–398. https://doi.org/10.1097/aco.0000000000000470.

Suleiman, M. Y., Passannante, A. N., Onder, R. L., Greene-Helms, W. F., & Perretta, S. G. (1997). Alteration of renal blood flow during epidural anesthesia in normal subjects. *Anesthesia and analgesia, 84*(5), 1076–1080. https://doi.org/10.1097/00000539-199705000-00022.

Süleymanlar, G., Utaş, C., Arinsoy, T., Ateş, K., Altun, B., Altiparmak, M. R., Ecder, T., Yilmaz, M. E., Çamsari, T., Başçi, A., Odabas, A. R., & Serdengeçti, K. (2011). A population-based survey of Chronic REnal Disease In Turkey--the CREDIT study. *Nephrology, dialysis, transplantation: official publication of the European Dialysis and Transplant Association - European Renal Association, 26*(6), 1862–1871. https://doi.org/10.1093/ndt/gfq656.

Tanaka, N., Nagata, N., Hamakawa, T., & Takasaki, M. (1997). The effect of dopamine on hepatic blood flow in patients undergoing epidural anesthesia. *Anesthesia and analgesia, 85*(2), 286–290. https://doi.org/10.1097/00000539-199708000-00008.

Tran, D. Q., Boezaart, A. P., & Neal, J. M. (2017). Beyond Ultrasound Guidance for Regional Anesthesiology. *Regional anesthesia and pain medicine, 42*(5), 556–563. https://doi.org/10.1097/AAP.0000000000000628.

Tripodi, A., & Mannucci, P. M. (2011). The Coagulopathy of Chronic Liver Disease. *New England Journal of Medicine, 365*(2), 147–156. https://doi.org/10.1056/nejmra1011170.

Tsuchiya, H., Mizogami, M., Ueno, T., & Shigemi, K. (2012). Cardiotoxic local anesthetics increasingly interact with biomimetic membranes under ischemia-like acidic conditions. *Biological & pharmaceutical bulletin, 35*(6), 988–992. https://doi.org/10.1248/bpb.35.988.

Tunney, R. K., Jr, Whyte, K., & DeAntonio, H. J. (2018). Lidocaine toxicity in the setting of HeartMate II left ventricular assist device. *Journal of clinical pharmacy and therapeutics, 43*(5), 733–736. https://doi.org/10.1111/jcpt.12717.

Turan, A., Bajracharya, G. R., Leung, S., Yazici Kara, M., Mao, G., Botsford, T., Ruetzler, K., Maheshwari, K., Ali Sakr Esa, W., Elsharkawy, H., & Sessler, D. I. (2019). Association of Neuraxial Anesthesia With Postoperative Venous Thromboembolism After Noncardiac Surgery: A Propensity-Matched Analysis of ACS-NSQIP Database. *Anesthesia and analgesia, 128*(3), 494–501. https://doi.org/10.1213/ANE.0000000000003394.

Vaja, R., McNicol, L., & Sisley, I. (2010). Anaesthesia for patients with liver disease. *Continuing Education in Anaesthesia Critical Care &Amp; Pain, 10*(1), 15–19. https://doi.org/10.1093/bjaceaccp/mkp040.

Van Dam, R. M., Hendry, P. O., Coolsen, M. M., Bemelmans, M. H., Lassen, K., Revhaug, A., Fearon, K. C., Garden, O. J., Dejong, C. H., & Enhanced Recovery After Surgery (ERAS) Group (2008). Initial experience with a multimodal enhanced recovery programme in patients undergoing liver resection. *The British journal of surgery, 95*(8), 969–975. https://doi.org/10.1002/bjs.6227.

Vasson, M. P., Baguet, J. C., Arveiller, M. R., Bargnoux, P. J., Giroud, J. P., & Raichvarg, D. (1993). Serum and urinary alpha-1 acid glycoprotein in chronic renal failure. *Nephron, 65*(2), 299–303. https://doi.org/10.1159/000187492.

Vasques, F., Behr, A. U., Weinberg, G., Ori, C., & Di Gregorio, G. (2015). A Review of Local Anesthetic Systemic Toxicity Cases Since Publication of the American Society of Regional Anesthesia Recommendations: To Whom It May Concern. *Regional anesthesia and pain medicine, 40*(6), 698–705. https://doi.org/10.1097/AAP.0000000000000320.

Wadlund D. L. (2017). Local Anesthetic Systemic Toxicity. *AORN journal, 106*(5), 367–377. https://doi.org/10.1016/j.aorn.2017.08.015.

Wagener, G., & Brentjens, T. E. (2010). Anesthetic concerns in patients presenting with renal failure. *Anesthesiology clinics, 28*(1), 39–54. https://doi.org/10.1016/j.anclin.2010.01.006.

Waldinger, R., Weinberg, G., & Gitman, M. (2020). Local Anesthetic Toxicity in the Geriatric Population. *Drugs & aging, 37*(1), 1–9. https://doi.org/10.1007/s40266-019-00718-0.

Wiklund R. A. (2004). Preoperative preparation of patients with advanced liver disease. *Critical care medicine, 32*(4 Suppl), S106–S115. https://doi.org/10.1097/01.ccm.0000115624.13479.e6.

Wu, T., Tang, L. V., & Hu, Y. (2022). Venous Thromboembolism in Kidney Diseases and Genetic Predisposition. *Kidney diseases (Basel, Switzerland), 8*(3), 181–189. https://doi.org/10.1159/000523777.

Xia, V. W., Messerlian, A. K., Mackley, J., Calmes, S. H., & Matevosian, R. (2006). Successful epidural anesthesia for cesarean section in a parturient with severe aortic stenosis and a recent history of pulmonary edema--a case report. *Journal of clinical anesthesia, 18*(2), 142–144. https://doi.org/10.1016/j.jclinane.2005.06.007.

Yamane, Y., Omae, T., Kou, K., & Sakuraba, S. (2017). Successful use of femoral nerve block with dexmedetomidine for fracture fixation of an intracapsular fracture of the femoral neck in a patient with severe aortic stenosis: a case report. *JA clinical reports, 3*(1), 1-4. https://doi.org/10.1186/s40981-017-0126-1.

Zhang, J., Wang, X., Zhang, H., Shu, Z., & Jiang, W. (2019). Comparison of combined lumbar and sacral plexus block with sedation versus general anaesthesia on postoperative outcomes in elderly patients undergoing hip fracture surgery (CLSB-HIPELD): study protocol for a prospective, multicentre, randomised controlled trial. *BMJ open, 9*(3), e022898. https://doi.org/10.1136/bmjopen-2018-022898.

Zinn, S. E., Fairley, H. B., & Glenn, J. D. (1985). Liver function in patients with mild alcoholic hepatitis, after enflurane, nitrous oxide-narcotic, and spinal anesthesia. *Anesthesia and analgesia, 64*(5), 487–490.

Chapter 3

Oncological Patients, Chemotherapeutics and Anesthesia

Sinan Yılmaz*, MD
and Kazim Karaaslan, MD
Department of Anesthesiology and Reanimation, Bezmialem Vakıf University, Istanbul, Turkiye

Abstract

Today, despite the advances in diagnosis and treatment methods, cancer is increasingly ranked second worldwide as the leading cause of morbidity and mortality after cardiovascular diseases and is becoming a health problem with increasing importance day by day. According to the World Health Organization 2020 report, approximately 20 million people are diagnosed with cancer and 10 million die from cancer or related complications. Every year, 3-4 out of 1000 people are diagnosed with new cancer and it causes death in 1-2 of them. Although lung, prostate, colorectal, and breast cancers are more common, obesity and smoking are important risk factors for cancer development. Distant metastases can occur even at the diagnosis stage of cancer patients. Metastases are essential to determine the prognosis according to the type of primary tumor, the characteristics of the tissue or organ in which metastasis is detected, and the location and number of metastases. Anesthesia applications are increasing in patients receiving cancer treatment. While some of these applications are for cancer treatment, some include noncancer surgeries, diagnostic and therapeutic interventions, and imaging. Multiple anesthesia applications are increasing, especially in pediatric and disabled patient groups. In these groups of patients, changes

* Corresponding Author's Email: siyilmaz@bezmialem.edu.tr.

In: Organ Failure and Anesthesia Practices
Editors: Ahmet Şen and Basar Erdivanli
ISBN: 979-8-89113-486-7

can develop in organ and system functions that may affect the anesthesia plan and application for many different reasons.

Keywords: cancer, anaesthesia, chemotherapy, hematological disorders, anaesthetics

Introduction

Cancer is a mass that occurs when cells in an organ or tissue change with some effects. They divide and multiply uncontrollably and irregularly locally and at distant points. These cells differ from normal tissues in terms of their high proliferation ability, insensitivity to factors that prevent their growth, the absence of cell death (apoptosis), the ability to form new vessels (angiogenesis) and the ability to invade and metastasize to tissues. Typically, cells multiply under a specific control by dividing according to the need. Cells are destroyed by programmed death or apoptosis; on the other hand, they multiply under the influence of growth factors. Oncogenes cause cells to grow too much by mutating some genes in DNA. Cancer is a group of diseases that affect many systems. Diagnosis and treatment require the cooperation of many specialties. It is difficult to treat. Early diagnosis is essential. (Wisley, 2020; Stewart, 2003; Arain & Buggy, 2007; Kurosawa, 2012; Longhini, 2020). Although surgery and radiotherapy are local treatment methods, they can be supported by systemic treatments such as chemotherapy and immunotherapy.

The first use of the word cancer in the medical literature; It is named after Hippocrates, who lived between 460-375 BC, with the Greek word "carcinos" meaning crab, with the image of tumoral masses surrounded by blood vessels in the tissues reminiscent of a crab. Later, in the Greek alphabet, the word carcinos was written in Latin letters, while "carcinoma" meaning "crab" was used. In the following centuries, the Greek pronunciation of this word was adopted in Latin works, and the Latin word cancer, meaning crab, continued to be used. In later years, the Greek word "oncos" meaning mass or load, gave the oncology branch its name. In documents dating back to ancient times, some articles describe cancer without knowing exactly what it is. "There is no cure" in the notes of the Egyptian physician Imhotep, who lived in the 27th century BC. The masses in the breast are mentioned, suggesting breast cancer (Temel, 2005).

Cancer Treatment

Cancer treatment aims to prevent metastasis formation with curative treatment while destroying the cell tumor and preventing its growth and proliferation. Although chemotherapy, radiotherapy, and surgery are the most widely used methods in cancer treatment, different approaches, such as hormone therapy and biological processes, can be used together or alone to support other methods. It is impossible to talk about a single definitive treatment method because each method has its advantages and disadvantages, cancer is a unique disease, and treatments can differ from person to person. (Chang et al., 2021; Nadler et al., 2019). Cancer treatment with drug therapy is called chemotherapy. The drugs used in chemotherapy are also called chemotherapeutics or antineoplastic drugs. Chemotherapy can be provided for a complete cure or used to prolong life or control symptoms. Normally, cells in the body multiply, grow, and die in a controlled manner. Cancer cells continue to multiply and grow uncontrollably. Chemotherapy kills cancer cells, blocking their effects, and slowing their growth. However, it can cause side effects by damaging healthy normal cells, especially the rapidly regenerating group. Cell influence level may vary depending on drug type, dose, and patient characteristics.

Surgical Treatment

Surgery is often used to make the initial diagnosis of the tumor and remove the tumor mass or metastases. In some cases, surgery can be performed for palliation or rehabilitation. Surgical removal of solid tumors is still considered the mainstay and best prognostic treatment (Kim, 2018). However, surgery can increase the likelihood of tumor spread and recurrence through many mechanisms. It is known that even in cases where the tumor is successfully excised and the surgical margins are histologically clean, minimal residual tumor tissue can remain. Cells enter the circulation during tumor manipulation and form micrometastases (Inoue et al., 2022; Huettemann & Sakka, 2005). In addition, immunosuppression, neuro-endocrine and angiogenic changes secondary to surgery may increase tumor development (Kim, 2018). After surgery, NK cell function, essential for preventing tumor development, is suppressed. (Wu et al., 2020; Gupta et al., 2002). There is a direct proportion between the magnitude of the stress and the prevalence of systemic changes.

It has been reported that NK cell functions return faster and tumor spread is reduced by suppressing surgical stress with the help of beta-blockers, opioids, or cyclooxygenase (COX) inhibitors (Ricon et al., 2016; Huettemann & Sakka, 2005).

Radiotherapy

Radiotherapy is a treatment method that focuses on killing cancer cells using ionizing rays. While it can be done by targeting only a specific part of the body, treatments targeting the whole body are also applied. Radiation therapy aims to shrink the tumor by using it before the surgical procedure. After the dosage calculations are performed by the radiation oncologist, the goal is to shrink the tumor area and kill the cancerous cells after the radiation is administered to the tissue or organ. However, one of the most significant disadvantages of RT is that it kills healthy cells while killing harmful cells. In addition, typical side effects such as vomiting, hair loss, fatigue, and loss of appetite can also affect the patient's quality of life. Therefore, other treatment modalities may be considered (Groenewold et al., 2022).

Stem Cell Therapy

Stem cells are extraordinary cells that can differentiate into other types of cells. Each stem cell has the potential to produce a new stem cell. When the stem cell divides, it either remains as a stem cell or can differentiate and become another cell. Unlike adult cells, they can renew themselves by dividing. Cells used in treatment should be able to transform into the desired cell type, survive and function properly in the host cell after transplantation, and not damage the surrounding tissues and organs. Stem cell therapies are divided into three basic types for treatment in humans. The first is allogeneic transplantation, where the donor is another person; the second is autologous transplantation using the individual's stem cells; and the third is syngeneic transplantation, where the donor is a twin or triplet of the recipient. The most significant advantage of using stem cells from another donor in treatment is that the donor has healthy cells and does not carry cancerous cells. However, the most significant disadvantage is that achieving tissue compatibility between the recipient and the donor can sometimes be challenging. Before or during the stem cell treatment, the effectiveness of the treatment can be increased by applying radiotherapy and/or chemotherapy to the patients, or this reaction can be reduced with potent immunosuppressive drugs (Groenewold et al., 2022).

Chemotherapy

The word "chemotherapy" actually entered the literature before cancer treatment. Paul Ehrlich first used it for the treatment of syphilis in the 1900s. The success of chemical agents developed over time has given hope to studies on the treatment of other diseases, such as cancer. Initially, there were two difficulties in developing the agent that could be used in therapy. The first is to identify those with the potential for anticancer effects among many chemicals, and the second is to conduct clinical trials that show that they are effective. Since it is impossible to determine the drugs to be used in the treatment of cancer in humans from among a large number of chemicals, many tumor models were developed in the laboratory environment, and the drugs to be used in humans were selected after animal experiments. After determining that a drug developed in this way was influential in treatment, it was started to be tested in appropriate patient groups. Examining the damage caused by chemicals such as mustard gas, which is exposed in situations such as war, in the body could accelerate the development of drugs to be used in cancer treatment (Temel, 2015; Groenewold et al., 2022; Navari, 2020).

There are types of chemotherapy. Most common are:

1. Adjuvant chemotherapy is administered after primary surgical treatment to kill any remaining cancer cells to reduce the chances of recurrence and kill micrometastatic disease. Increases disease-free survival.
2. Neoadjuvant therapy is a type of induction therapy. It is administered before surgery to shrink a tumor or stop the spread of cancer, making surgery less invasive and more effective. Neoadjuvant therapy is applied before primary treatment.
3. Palliative chemotherapy is administered to control symptoms or prolong life in a patient in whom a cure is unlikely.
4. Maintenance chemotherapy is long-term, low-dose, single, or combination chemotherapy to delay the regrowth of residual tumor cells in a patient who has achieved complete remission with treatment.

Chemotherapeuthetics

Although people have treated diseases with plants found in nature for hundreds of years, the development of cancer drugs accelerated in the 20th century (Temel, 2015). Chemical substances isolated from nature, chemicals extracted in the laboratory, or synthesized and produced in factories have taken their place in today's cancer treatment after severe testing stages. Studies continue to increase. These drugs; can be classified according to their chemical structure, source of origin, mechanism of action, or potential for damage in the tissue. They can be toxic to the cell directly and effective in treatment by damaging cells at a particular stage of the cell cycle, inhibiting some cellular functions and cell division, or by inducing apoptotic or necrotic cell death.

Classification of antineoplastic drugs:

1. Alkylating Drugs; All are pro-drugs. They show their effects by binding to nucleophilic groups in cell structures. With the intra- and interchain bonds in DNA, DNA transcription and cell proliferation are stopped. Alkylating agents damage the DNA of cells, preventing them from replicating themselves. Treats hematological malignancies such as leukemia, Hodgkin lymphoma, multiple myeloma, and breast, lung, and ovarian cancers. These drugs can damage the bone marrow, as well as cancer cells. Alkylating drugs are divided into several groups.
    a. Mechlorethamine: It was developed from nitrogenous mustard gas, which is banned. It is used in the treatment of Hodgkin's disease and some solid tumors because it causes lymphocytopenia.
    b. Cyclophosphamide is a synthetic alkylating agent. It is related to nitrogen mustards with antineoplastic and immunosuppressive activities. In the liver, it is converted to the active metabolites aldophosphamide and phosphoramide mustard. They bind to DNA, inhibit DNA replication, and initiate cell death. It is used in chemotherapy to suppress the immune system and treat lymphoma, multiple myeloma, leukemia, ovarian cancer, breast cancer, small cell lung cancer, neuroblastoma, and sarcoma. In addition to cancer treatment, it is immunosuppressive in progressive autoimmune diseases, nephrotic syndrome, and after organ transplantation.

c. Ethyleneims: Triethylene methamine, Thiotepa, and Alteramin are in this group of drugs.
d. Alkyl sulfonates: Busulfan has a potent cytotoxic effect. Removing existing bone marrow before transplantation is most commonly applied in treatment.
e. Nitrosourea group drugs: This group of drugs is used primarily in the treatment of tumors due to their transmission to the central nervous system.
f. Triazene and Hydrazine Derivatives: Dacarbazine and Procarbazine are drugs in this group.

2. Antimetabolites: They stop growth by interfering with the normal metabolism of cells. This group of drugs is often used to treat leukemia and cancers of the breast, ovary, and colon. Antimetabolites include 5-fluorouracil, 6-mercaptopurine, cytarabine, gemcitabine, and methotrexate. The drugs in this group are:
   a. Folic acid antimetabolites: prevent the development of cancer cells. DNA suppresses RNA protein synthesis, leading to cell death.
   b. Purine antimetabolites: Used in the maintenance treatment of acute lymphoblastic leukemia (ALL).
   c. Pyrimidine antimetabolites: They stop the synthesis of pyrimidine in the cancer cell and cause the loss of one of the building blocks required for DNA synthesis in the cell.
3. Herbal Anticarcinogens: These are drugs obtained from some plants and used to treat cancer. It affects cell microtubules. It stops the cancer cell in metaphase. Vincristine, Vinblastine, Paclitaxel, Podophyllotoxin, Etoposide, and Teniposide are some plant-derived anticarcinogens.
   a. Vinca alkaloids: Vincristine, Vinblastine: They inhibit polymerization by binding to microtubules; Mitosis stops at metaphase. DNA synthesis and DNA structure are not affected. They also inhibit leukocyte phagocytosis, chemotaxis, and axonal conduction in neurons. They are extensively bound to plasma proteins and formed blood elements. They are mainly metabolized and excreted by the hepatobiliary system. They are metabolized by cytochrome P450. Their toxicity is less than that of other antineoplastics. However, it can cause neuromuscular side effects. Peripheral neuropathy is the most common side effect. In practice, extravasations can cause local damage.

Vincristine treats acute lymphocytic leukemia, soft tissue tumors, and Hodgkin's and Non-Hodgkin's lymphoma.

b. Taxanes: Paclitaxel is of herbal origin; it does not prevent tubulin polymerization. However, they disrupt the tubulin-microtubule balance by preventing depolymerization. The tubules are stable but dysfunctional. The cytotoxic effect occurs. Caution should be exercised in the concomitant use of drugs metabolizing by cytochrome p450 enzymes. It is used in ovarian and metastatic breast cancer, small cell lung cancer, and some head and neck cancers.

4. Antibiotics: They act by disrupting DNA functions of cancer cells. Dactinomycin, Doxorubusin, Daunorubicin, Bleomycin, and Plikamycin (Mithramycin) are some antibiotics used in cancer treatment.
   a. Dactinomycin: Used with other drugs in some soft tissue cancers, Willm's tumor.
   b. Doxorubicin, Daunorubicin: Doxorubicin treats sarcoma, breast and lung cancer, lymphoma, and acute lymphocytic leukemia. Daunorubicin is used in the treatment of acute lymphocytic and myelocytic leukemia.
   c. Bleomycin: Bleomycin is combined with some drugs to treat testicular tumors.
   d. Plikamycin reduces calcium levels in patients with bone tumors and hypercalcemia.
5. Hormone and Hormone Antagonists: Tumor development and tumor growth rate may slow down and patient complaints decrease due to treatment in tumors that are sensitive to hormones. Glucocorticoid hormones, antiandrogens, gonadotropin-releasing hormone, progestins, estrogens, and hormone antagonists are used in cancer treatment.
   a. Glucocorticoid hormones: Prednisone, one of the glucocorticoid hormones, is a drug used to treat cancer.
   b. Antiandrogens: Used in the treatment of prostate cancer.
   c. Gonodotropin releasing hormone Leuprolide and Goserelin from this group of drugs are used to treat prostate cancer.
   d. Progestins: Used in endometrial carcinoma, metastatic renal carcinoma, and breast cancer.

   e. Estrogens: Used in the treatment of prostate cancer. Tamoxifen is an estrogen antagonist drug. It is used in the treatment of breast cancer.
6. Other Antineoplastic Drugs: Cisplatin, Carboplatin, Etoposide, Procarbazine, L-Asparaginase, Thalidomide, and Interferons are drugs used in cancer treatment.
   a. Cisplatin, Carboplatin: It is used with some antineoplastic drugs in the treatment of solid tumors such as metastatic testicular carcinoma.
   b. Etoposide (VP–6) and Procarbazine: Etoposide (VP–6) treats lung carcinoma and testicular carcinomas, and Procarbazine treats Hodgkin and other cancers.
   c. L-Asparaginase: Treats acute lymphocytic leukemia in childhood with L-asparaginase, Vincristine, and Prednisone.
   d. Thalidomide: Cancer cells increase blood vessel formation (angiogenesis) while tumors form. Thalidomide prevents the formation of the blood vessels needed to develop cancer cells. Thus, it affects the growth and development of the cancer cell.

Chemotherapy Complications

Nausea-vomiting; chemotherapeutics can trigger nausea and vomiting. It is produced by stimulation of the chemoreceptor trigger zone. In addition, opioid analgesics used to treat pain, metabolic disorders, hemodynamic instability, uremia, hypoxia, and ketoacidosis may increase complaints (Navari, 2020).

Cardiotoxicity; it can be observed in different clinics, such as arrhythmias, ischemic changes, congestive heart failure, and cardiomyopathy due to drugs after chemotherapy. It can be seen early during treatment or even years after treatment. Anthracycline group drugs are the most responsible drugs for cardiotoxicity. While the examination of the patients is regular at rest after chemotherapy, it becomes evident with effort. The application of anesthesia makes it easier to see the clinic. Cardiotoxicity; the total dose of the drug administered, the administration rate, the administration route, the administration of additional mediastinal radiotherapy, advanced age, female gender, concomitant cardiac diseases, anemia, and electrolyte disorders are the factors that characterize the clinic. The risk of cardiac complications increases in patients who received cardiotoxic chemotherapy in childhood. In the preoperative evaluation, patients who receive chemotherapy should be carefully evaluated and, if necessary, they should be examined by Cardiology with ECG and echocardiography. Care should be taken in the induction and maintenance of anesthesia and closely followed with respect to hemodynamic stabilization (Choksey & Timm, 2021; Huettemann et al., 2004).

Pulmonary toxicity; pulmonary system findings can be seen in 5-10% of patients receiving chemotherapy. The severity of the results varies according to the drugs used in chemotherapy. Although pulmonary edema, bronchospasm, pleural effusion,and inflammatory reactions may be seen early, pulmonary fibrosis may be observed later. Often, bleomycin, busulfan, carmustine, and mitomycin are involved in developing pulmonary fibrosis. Advanced age, drug dosage, renal failure, and simultaneous thoracic radiotherapy exacerbate the findings (Boopathi & Thangavel, 2021).

Nephrotoxicity; renal damage can develop secondary to nephrotoxic chemotherapeutic agents such as cisplatin, paclitaxel, cyclophosphamide, vincristine, and carboplatin. However, renal functions can be altered due to cancer and prerenal causes such as dehydration due to chemotherapy-induced anorexia, vomiting and diarrhea, hypovolemia, sepsis, or cardiac-related perfusion impairment, and postrenal causes, mainly due to mechanical compression of the tumor located in the pelvis and abdomen. Adaptive hydration should be considered before and during chemotherapy. The use of ureteral catheters should be considered in patients who may develop postrenal insufficiency due to mechanical compression. Multiple myeloma and developing tumor lysis syndrome can exacerbate the findings with antibiotics and drugs from the NSAID group used in treatments (Malyszko et al., 2017).

Hepatotoxicity; hepatotoxicity due to chemotherapeutics may be observed. The findings may be exacerbated in patients with liver metastasis, primary hepatic disease, systemic infections, hepatosteatosis, cholestasis, cholangitis, cirrhosis, and hepatic necrosis. It is recommended to use minimally metabolized agents for the anesthesia of patients (Aloia & Fay, 2010).

Neurotoxicity; central, autonomic, or peripheral neuropathies may develop secondary to chemotherapy. Nerves may be involved. Peripheral neuropathy develops at a high rate with the use of cisplatin. In chemotherapy patients, damage to neural tissues develops more easily after block applications for anesthesia. If regional anesthesia is applied, it is recommended to inform patients and record detailed sensory and motor examinations prior to the procedure (Tailliber et al., 2016; Magge & DeAngelis, 2015).

Myelosuppression; bone marrow suppression may be due to multiple factors. Tumor metastasis to the bone marrow and some factors secreted by the tumor can cause suppression in the bone marrow. In addition, chemautherapeutics can cause hematological problems by suppressing the bone marrow. Anemia is prevalent. Leukopenia, neutropenia, and thrombocytopenia may accompany them. Sometimes, hematologic problems due to myelosuppression may cause the patient to die. In addition to chemotherapy, factors such as malnutrition and sepsis can increase symptoms. The risk of thrombosis increases with smoking and major surgery in cancer patients. Prophylaxis and mobilization should be applied in the most appropriate and early postoperative period (Huettemann & Sakka, 2005).

Table 1. Common complications and treatment of chemautherapatics

TOXICITY	DRUG-INDUCED	ANTIDOTE
Nausea-vomitting	Platinum Anthracyclines Alkylatings	1. Serotonin receptor antagonists 2. NK 1 receptor antagonists 3. Tacykinin, 4. Olanzapine
Alopecia	Anthracyclines Taxanes	Scalp-cooling techniques (not universally accepted)
Cardiotoxicity	Anthracyclines Cyclophosphamide 5-FU.	Early detection Dexrazoxane
Pulmonary toxicity	Bleomycin Alkylatings Gemcitabine.	Early detection corticosteroids
Nephrotoxicity	Platinum Methotrexate (↑dose)	Adequate hydration
Neurotoxicity	Alkaloids Platinum Taxanes	Early detection
Gonadal damage	Alkylatings Others	Sperm preservation
Second malignancies	Alkylatings	Avoid, if possible, responsible drugs and/or RT in curable diseases.

Metabolic disorders; hypercalcemia is expected due to bone metastasis, hormonal factors, and renal involvement. Increased arginine-vasopressin activity, syndrome of inappropriate antidiuretic hormone secretion, or dilutional hyponatremia due to water retention are common. More than one metabolic disorder can be seen together (Hyperuricemia, hyperphosphatemia, hyperkalemia, hypocalcemia). Acute renal failure and tumor lysis syndrome can worsen the general condition (Huettemann & Sakka, 2005).

Changes in drug metabolism; multiple drug use is common in cancer patients due to comorbidities and cancer treatment. While some of the drugs used may increase the effect of other medications and cause accumulation, others may increase the metabolism of others. For these reasons, drug interactions should be considered, and dose adjustments should be made during concomitant drug use (Alnaim et al., 2022; Beijnen & Schellens, 2004) (Table 1).

Pre-Anesthesia Evaluation

Patients diagnosed with cancer who are scheduled to receive anesthesia should carefully evaluate whether they have received treatment or not. Changes due to the patient, disease, treatment, or other reasons are recorded and considered in the anesthesia application. In this period, routine evaluations such as demographic data, systemic disorders, medications, allergies, and anesthesia history of patients are similar to classical anesthesia applications. However, these patients have more psychological and physical problems than other individuals. Depression, general condition disorder, indulgence, and weight loss are more common (Arain & Buggy, 2007; Kurosawa, 2012).

Hormonal changes, previous chemotherapy and steroid treatments, anemia, thrombocytopenia, leukopenia, immunodeficiency findings, organ failures, treatment-related side effects (nausea, vomiting, diarrhea, electrolyte and acid-base imbalances, hair loss, anorexia), pain and drugs used for pain management should be examined. While evaluating, the current findings should be evaluated and interpreted considering previous results. Good values at that time may not mean that the patient's systemic condition is always good. The reasons stated may require changes during anesthesia management in terms of anesthesia administration and monitoring perspective (Arain & Buggy, 2007; Kurosawa, 2012).

Severe depression is common in cancer patients (Bortolato et al., 2017). Complaints such as fear of death, indulgence, weight loss, metabolic changes, hair loss, and loss of appetite may cause depression. Stress itself directly or indirectly affects the course of the disease, quality of life, and duration. A study carried out with breast cancer patients showed that the presence of depression and anxiety increases the frequency of recurrence and shortens the life of the patient (Wang et al., 2020). Anxiety and stress increase the production of glucocorticoids, endogenous opioids and catecholamines via the hypothalamic-pituitary-adrenal (HPA) axis and the sympathetic nervous system, increasing tumor spread and metastasis development. The preoperative evaluation aims to relieve the patient's worries and stress and relieve pain, if any. Even just informing the patient can suppress excitement and anxiety in the patient. In this way, sympathetic discharge and cytokine release can be reduced. Patients can be premedicated with combinations of opioids, benzodiazepines, antihistamines, and antiemetics. Pain is very common in chronic patients. Even newly diagnosed patients may have pain complaints. Opioid analgesics can be added to the premedication in patients with pain. The severity of their illness does not always parallel each other. Therefore, there is no standard dose for patients. It is recommended to make a patient-specific application by evaluating each patient separately. Hemodynamic and neurological disorders that may develop due to anorexia, rapid weight loss, nausea, vomiting, diarrhea, or fluid electrolyte and acid base changes due to endocrine reasons should be carefully examined beforehand. Conditions such as superior vena cava syndrome, spinal cord compression, and circulatory disorders that may occur due to mechanical and local compression of the tumor can complicate the monitoring and interventions or require advanced stages. The location and dimensions of the mass, its relationship to surrounding tissues, the presence and localization of distant metastases, anatomical changes that may occur due to previous treatments, immunodeficiency, bleeding diathesis, anemia, steroid use, signs of secondary organ failure, characteristics of previous surgeries and procedures should be carefully evaluated. During preoperative evaluation, it is essential to examine organ and system functions and perform surgery under the most appropriate conditions. Cardiopulmonary, hematological, hepatic, and renal systems should be primarily evaluated and if there is a deterioration of functions, they should be optimized. According to the operation and the expected bleeding risk, preparations for erythrocyte concentrate and other blood products should be made. If necessary, additional consultation, further examination, and imaging can be performed. However, surgery and preparation for anesthesia should not be delayed to prevent the prognosis of the disease and the development of metastases. It should be considered that operating without preparing the appropriate conditions will increase morbidity and complications.

Many endocrine diseases, such as accompanying Diabetes Mellitus (DM), Diabetes Insipidus (DI), hypopituitarism, thyroid diseases, adrenal cortex, medulla diseases, and paraneoplastic syndromes, can lead to perioperative morbidity and mortality. If control and follow-up of these problems are not performed correctly, they can cause significant perioperative morbidity and mortality.

Anesthesia preparation should be carefully planned according to the patient's age, height, and weight. Possible accompanying diseases should be examined according to age. Height and weight changes due to endocrine disorders should be questioned. The general condition may be impaired due to fluid and electrolyte imbalances due to cancer and its treatment. Chemotherapy and skin changes related to treatment may cause difficulties in establishing new vascular access with vascular interventions, position-related injuries, and decubitus. Head and neck tumors and radiation therapy can cause mouth opening restriction, difficult intubation, and mask ventilation. Laboratory values should be carefully studied in patients who have recently received chemotherapy. The duration of the changes that will occur secondary to chemotherapy should be considered and blood tests should be repeated if necessary (Table 2).

Table 2. ASA Physical Status Classification

ASA	Definition
ASA I	A normal healthy patient
ASA II	A patient with mild systemic disease
ASA III	A patient with severe systemic disease
ASA IV	A patient with severe systemic disease that is a constant threat to life
ASA V	A moribund patient who is not expected to survive without the operation
ASA VI	A declared brain dead patient whose organs are being removed for donor purposes.

Special Conditions Related to Anesthesia in Cancer Patients

Hypothermia

Perioperative hypothermia, which can develop due to many reasons such as operating room air conditioning, ambient temperature, the width of the surgical field, anesthetic fluid and drugs, and washing, is frequently observed if appropriate precautions are not taken. Hypothermia directly alters cellular and humoral immunity and decreases cytokine release. Furthermore, it increases the need for bleeding and transfusion through hemostasis and coagulation mechanisms, activates the sympathetic system, and increases glucocorticoid release. These adverse conditions facilitate the development of cancer cells (Snyder & Greenberg, 2010). In the study by Moslemi-Kebria et al., in which they compared those with postoperative body temperature below and above 36° C in patients who underwent debulking surgery for ovarian cancer, they found that postoperative survival in hypothermic patients was ten months longer than the average lifespan of patients without hypothermia (Moslemi-Kebria et al., 2012). In addition, wound infection increases in patients with hypothermia, and the possibility of cardiac event development increases.

Postoperative Analgesia

The stress response with postoperative pain increases the frequency of metastasis and recurrence. In animal experiments, untreated postoperative pain has been shown to reduce NK cell activity and the frequency of metastases. More than half of cancer patients complain of severe pain, and the vast majority of these patients receive various pain treatments. Opioid analgesics are often preferred at this time. Postoperative pain management is different from chronic pain management. During this period, patients may have developed tolerance to opioid painkillers that they already use and drug doses may need to be modified during anesthesia. (Snyder & Greenberg 2010)

Blood Transfusion

Blood transfusions secondary to anemia are frequently applied in cancer patients. In retrospective studies of cancer patients, there are indications of a possible relationship between blood transfusion and increased morbidity. In these studies, blood transfusion can increase the likelihood of cardiovascular complications or ischemic stroke (Tauriainen et al., 2022). It draws attention to studies on a possible relationship between blood transfusion and increased tumor recurrence (Petrelli et al., 2021; Atzil et al., 2008). In addition to existing anemia, unnecessary blood loss increases the likelihood of blood transfusions and the associated risks. Different values are used in terms of transfusion according to the characteristics and clinical symptoms of the patients. However, the threshold level of hemoglobin (Hb) is considered to be <9 g/d most often. After administering one unit of red blood cells (RBC), the Hb increases by 1 g/dL. Erythrocyte transfusions have been associated with an increased risk of developing non-Hodgkin lymphoma and chronic lymphocytic leukemia.

Anemia is the most common hematological problem in cancer patients. Anemia is observed in approximately half of the patients at follow-up. It can occur for a variety of reasons. Therefore, a detailed physical examination and history of the patient should be taken. Previous blood tests, drugs used, and chemotherapeutics are essential to determine the etiology. Anemia reflects a decrease in circulating erythrocyte mass due to a decrease in hemoglobin. Bleeding, decreased erythrocyte production, or increased destruction can cause this condition. The peripheral blood smear shows erythrocyte morphology. It distinguishes between normochromic normocytic, hypochromic microcytic, or macrocytic anemias. The erythrocyte volume (MCV) and hemoglobin indices help to distinguish the type of anemia. In a patient with an increased reticulocyte count, anemia suggests that the problem is not in the bone marrow, but due to hemolysis or bleeding. In cases where the reticulocyte count is low, it indicates a problem in the bone marrow. The most common causes of anemia in cancer patients are; anemia of chronic anemia, anemia due to bone marrow involvement, anemia due to iron deficiency, and anemia that develops after chemotherapy or radiotherapy. In chronic disease anemia, the mean erythrocyte volume (MCV) is average or decreases. The serum iron and iron binding capacity are low. Serum ferritin may be normal or even increased. Iron stores are regular. Due to bone marrow involvement, early forms of erythroid series are seen in peripheral blood smears in anemia. Depending on the severity of the participation, leukopenia and thrombocytopenia accompanied by pancytopenia can be seen. Frequent blood sampling, bleeding, and gastrointestinal system cancers in which iron absorption is impaired may cause iron deficiency anemia. Anemia secondary to chemotherapy and radiotherapy is due to bone marrow depression. Hemolytic anemia can be seen as immune-induced, drug-induced, or due to hemophagocytic syndrome. With the increase in reticulocytes and indirect bilirubin due to erythrocyte destruction, plasma haptoglobin decreases, hemoglobin in plasma, hemosiderin, and hemoglobin in urine appear. Clinically, jaundice and splenomegaly are seen (Schrijvers, 2011; Gilreath & Rodgers, 2020).

Anesthesia Method and Cancer

The relationship between anesthesia methods and cancer development has been the subject of many studies, as it directly concerns patient morbidity and mortality. The use of regional anesthesia applications directly or in addition to general anesthesia has been investigated in many studies, primarily due to the properties of drugs used in general anesthesia to increase tumor and metastasis development (Heaney & Buggy, 2012; Bar-Yosef et al., 2001). In most studies, it has been stated that regional anesthesia methods reduce recurrence and improve patient survival in more than one cancer type such as breast, prostate, ovarian, malignant melanoma, and colon cancers (Exadaktylos et al., 2006; Wada et al., 2007). Biki et al. reported that epidural anesthesia applied with general anesthesia in prostate cancer, compared to general anesthesia using opioids, made a 57% difference in survival with regional anesthesia (Gottschalk et al., 2010; Tavare et al., 2012; Biki et al., 2008). However, it is accepted that prospective further studies should support these data for many reasons, such as the often-retrospective nature of the studies, differences in tumor types, disease stages, postoperative treatment methods, and patient clinics. Myles et al. examined the control of epidural and general anesthesia on recurrence in various major abdominal oncologic resections and found no change in recurrence-free survival (Myles et al., 2011). It should be noted that some analyses show no benefit after an effect not intended as an exclusion or limitation of other risk factors. Few studies evaluate the relationship between cancer and anesthesia method and are primarily experimental studies. Although regional anesthesia methods seem more functional, they do not have a definite general validity. In regional anesthesia applications, it is aimed at using local anesthetic drugs with antineoplastic properties with blocks made from various regions and to reduce the use of general anesthetics that facilitate tumor development (Biki et al., 2008). In addition, with regional anesthesia, patients' pain scores are reduced, and immunosuppression is less common. However, there are some difficulties in applying regional anesthesia to cancer patients. It may be difficult to perform the procedures due to anatomical changes in patient physical characteristics, lymphadenopathies, distant metastases, increased pain sensation, existing catheters, drains, or other foreign bodies. Assistive imaging devices, such as ultrasonography and fluoroscopy, can facilitate the procedures and reduce possible complications. Due to bleeding diathesis and susceptibility to infection, it is essential to perform the procedures by experienced people, prepare for the appropriate conditions and take precautions for possible complications.

Anesthesia Drugs and Cancer

It is also essential to know what kind of change the anesthesia method to be applied during the operation may cause in the development of cancer and metastasis in cancer patients. In experimental studies, it is known that anesthetics added to antineoplastic drugs in vitro have tumoricidal effects on tumor cells. However, in animal models, the findings supporting this could not be reached. Intravenous and inhalation anesthetics have been emphasized to increase metastasis development by decreasing NK cell activity, induce apoptosis by altering B lymphocyte function, and stimulate angiogenesis by increasing the level of hypoxia-inducible factor (HIF 1-alpha) level and worsen the prognosis (Arain & Buggy, 2007; Beijnen & Schellens, 2004; Tavare et al., 2012; Kim, 2018; Seo et al., 2022; Mao et al., 2013).

Intravenous Anesthetics

Benzodiazepines are often preferred, especially for premedication, as they provide amnesia with their anxiolytic, sedative, and hypnotic properties. They reduce cytokine release due to their central immunomodulatory effects and reduce surgical stress (Arain & Buggy, 2007).

Propofol is often used as an induction agent. It can be used safely in cancer patients. It is an advantage to have antiemetic properties for nausea and vomiting complaints. As a result of its inhibition of the cyclooxygenase enzyme, it reduces tumor development. Its significant advantages are that it reduces the release of PGE2 from monocytes and ensures that NK cell functions remain stable. Reduces the development of metastasis by reducing adhesion, migration, and apoptosis in cancer cells (Arain & Buggy, 2007; Gottschalk et al., 2010; Heaney & Buggy, 2012; Bar-Yosef et al., 2001; Karami et al., 2022; Oh et al., 2022; Jansen et al., 2022; Yap et al., 2019; Oh et al., 2018).

Ketamine has pronounced adrenergic activity and exhibits immunosuppressive activity. The viability of tumor cells was observed to increase more than twofold with the combination of ketamine and thiopental in rats. It reduces the production of pro-inflammatory cytokines. They adversely affect the prognosis by suppressing macrophage, lymphocyte, mast cell, and NK cell functions. An animal experiment determined that the administration of ketamine, thiopental, and halothane decreased NK cell activity and increased lung metastases (Tavare et al., 2012; Biki et al., 2008; Heaney & Buggy, 2012).

Thiopental sodium reduces the chemotaxis of NK cells and their number in the circulation. Etomidate reduces basal cortisol secretion (Arain & Buggy, 2007).

Opioids are used in anesthesia, as well as in the treatment of acute and chronic pain. In addition to its analgesic effects, it also has immunomodulatory effects. They inhibit the cellular and humoral immune response in humans. They increase tumor growth by reducing NK cell activity, phagocytic development, or the production of antibodies and cytokines. High doses of morphine and fentanyl alter NK cell activation for 24-48 hours (Li et al., 2015). The overall effects vary depending on the mode of use, amount, duration, and type of opioid. The effects of opioids can be seen directly by binding to opioid receptors (mainly mu-opioid receptors) in immune cells or indirectly through the hypothalamic-pituitary-adrenal (HPA) axis or the autonomic nervous system. The opioid receptors of Mu may be overexpressed in other than small cell lung cancers. If these receptors are blocked in vitro, opioid-assisted tumor growth is reduced by 35-50% and metastases by 45-70% (Mathew et al., 2011). Studies show that administering opioids in the preoperative period reduces or increases the incidence of postoperative metastases. Increase angiogenesis by increasing the number of COX-II receptors and the production of PGE2 (Tavare et al., 2012; Heaney & Buggy, 2012). In particular, morphine facilitates the formation of metastases by increasing urokinase activity in tumor cells (Tavare et al., 2012). Tramadol is a weak opioid. Prevents tumor development by increasing the activity of noradrenergic and serotonergic cells and the activity of NK cells. In vitro, it increases tumor cell proliferation, migration, and cancer gene expression in human cells. As a result, pain treatment reduces the stress response and reduces metastasis formation while reducing the use of inhalation agents that reduce NK cells and their function (Gottschalk et al., 2010; Tavare et al., 2012; Biki et al., 2008; Gupta et al., 2002; Juneja, 2014; Bimonte et al., 2013; Afsharimani et al., 2011 Connoly & Buggy, 2016).

Local Anesthetics

Local anesthetics block voltage-gated sodium channels (VGSC) in excitable cells. VGSC is highly expressed in many cancers in vitro and in vivo. Down-regulation of VGSC gene expression suppresses migration and invasion of multiple tumor cells. Local anesthetics have been reported to show antineoplastic properties when used systemically. They have antiproliferative and cytotoxic effects on tumor cells. They decrease the endothelial growth factor, which is secreted from these cells, and the invasion ability of the cells. They also reduce mesenchymal cell proliferation and activate tumor suppressor factors. (Huettemann & Sakka 2005; Snyder & Greenberg 2010; Heaney & Buggy 2012) In the study of Mammato et al., it was shown that lidocaine infiltration, which suppresses the immune response in vitro, prevents cancer cell invasion by partially modulating HB-EGF ectodomain shedding from the cell surface (Mammato et al., 2002). Yoon et al.'s study showed that tetracaine decreased intracellular GFP-kinesin motility and caused the collapse of tubulin microtentacles (McTNs), thereby reducing tumor aggregation and metastatic progression (Yoon et al., 2011). The study by Lirk et al. showed that *in vitro*, lidocaine demethylates the DNA of breast cancer cell lines in a dose-dependent manner, sensitizing tumor cells to the cytotoxic effects of chemotherapeutics (Lirk et al., 2012).

Inhalation Anesthetics

Inhalation anesthetics have suppressive effects on the immune system. It reduces NK cell function by up to 90%. In orthopedic surgery performed under general anesthesia, inhalation anesthetics have been shown to suppress cell immunity and increase apoptosis in lymphocytes. Similarly, propofol-N_2O combination has been reported to produce a more favorable prognosis than sevoflurane-N_2O combination in glioblastoma surgery. It has also been stated that the removal of lesions with local anesthesia instead of general anesthesia increases patient survival in patients with malignant melanoma. An experimental study stated that liver metastases decreased in the second group when the groups were compared after laparotomy performed with only sevoflurane anesthesia and spinal anesthesia in addition to sevoflurane anesthesia in mice injected with tumors intravenously. However, there are no definitive data on the superiority of inhalation agents over each other in malignant anesthesia (Arain & Buggy, 2007; Huettemann & Sakka, 2005; Snyder & Greenberg, 2010; Biki et al., 2008; Karami et al., 2022; Yan et al., 2018). In patients undergoing inhalation anesthesia, neurocognitive functions were delayed after cancer surgery compared to intravenous anesthesia (Ding et al., 2022).

Nitrous oxide (N_2O) Nitrous oxide is used with oxygen during anesthesia. It interacts with DNA by altering purine and thymidylate synthesis, suppresses NK cell function, and affects neutrophil chemotaxis and monocyte production. It is known to have immunomodulatory effects. Tumor recurrence was found to be similar between the groups using a mixture of 65% N_2O-O_2 and 65% Air-O_2 in colorectal cancer surgery anesthesia. In experimental studies, the use of intraoperative N_2O has been shown to increase lung and liver metastases. The cytotoxic effect of methotrexate increases in patients using N_2O. For methotrexate, the lethal dose is reduced by 50%. This effect may be due to the effects of both agents on folate metabolism (Arain & Buggy, 2007; Huettemann et al., 2004; Snyder & Greenberg, 2010; Heaney & Buggy, 2012).

Cyclooxygenase (COX) Inhibitors

The cyclooxygenase enzyme is the critical enzyme in the transporter of prostaglandin (PG) from arachidonic acid. In the case of inflammation, PG production increases and cytotoxic T cells and antineoplastic cytotoxins decrease. At the same time, there is a significant decrease in immunosuppressive cytokines. As a result of increased PG; cancer growth, adhesion, migration, and invasion ability, they also inhibit the cytotoxic properties of NK growth. It has been reported that morphine-induced angiogenesis, tumor growth, metastasis, and mortality are reduced in patients receiving celecoxib for a long time (Xu et al., 2014). In the study by Glassner et al., both of the melanoma and lung cancer models created in rats, the combination of propranolol and etodolac significantly improved survival rates (Glasner et al., 2010). In the study of Yang et al., after using selective COX-2 inhibitors for 1-5 years, the risk of developing colorectal cancer decreased by at least 10% compared to the average population in controls of 6 months, 3 years and five years controls (Yang et al., 2012).

Conclusion

With the available data and evidence, the answers to questions such as the ideal anesthesia method or anesthetic agent that will change routine anesthesia practices in cancer patients have not been clarified. Optimization of preanesthesia evaluation, perioperative follow-up, and postoperative care of the cancer patient will positively contribute to patient treatment (Horowitz et al., 2015). The effect of anesthetic techniques on the long-term cancer outcome in surgical cancer treatment continues to be investigated. There seems to be a need for randomized, controlled, multicenter, prospective, multicenter, randomized controlled clinical studies, and large case series in this regard.

Our recommendations on cancer surgery anesthesia:

- When evaluating patients who have previously undergone surgery, chemotherapy, or radiotherapy for cancer treatment, possibilities such as bleeding and coagulation disorders, immune system, nutritional disorders, psychological status, changes in organ function, and airway difficulties should be considered.
- The impact of cancer and its treatment on the functional reserve of all major organ systems, such as the heart, lung, kidney, and liver, must be evaluated in each patient.
- Intravenous propofol anesthesia should be preferred and inhalation anesthetics should be reduced as much as possible.
- COX inhibitors should be used for pain in the intraoperative and postoperative periods.
- The use of regional anesthesia techniques in combination with general anesthesia should be increased.
- Precautions should be taken to ensure intraoperative normothermia in patients.
- While performing a blood transfusion, the transfusion should be reduced as much as possible, considering the characteristics of the patient.
- Psychological support should be provided to patients during the treatment process.

References

Afsharimani, B., Cabot, P., & Parat, M. O. (2011). Morphine and tumor growth and metastasis. *Cancer metastasis reviews*, *30*(2), 225–238. https://doi.org/10.1007/s10555-011-9285-0.

Alnaim, L. S., Almalki, H. M., Almutairi, A. M., & Salamah, H. J. (2022). The prevalence of drug-drug interactions in cancer therapy and the clinical outcomes. *Life sciences*, *310*, 121071. https://doi.org/10.1016/j.lfs.2022.121071.

Aloia, T. A., & Fahy, B. N. (2010). Chemotherapy-associated hepatotoxicity: how concerned should we be?. *Expert review of anticancer therapy*, *10*(4), 521–527. https://doi.org/10.1586/era.09.185.

Arain, M. R., & Buggy, D. J. (2007). Anaesthesia for cancer patients. *Current opinion in anaesthesiology*, *20*(3), 247–253. https://doi.org/10.1097/ACO.0b013e32814f1c34.

Atzil, S., Arad, M., Glasner, A., Abiri, N., Avraham, R., Greenfeld, K., Rosenne, E., Beilin, B., & Ben-Eliyahu, S. (2008). Blood transfusion promotes cancer progression: a critical role for aged erythrocytes. *Anesthesiology*, *109*(6), 989–997. https://doi.org/10.1097/ALN.0b013e31818ddb72.

Bar-Yosef, S., Melamed, R., Page, G. G., Shakhar, G., Shakhar, K., & Ben-Eliyahu, S. (2001). Attenuation of the tumor-promoting effect of surgery by spinal blockade in rats. *Anesthesiology*, *94*(6), 1066–1073. https://doi.org/10.1097/00000542-200106000-00022.

Beijnen, J. H., & Schellens, J. H. (2004). Drug interactions in oncology. *The Lancet. Oncology*, *5*(8), 489–496. https://doi.org/10.1016/S1470-2045(04)01528-1.

Biki, B., Mascha, E., Moriarty, D. C., Fitzpatrick, J. M., Sessler, D. I., & Buggy, D. J. (2008). Anesthetic technique for radical prostatectomy surgery affects cancer recurrence: a retrospective analysis. *Anesthesiology*, *109*(2), 180–187. https://doi.org/10.1097/ALN.0b013e31817f5b73.

Bimonte, S., Barbieri, A., Palma, G., & Arra, C. (2013). The role of morphine in animal models of human cancer: does morphine promote or inhibit the tumor growth?. *BioMed research international*, *2013*, 258141. https://doi.org/10.1155/2013/258141.

Boopathi, E., & Thangavel, C. (2021). Dark Side of Cancer Therapy: Cancer Treatment-Induced Cardiopulmonary Inflammation, Fibrosis, and Immune Modulation. *International journal of molecular sciences*, *22*(18), 10126. https://doi.org/10.3390/ijms221810126.

Bortolato, B., Hyphantis, T. N., Valpione, S., Perini, G., Maes, M., Morris, G., Kubera, M., Köhler, C. A., Fernandes, B. S., Stubbs, B., Pavlidis, N., & Carvalho, A. F. (2017). Depression in cancer: The many biobehavioral pathways driving tumor progression. *Cancer treatment reviews*, *52*, 58–70. https://doi.org/10.1016/j.ctrv.2016.11.004.

Buckley, A., McQuaid, S., Johnson, P., & Buggy, D. J. (2014). Effect of anaesthetic technique on the natural killer cell anti-tumour activity of serum from women undergoing breast cancer surgery: a pilot study. *British journal of anaesthesia*, *113 Suppl 1*, i56–i62. https://doi.org/10.1093/bja/aeu200.

Cassinello, F., Prieto, I., del Olmo, M., Rivas, S., & Strichartz, G. R. (2015). Cancer surgery: how may anesthesia influence outcome? *Journal of clinical anesthesia*, *27*(3), 262–272. https://doi.org/10.1016/j.jclinane.2015.02.007.

Chang, C. Y., Wu, M. Y., Chien, Y. J., Su, I. M., Wang, S. C., & Kao, M. C. (2021). Anesthesia and Long-term Oncological Outcomes: A Systematic Review and Meta-analysis. *Anesthesia and analgesia*, *132*(3), 623–634. https://doi.org/10.1213/ANE.0000000000005237.

Choksey, A., & Timm, K. N. (2021). Cancer Therapy-Induced Cardiotoxicity-A Metabolic Perspective on Pathogenesis, Diagnosis and Therapy. *International journal of molecular sciences*, *23*(1), 441. https://doi.org/10.3390/ijms23010441.

Connolly, C., & Buggy, D. J. (2016). Opioids and tumour metastasis: does the choice of the anesthetic-analgesic technique influence outcome after cancer surgery?. *Current opinion in anaesthesiology*, *29*(4), 468–474. https://doi.org/10.1097/ACO.0000000000000360.

Ding, Y., Yu, J., Cui, F., & Li, J. (2022). Comparison of Intravenous and Inhalational Anesthetic on Postoperative Cognitive Outcomes in Elderly Patients Undergoing Cancer Surgery: Systematic Review and Meta-analysis. *Journal of perianesthesia nursing : official journal of the American Society of PeriAnesthesia Nurses*, *37*(5), 683–690. https://doi.org/10.1016/j.jopan.2021.11.017.

Exadaktylos, A. K., Buggy, D. J., Moriarty, D. C., Mascha, E., & Sessler, D. I. (2006). Can anesthetic technique for primary breast cancer surgery affect recurrence or metastasis? *Anesthesiology*, *105*(4), 660–664. https://doi.org/10.1097/00000542-200610000-00008.

Gilreath, J. A., & Rodgers, G. M. (2020). How I treat cancer-associated anemia. *Blood*, *136*(7), 801–813. https://doi.org/10.1182/blood.2019004017.

Glasner, A., Avraham, R., Rosenne, E., Benish, M., Zmora, O., Shemer, S., Meiboom, H., & Ben-Eliyahu, S. (2010). Improving survival rates in two models of spontaneous postoperative metastasis in mice by combined administration of a beta-adrenergic antagonist and a cyclooxygenase-2 inhibitor. *Journal of immunology (Baltimore, Md.: 1950)*, *184*(5), 2449–2457. https://doi.org/10.4049/jimmunol.0903301.

Gottschalk, A., Sharma, S., Ford, J., Durieux, M. E., & Tiouririne, M. (2010). Review article: the role of the perioperative period in recurrence after cancer surgery. *Anesthesia and analgesia*, *110*(6), 1636–1643. https://doi.org/10.1213/ANE.0b013e3181de0ab6.

Groenewold, M. D., Olthof, C. G., & Bosch, D. J. (2022). Anaesthesia after neoadjuvant chemotherapy, immunotherapy or radiotherapy. *BJA education*, *22*(1), 12–19. https://doi.org/10.1016/j.bjae.2021.08.002.

Gupta, K., Kshirsagar, S., Chang, L., Schwartz, R., Law, P. Y., Yee, D., & Hebbel, R. P. (2002). Morphine stimulates angiogenesis by activating proangiogenic and survival-promoting signaling and promotes breast tumor growth. *Cancer research*, *62*(15), 4491–4498.

Heaney, A., & Buggy, D. J. (2012). Can anaesthetic and analgesic techniques affect cancer recurrence or metastasis?. *British journal of anaesthesia*, *109 Suppl 1*, i17–i28. https://doi.org/10.1093/bja/aes421.

Horowitz, M., Neeman, E., Sharon, E., & Ben-Eliyahu, S. (2015). Exploiting the critical perioperative period to improve long-term cancer outcomes. *Nature reviews. Clinical oncology*, *12*(4), 213–226. https://doi.org/10.1038/nrclinonc.2014.224.

Huettemann, E, Sakka, S. G. (2005). Anaesthesia and anti-cancer chemotherapeutic drugs. *Current opinion in anaesthesiology*, *18*(3), 307–314. https://doi.org/10.1097/01.aco.0000169240.14056.19.

Huettemann, E., Junker, T., Chatzinikolaou, K. P., Petrat, G., Sakka, S. G., Vogt, L., & Reinhart, K. (2004). The influence of anthracycline therapy on cardiac function during anesthesia. *Anesthesia and analgesia*, *98*(4), 941–947. https://doi.org/10.1213/01.ANE.0000108135.52036.48.

Inoue, G. N. C., Pimenta, R., Camargo, J. A., Viana, N. I., Guimarães, V. R., Srougi, M., Nahas, W. C., Leite, K. R. M., & Reis, S. T. (2022). Combined spinal and general anesthesia attenuate tumor promoting effects of surgery. An experimental animal study. *Annals of medicine and surgery (2012)*, *75*, 103398. https://doi.org/10.1016/j.amsu.2022.103398.

Jansen, L., Dubois, B. F. H., & Hollmann, M. W. (2022). The Effect of Propofol versus Inhalation Anesthetics on Survival after Oncological Surgery. *Journal of clinical medicine*, *11*(22), 6741. https://doi.org/10.3390/jcm11226741.

Juneja R. (2014). Opioids and cancer recurrence. *Current opinion in supportive and palliative care*, *8*(2), 91–101. https://doi.org/10.1097/SPC.0000000000000056.

Karami, M. Y., Dehghanpisheh, L., Karami, A., Sabzloun, Z., Niazkar, H. R., Mojarad, N., Panah, A., Talei, A., & Tahmasebi, S. (2022). Comparison of volatile/inhalational and IV anesthesia in long-term survival of patients with breast cancer: a retrospective study. *European journal of medical research*, *27*(1), 271. https://doi.org/10.1186/s40001-022-00911-9.

Kim R, (2018) Anesthetic technique for cancer surgery: Harm or benefit for cancer recurrence?, *European Journal of Surgical Oncology*, Volume 44, Issue 5, https://doi.org/10.1016/j.ejso.2018.02.207.

Kim R. (2018). Effects of surgery and anesthetic choice on immunosuppression and cancer recurrence. *Journal of translational medicine*, *16*(1), 8. https://doi.org/10.1186/s12967-018-1389-7.

Kurosawa S. (2012). Anesthesia in patients with cancer disorders. *Current opinion in anaesthesiology*, *25*(3), 376–384. https://doi.org/10.1097/ACO.0b013e328352b4a8.

Li, A. X., Xin, W. Q., & Ma, C. G. (2015). Fentanyl inhibits the invasion and migration of colorectal cancer cells via inhibiting the negative regulation of Ets-1 on BANCR. *Biochemical and biophysical research communications*, *465*(3), 594–600. https://doi.org/10.1016/j.bbrc.2015.08.068.

Lirk, P., Berger, R., Hollmann, M. W., & Fiegl, H. (2012). Lidocaine time- and dose-dependently demethylates deoxyribonucleic acid in breast cancer cell lines in vitro. *British journal of anaesthesia*, *109*(2), 200–207. https://doi.org/10.1093/bja/aes128.

Longhini, F., Bruni, A., Garofalo, E., De Sarro, R., Memeo, R., Navalesi, P., Navarra, G., Ranieri, G., Currò, G., & Ammendola, M. (2020). Anesthetic Strategies in Oncological Surgery: Not Only a Simple Sleep, but Also Impact on Immunosuppression and Cancer Recurrence. *Cancer management and research*, *12*, 931–940. https://doi.org/10.2147/CMAR.S237224.

Looney, M., Doran, P., & Buggy, D. J. (2010). Effect of anesthetic technique on serum vascular endothelial growth factor C and transforming growth factor β in women undergoing anesthesia and surgery for breast cancer. *Anesthesiology*, *113*(5), 1118–1125. https://doi.org/10.1097/ALN.0b013e3181f79a69.

Magge, R. S., & DeAngelis, L. M. (2015). The double-edged sword: Neurotoxicity of chemotherapy. *Blood reviews*, *29*(2), 93–100. https://doi.org/10.1016/j.blre.2014.09.012.

Malyszko, J., Kozlowska, K., Kozlowski, L., & Malyszko, J. (2017). Nephrotoxicity of anticancer treatment. *Nephrology, dialysis, transplantation : official publication of the*

European Dialysis and Transplant Association - European Renal Association, *32*(6), 924–936. https://doi.org/10.1093/ndt/gfw338.

Mammoto, T., Higashiyama, S., Mukai, M., Mammoto, A., Ayaki, M., Mashimo, T., Hayashi, Y., Kishi, Y., Nakamura, H., & Akedo, H. (2002). Infiltration anesthetic lidocaine inhibits cancer cell invasion by modulating ectodomain shedding of heparin-binding epidermal growth factor-like growth factor (HB-EGF). *Journal of cellular physiology*, *192*(3), 351–358. https://doi.org/10.1002/jcp.10145.

Mao, L., Lin, S., & Lin, J. (2013). The effects of anesthetics on tumor progression. *International journal of physiology, pathophysiology and pharmacology*, *5*(1), 1–10.

Mathew, B., Lennon, F. E., Siegler, J., Mirzapoiazova, T., Mambetsariev, N., Sammani, S., Gerhold, L. M., LaRiviere, P. J., Chen, C. T., Garcia, J. G., Salgia, R., Moss, J., & Singleton, P. A. (2011). The novel role of the mu opioid receptor in lung cancer progression: a laboratory investigation. *Anesthesia and analgesia*, *112*(3), 558–567. https://doi.org/10.1213/ANE.0b013e31820568af.

Moslemi-Kebria, M., El-Nashar, S. A., Aletti, G. D., & Cliby, W. A. (2012). Intraoperative hypothermia during cytoreductive surgery for ovarian cancer and perioperative morbidity. *Obstetrics and gynecology*, *119*(3), 590–596. https://doi.org/10.1097/AOG.0b013e3182475f8a.

Myles, P. S., Peyton, P., Silbert, B., Hunt, J., Rigg, J. R., Sessler, D. I., & ANZCA Trials Group Investigators (2011). Perioperative epidural analgesia for major abdominal surgery for cancer and recurrence-free survival: randomised trial. *BMJ (Clinical research ed.)*, *342*, d1491. https://doi.org/10.1136/bmj.d1491.

Nadler, J. W., Quinn, T. D., & Bennett-Guerrero, E. (2019). Can anesthesiologists affect cancer outcomes? Les anesthésiologistes peuvent-ils avoir un impact sur les pronostics du cancer?. *Canadian journal of anaesthesia = Journal canadien d'anesthesie*, *66*(5), 491–494. https://doi.org/10.1007/s12630-019-01331-w.

Navari R. M. (2020). Nausea and Vomiting in Advanced Cancer. *Current treatment options in oncology*, *21*(2), 14. https://doi.org/10.1007/s11864-020-0704-8.

Oh, C. S., Hong, S. W., Park, S., Kwon, Y., & Kim, S. H. (2022). Effect of equipotent doses of propofol and sevoflurane on endoplasmic reticulum stress during breast cancer surgery. *Korean journal of anesthesiology*, *75*(6), 487–495. https://doi.org/10.4097/kja.21569.

Oh, T. K., Kim, K., Jheon, S., Lee, J., Do, S. H., Hwang, J. W., & Song, I. A. (2018). Long-Term Oncologic Outcomes for Patients Undergoing Volatile Versus Intravenous Anesthesia for Non-Small Cell Lung Cancer Surgery: A Retrospective Propensity Matching Analysis. *Cancer control : journal of the Moffitt Cancer Center*, *25*(1), 1073274818775360. https://doi.org/10.1177/1073274818775360.

Petrelli, F., Ghidini, M., Ghidini, A., Sgroi, G., Vavassori, I., Petrò, D., Cabiddu, M., Aiolfi, A., Bonitta, G., Zaniboni, A., & Rausa, E. (2021). Red blood cell transfusions and the survival in patients with cancer undergoing curative surgery: a systematic review and meta-analysis. *Surgery today*, *51*(10), 1535–1557. https://doi.org/10.1007/s00595-020-02192-3.

Ricon, I., Hiller, J. G., & Ben-Eliyahu, S. (2016). The Combined Blockade of β-Adrenoceptor and COX-2 During the Perioperative Period to Improve Long-term

Cancer Outcomes. *International anesthesiology clinics*, *54*(4), 72–91. https://doi.org/10.1097/AIA.0000000000000116.

Schrijvers D. (2011). Management of anemia in cancer patients: transfusions. *The oncologist*, *16 Suppl 3*, 12–18. https://doi.org/10.1634/theoncologist.2011-S3-12.

Seo, K. H., Hong, J. H., Moon, M. H., Hwang, W., Lee, S. W., Chon, J. Y., Kwon, H., Hong, S. H., & Kim, S. (2022). Effect of total intravenous anesthesia versus inhalation anesthesia on long-term oncologic outcomes in patients undergoing curative resection for early-stage non-small cell lung cancer: A retrospective cohort study. *Korean journal of anesthesiology*, 10.4097/kja.22584. Advance online publication. https://doi.org/10.4097/kja.22584.

Snyder, G. L., & Greenberg, S. (2010). Effect of anaesthetic technique and other perioperative factors on cancer recurrence. *British journal of anaesthesia*, *105*(2), 106–115. https://doi.org/10.1093/bja/aeq164

Stewart B. W. and Kleihues P. (2003): World Cancer Report. IARCPress. Lyon. https://www.iarc.who.int/wp-content/uploads/2018/07/WorldCancerReport.pdf.

Taillibert, S., Le Rhun, E., & Chamberlain, M. C. (2016). Chemotherapy-Related Neurotoxicity. *Current neurology and neuroscience reports*, *16*(9), 81. https://doi.org/10.1007/s11910-016-0686-x

Tauriainen, T., Juvonen, T., Anttila, V., Maaranen, P., Niemelä, M., Eskola, M., Ahvenvaara, T., Husso, A., Virtanen, M. P. O., Kinnunen, E. M., Dahlbacka, S., Jalava, M., Laine, M., Valtola, A., Raivio, P., Vento, A., Airaksinen, J., Mäkikallio, T., & Biancari, F. (2022). Perioperative Bleeding Requiring Blood Transfusions is Associated With Increased Risk of Stroke After Transcatheter and Surgical Aortic Valve Replacement. *Journal of cardiothoracic and vascular anesthesia*, *36*(8 Pt B), 3057–3064. https://doi.org/10.1053/j.jvca.2022.04.029.

Tavare, A. N., Perry, N. J., Benzonana, L. L., Takata, M., & Ma, D. (2012). Cancer recurrence after surgery: direct and indirect effects of anesthetic agents. *International journal of cancer*, *130*(6), 1237–1250. https://doi.org/10.1002/ijc.26448.

Temel M. K. (2015). Sitotoksik kemoterapötiklerin yirminci yüzyıldaki gelişimi [The development of cytotoxic chemotherapeutics in the twentieth century], *Türk Onkoloji Dergisi, 30*(2):96-108. https://doi.org/10.5505/tjoncol.2015.1151.

Villet R. (2021). The surgery and surgeons of tomorrow in the treatment of cancer. *Journal of visceral surgery*, *158*(6), 459–461. https://doi.org/10.1016/j.jviscsurg.2021.11.011.

Wada, H., Seki, S., Takahashi, T., Kawarabayashi, N., Higuchi, H., Habu, Y., Sugahara, S., & Kazama, T. (2007). Combined spinal and general anesthesia attenuates liver metastasis by preserving TH1/TH2 cytokine balance. *Anesthesiology*, *106*(3), 499–506. https://doi.org/10.1097/00000542-200703000-00014.

Wang, X., Wang, N., Zhong, L., Wang, S., Zheng, Y., Yang, B., Zhang, J., Lin, Y., & Wang, Z. (2020). Prognostic value of depression and anxiety on breast cancer recurrence and mortality: a systematic review and meta-analysis of 282,203 patients. *Molecular psychiatry*, *25*(12), 3186–3197. https://doi.org/10.1038/s41380-020-00865-6.

Wisley I· (2020). WHO report on cancer: setting priorities, investing wisely and providing care for all. Geneva: World Health Organization; 2020. Licence: CC BY-NC-SA 3.0 IGO. https://apps.who.int/iris/rest/bitstreams/1267643/retrieve.

Wu, S. Y., Fu, T., Jiang, Y. Z., & Shao, Z. M. (2020). Natural killer cells in cancer biology and therapy. *Molecular cancer*, *19*(1), 120. https://doi.org/10.1186/s12943-020-01238-x.

Xu, L., Stevens, J., Hilton, M. B., Seaman, S., Conrads, T. P., Veenstra, T. D., Logsdon, D., Morris, H., Swing, D. A., Patel, N. L., Kalen, J., Haines, D. C., Zudaire, E., & St Croix, B. (2014). COX-2 inhibition potentiates antiangiogenic cancer therapy and prevents metastasis in preclinical models. *Science translational medicine*, *6*(242), 242ra84. https://doi.org/10.1126/scitranslmed.3008455.

Yan, T., Zhang, G. H., Wang, B. N., Sun, L., & Zheng, H. (2018). Effects of propofol/remifentanil-based total intravenous anesthesia versus sevoflurane-based inhalational anesthesia on the release of VEGF-C and TGF-β and prognosis after breast cancer surgery: a prospective, randomized and controlled study. *BMC anesthesiology*, *18*(1), 131. https://doi.org/10.1186/s12871-018-0588-3.

Yang, Y. H., Yang, Y. H., Cheng, C. L., Ho, P. S., & Ko, Y. C. (2012). The role of chemoprevention by selective cyclooxygenase-2 inhibitors in colorectal cancer patients - a population-based study. *BMC cancer*, *12*, 582. https://doi.org/10.1186/1471-2407-12-582.

Yap, A., Lopez-Olivo, M. A., Dubowitz, J., Hiller, J., Riedel, B., & Global Onco-Anesthesia Research Collaboration Group (2019). Anesthetic technique and cancer outcomes: a meta-analysis of total intravenous versus volatile anesthesia. Technique d'anesthésie et pronostics de cancer: une méta-analyse analyse comparant l'anesthésie intraveineuse totale et l'anesthésie par inhalation. *Canadian journal of anaesthesia = Journal canadien d'anesthesie*, *66*(5), 546–561. https://doi.org/10.1007/s12630-019-01330-x.

Yoon, J. R., Whipple, R. A., Balzer, E. M., Cho, E. H., Matrone, M. A., Peckham, M., & Martin, S. S. (2011). Local anesthetics inhibit kinesin motility and microtentacle protrusions in human epithelial and breast tumor cells. *Breast cancer research and treatment*, *129*(3), 691–701. https://doi.org/10.1007/s10549-010-1239-7.

Chapter 4

Anesthesia in Cardiovascular Failures

Leman Gökçenur Aydın*, MD
and Remzi İşçimen, MD
Department of Medicine, Bursa Uludag University, Bursa, Turkiye

Abstract

In simple terms, heart failure means a mismatch between filling the ventricle with blood and its injection. Basically, it is defined as heart failure with low ejection fraction (HFrEF), heart failure with preserved ejection fraction (HFpEF), and HF with mildly reduced EF (HFmrEF). Heart failure patients must be well evaluated in the preoperative period and operated under hemodynamically optimal conditions. These patients must be meticulously followed during the perioperative and postoperative periods. Individuals with peripheral vascular disease represent a group with important characteristics for anesthesiologists due to the additional comorbidities that occur as a result of the primary disease or have.

Keywords: heart failure, peripheral arterial diseases, peripheral vein diseases, anesthesia

Introduction

It has been calculated that about 300 million patients worldwide undergo major surgery annually. According to a report published in the USA, almost

* Corresponding Author's Email: lemangokcenur@gmail.com.

In: Organ Failure and Anesthesia Practices
Editors: Ahmet Şen and Basar Erdivanli
ISBN: 979-8-89113-486-7

half of patients over 45 years of age who underwent major surgery between 2012 and 2013 had at least two cardiovascular risk factors. Patients over 75 years of age have a higher risk of developing perioperative major adverse cardiovascular events (MACEs). Although age is considered the reason for the increased risk of complications, the greater risk appears to be associated with the urgency of surgery and cardiovascular, renal or pulmonary diseases. According to calculations, one fifth of patients over the age of 75 will undergo surgery every year by 2030. The number of surgical procedures will also increase with increasing age. Over the next 30 years, population aging will have a significant effect on perioperative patient management (Halvorsen et al., 2022).

About 10% of the population in the United States has peripheral arterial disease (Nehler et al., 2014). Individuals with peripheral arterial disease have a 3-5 times higher risk of developing cardiovascular ischemic events than the general population. Critical limb ischemia is associated with very high morbidity and mortality (Taylor Piliae et al., 2011). Anesthesiologists frequently encounter this group of patients during surgeries related to various systems or surgical treatment of vascular complications due to the disease. This chapter includes general information about heart failure, vascular diseases, and the anesthesia management of these patients.

Heart Failure

Definition

In simple terms, heart failure means a mismatch between filling the ventricle with blood and its injection. It results in clinical manifestations such as tissue hypoperfusion, fatigue, dyspnea, edema, and weight gain. Anomaly of the pericardium, myocardium, endocardium, heart valves, or great vessels can result in heart failure. However, heart failure, which develops with deterioration in systolic or diastolic myocardial function, is more common in practice. Heart failure with low ejection fraction (HFrEF) is defined as an ejection fraction (EF) of 40% or less, while heart failure with preserved ejection fraction (HFpEF, previously defined as diastolic heart failure) is defined as an ejection fraction of 50% or more. Individuals with an ejection fraction between 41% and 49% are defined as HFmrEF (HF with mildly reduced EF). The distinction between these two basic types of heart failure based on the EF calculation is a virtual definition; these are groups that are phenotypically similar, although their causes are different. Both HFrEF and HFpEF-type heart failure have diastolic dysfunction. In the HFpEF type, myocardial contractility is abnormal despite calculating relatively normal EF (Heidenreich et al., 2022; Hines & Jones, 2022a).

Pathophysiology

Cardiac output decreases in heart failure due to decreased stroke volume. Starling's law explains the relationship between end-diastolic ventricular volume and stroke volume. Failure of the heart does not increase stroke volume, heart rate increases to increase preload, which can cause myocardial ischemia (Delicce & Makaryus, 2022).

While the main characteristic of HFrEF is the abnormality of contractile functions, it is left ventricular diastolic dysfunction in HFpEF. Factors determining left ventricular diastole, such as venous blood flow, left atrial function, mitral valve dynamics, pericardial restraint, active relaxation, and passive compliance elastic properties of the left ventricle during diastole, determine the ability of the left ventricle to fill properly. Higher filling pressures are required for normal end-diastolic volume in patients with HFpEF. Myocardial relaxation is an active and energy-consuming process. This active relaxation slows down in heart failure caused by myocardial dysfunction for various reasons. Left ventricular relaxation depends on the afterload, which is more pronounced in the failing heart. Left ventricular relaxation is delayed. Therefore, tolerance to conditions such as hypovolemia, tachycardia, and exercise decreases.

Acute myocardial ischemia, myocardial stunning, post-infarct ventricular remodeling, high-pressure hypertrophy (e.g., aortic stenosis), high-volume hypertrophy (e.g., aortic valve regurgitation), hypertrophic obstructive cardiomyopathy, dilated cardiomyopathy, restrictive cardiomyopathy, and pericardial diseases can be listed as the most frequent causes of left ventricular diastolic dysfunction (Hines & Jones, 2022a).

HFrEF is usually characterized by a decrease in myocardial contractility as a result of ischemia, infarction, or cardiomyopathies. Dilatation and volume increase are observed in the left ventricle. Stroke volume and cardiac output are maintained at the cost of increased left ventricular end-diastolic volume, high filling pressures, and the development of pulmonary venous congestion. Chronic neurohormonal activation is followed to prevent decrease in cardiac output decrease; this response can increase heart rate, left ventricular afterload, and myocardial oxygen consumption (Hines & Jones, 2022a).

Diagnosis

Signs and Symptoms

The definition of acute heart failure is employed for the worsening of the patient's preexisting condition (acute decompensated heart failure) and for individuals with symptoms of heart failure observed for the first time (de novo acute heart failure). Symptoms of fluid retention due to congestion are observed with impaired compensation in acute decompensated heart failure. On the other hand, in de novo heart failure, peripheral perfusion decreases, and pulmonary edema develops, as no compensatory mechanism for acute changes is formed. De novo heart failure is most commonly caused by cardiac ischemia due to coronary artery occlusion. Viral, drug-related, or toxic peripartum cardiomyopathies are its less common causes (Hines & Jones, 2022a).

Tachypnea, fatigue, dyspnea, paroxysmal nocturnal dyspnea, orthopnea, exercise intolerance, S3 gallop rhythm in auscultation, jugular venous distention, peripheral edema, and decreased tissue perfusion are the most common signs and symptoms of heart failure. While paroxysmal nocturnal dyspnea and pulmonary edema are observed more frequently in patients with HFpEF, S3 gallops in auscultation are more common in patients with HFrEF (Hines & Jones, 2022a).

Imaging

Chest radiography helps with the imaging of cardiomegaly, pulmonary venous congestion, pulmonary edema, and existing lung disease. Distention of the pulmonary veins, an early sign of left ventricular failure and pulmonary venous hypertension, can be observed in the upper lobes of the lungs. Perivascular edema presents as hilar or perihilar haze and the hilum is enlarged. Kerley lines A, B, and C are visible. The chest radiograph can show pericardial and pleural effusion. Approximately 12 hours after the development of pulmonary edema, the findings become visible on chest radiography, and the findings may continue to be visible for a few days after the symptoms have resolved.

Transthoracic echocardiography plays an essential role in determining the type of heart failure. Repeated measurements are useful in patients with marked changes in their clinical condition. Transesophageal echocardiography should be considered when the patient's clinical signs are not compatible with transthoracic echocardiography in severe mitral and aortic valve diseases (van der Meer et al., 2019).

Noninvasive stress imaging methods are recommended for some conditions to detect ischemia in de novo heart failure. Cardiac magnetic resonance imaging is recommended in cases where inflammatory or infiltrative diseases are suspected for which the definition of myocardial tissue is required and in complex congenital heart diseases. Coronary angiography is recommended in individuals with a history of angina pectoris, ventricular arrhythmia, or aborted cardiac death together with heart failure (van der Meer et al., 2019).

Electrocardiography

ECG abnormalities are frequently observed in patients with heart failure. Left ventricular hypertrophy and previous findings of myocardial infarction (MI) may be observed according to the underlying cause. Electrocardiography has a low predictive value in the diagnosis and prediction of the risk of heart failure (Hines & Jones, 2022a).

Laboratory

Natriuretic peptide measurement (BNP or NT-proBNP) can be performed in incipient heart failure. Its use is recommended by the ACC/AHA (ACC: American College of Cardiology; AHA: American Heart Association) and ESC (European Society of Cardiology) in the diagnosis or exclusion of heart failure in the case of acute dyspnea. Its use is suggested for the classification of risk in chronic heart failure and for the prognosis in hospitalized patients with heart failure. The use of ST2 and galectin, biomarkers for myocardial stress and fibrosis, has been recommended, but their level of evidence is low (van der Meer et al., 2019; Heidenreich et al., 2022).

Heart Failure Classification

The New York Heart Association (NYHA) and the ACC/AHA have prepared classifications for heart failure. The NYHA classification focuses on physical activity restriction, while the ACC/AHA provides information on the presence and severity of the disease. Clinicians determine the NYHA classification at the first diagnosis and re-evaluate it after treatment. For example, a patient with symptomatic heart failure (stage C) can become asymptomatic after treatment (NYHA class I), but this patient is still classified as stage C (Table 1 and Table 2) (Heidenreich et al., 2022).

Treatment

Medical Treatment in Chronic Heart Failure

In chronic heart failure, the survival of patients with HFrEF has increased over the past 30 years. However, mortality in patients with HFpEF has not changed. The aggressive treatment of related conditions such as hypertension and diabetes, weight loss, and exercise constitute the main treatment goals in patients with HFpEF. Drugs forming the basis of HFrEF therapy, such as beta-blockers and renin-angiotensin-aldosterone system (RAAS) blockers, have been shown not to have a consistent effect on HFpEF. Furosemide and other loop diuretics reduce left ventricular filling pressures, decrease pulmonary venous congestion, and improve clinical symptoms in patients with acute and chronic HFrEF and HFpEF. The mentioned drugs are strongly recommended by the ACC/AHA and ESC guidelines (van der Meer et al., 2019).

Numerous studies have shown that beta-blockers are beneficial in the treatment of patients with HFrEF. Beta-blockers are recommended by the ACC/AHA and ESC guidelines for this indication. However, beta-blockers have been shown to have no effect on long-term hospitalization rates in patients with HFpEF, and their use has been limited for other indications such as myocardial infarction, and rate control in atrial fibrillation. Angiotensin receptor blockers (ARBs) and angiotensin-converting enzyme (ACE) inhibitors, identified as RAAS inhibitors, constitute the main therapy for HFrEF (van der Meer et al., 2019).

It is vital to make lifestyle changes and control underlying diseases, such as diabetes and hypertension, in the prognosis of heart failure. Some dietary changes, for example, sodium restriction, may ensure partial hemodynamic improvements in patients with heart failure. Taking hypertension under control reduces the incidence and severity of heart failure (Halvorsen et al., 2022).

Atrial fibrillation is frequently observed in patients with heart failure and is associated with conditions such as right ventricular dysfunction and tricuspid regurgitation. The treatment aims to ensure sinus rhythm, but it may not always be possible to apply it in practice. Ensuring rate control is an acceptable goal in such cases (Hines & Jones, 2022a).

Table 1. The New York Heart Association classification system (Raphael et al., 2007)

NYHA functional classification	
I	Patients with cardiac disease but without the limitations of physical activity resulting from them. Ordinary physical activity does not cause excessive fatigue, palpitation, dyspnea, or anginal pain.
II	Patients with cardiac disease that results in a slight limitation of physical activity. They are comfortable at rest. Ordinary physical activity results in fatigue, palpitation, dyspnea, or anginal pain.
III	Patients with cardiac disease that results in marked limitation of physical activity. They are comfortable at rest. Less-than-ordinary physical activity causes fatigue, palpitation, dyspnea, or anginal pain.
IV	Patients with cardiac disease that results in the inability to perform any physical activity without discomfort. Symptoms of cardiac failure or anginal syndrome may be present even at rest. If physical activity is carried out, discomfort increases.

Medical Treatment in Acute Heart Failure

Anesthesiologists may encounter acute heart failure during surgery in the form of de novo heart failure or acute decompensated heart failure. It is necessary to quickly administer loop diuretics such as furosemide, bumetanide, and torsemide to patients who are considered to have fluid overload. The decreased intravascular volume reduces pulmonary congestion by lowering central venous pressure and pulmonary capillary wedge pressure. It is recommended to use vasodilator drugs to increase filling pressure by reducing afterload. Nitroprusside and nitroglycerin effectively reduce left ventricular afterload. Vasopressin receptor antagonists such as tolvaptan can be used as an adjunct to therapy (Hines & Jones, 2022a).

It is necessary to administer inotropic agents in cases of cardiogenic shock or acute reduction in contractility. Catecholamines (adrenaline, noradrenaline, dopamine, and dobutamine) directly stimulate beta receptors in the myocardium and increase cAMP (cyclic adenosine monophosphate) by activating adenyl cyclase. Phosphodiesterase inhibitors (milrinone) show an indirect effect by inhibiting the degradation of cAMP. Levosimendan, a calcium sensitizer, provides vasodilation in addition to this effect and inhibits phosphodiesterase in high doses. Levosimendan can be used as a bridge therapy in patients with heart failure and transplant candidates (Masarone et al., 2022).

Table 2. The ACC/AHA stages of HF are shown (ACC: American College of Cardiology; AHA: American Heart Association; CVD: cardiovascular disease; GDMT: guideline-directed medical therapy; and HF: heart failure) (van der Meer et al., 2019)

STAGE A: At Risk for Heart Failure	STAGE B: Pre-Heart Failure	STAGE C: Symptomatic Heart Failure	STAGE D: Advenced Heart Failure
Patients at risk for HF, but without current or previous symptoms/signs of HF and without structural/functional heart disease or abnormal biomarkers Patients with hypertension, CVD, diabetes, obesity, exposure to cardiotoxic agents, genetic variant for cardiomyopathy, or family history of cardiomyopathy	Patients without current or previous symptoms/signs of HF but evidence of 1 of the following: – Structural heart disease – Evidence of increased filling pressures – Risk factors and ○ increased levels of natriuretic peptides or ○ persistently elevated cardiac troponin – in the absence of competing diagnoses	Patients with current or previous symptoms/ signs of HF	Marked HF symptoms that interfere with daily life and recurrent hospitalizations despite attempts to optimize GDMT

Surgical Treatment in Heart Failure

Increased ventricular chamber volume and chamber dilatation affect the contractile function of the ventricle. The pathological change in the shape of the heart mentioned above causes an increase in ventricular wall tension, a decrease in subendocardial blood flow, and arrhythmias. The purpose of surgical treatments is to prevent ventricular remodeling and try to preserve the normal anatomical shape of the heart.

Revascularization therapies consisting of coronary artery bypass graft (CABG) and percutaneous coronary intervention (PCI) procedures are very effective in improving left ventricular function after myocardial infarction. Cardiac resynchronization therapy (CRT) is a dual chamber cardiac pacemaker that consists of two electrodes placed in the right atrium and right ventricle. It is utilized in patients with heart failure with ventricular conduction delay. Implantable cardioverter defibrillators (ICDs) are used to prevent dysrhythmias in patients with advanced heart failure. Left ventricular assist devices (LVADs) are used as a bridge therapy in cases where heart function is expected to be restored and in patients awaiting cardiac transplantation and as a destination therapy for patients with advanced heart failure and who are not candidates for transplantation. Devices such as intraaortic balloon pump, impella, peripheral and central ventricular assist device/extracorporeal membrane oxygenation (ECMO), and biventricular assist device (BiVAD) are methods that can be used in acute heart failure (Hines & Jones, 2022a).

Anesthesia Method

Preoperative Evaluation

There is an increased risk of pneumonia, renal failure, sepsis, and cardiac arrest in patients with heart failure. Therefore, a good preoperative evaluation is crucial in patients with heart failure. In patients with heart failure, it must be evaluated whether the patient is compensated. The level of heart failure must be identified by evaluating the functional status. Even if the patient is stable, risk factors such as blood pressure and dyslipidemia must be kept under control (Halvorsen et al., 2022).

High-risk noncardiac surgeries should probably be avoided in patients with severe heart failure (NYHA class IV), cardiogenic shock, severe pulmonary hypertension, and severe frailty. Metabolic equivalents (METs) <4, a classification based on the patient's statement, suggest poor functional capacity. However, studies could not prove the value of METs (Halvorsen et al., 2022).

A 12-lead ECG should be observed in the preoperative evaluation (Halvorsen et al., 2022). Transthoracic echocardiography (TTE) evaluation must be performed in patients with worsening symptoms, and TTE should not be older than 6 months. In emergencies, the FOCUS (focused cardiac ultrasound) method can be used as an alternative to TTE to prevent delay in surgery. The chest radiograph can show the symptoms of decompensated heart failure. Current electrolyte values, liver function tests, coagulation test, and complete blood count should be seen from laboratory tests (Halvorsen et al., 2022).

It is necessary to plan the medications used by patients with heart failure prior to surgery. Diuretics should not be used on the day of surgery. The use of beta-blockers should be continued, as continued treatment in patients using beta-blockers reduces perioperative morbidity and mortality. It is not recommended to administer beta-blockers perioperatively to patients who do not use beta-blockers. Patients using statins are suggested to continue their use in the perioperative period. The ICD and pacemaker status of patients must be questioned (Halvorsen et al., 2022).

The blocked Renin Angiotensin Aldosterone System (RAAS) increases the risk of intraoperative hypotension. It is recommended that RAAS inhibitors be discontinued prior to surgery in patients without heart failure. However, studies have not observed a relationship between cardiac events and mortality in patients with heart failure in whom the use of RAAS inhibitors was interrupted on the day of surgery, and has not been proven to cause less intraoperative hypotension. Therefore, the ESC stated in the guide published in 2022 that the use of RAAS inhibitors could continue (Halvorsen et al., 2022).

Patients with heart failure are at risk for perioperative venous thromboembolism (VTE). If the perioperative risk of VTE and thrombophylaxis is required, drug selection should be based on the type of surgery, the length of time the patient will remain immobilized, and other additional factors (Halvorsen et al., 2022).

Intraoperative Management

Monitoring

Routine cardiovascular monitoring involves ECG, automatic intermittent noninvasive blood pressure measurement, and peripheral oxygen saturation monitoring. The monitoring methods employed vary according to the characteristics of the patient and the type of surgery. Intraarterial catheter placement for invasive arterial blood pressure monitoring provides instantaneous blood pressure monitoring and can guide fluid management by showing reciprocal variations. Continuous ECG and ST-segment analysis enable the detection of ischemia and arrhythmias in the heart. Temperature monitoring can help prevent the development of hypothermia. The central venous catheter allows monitoring of the central venous pressure and is used to administer fluid replacement and vasoactive drug infusions in cases with a risk of significant blood or fluid loss. Near-infrared spectroscopy shows regional tissue perfusion and oxygenation. The pulmonary artery catheter ensures the measurement of the pulmonary artery pressure and the measurement of cardiac output using the thermodilution method. Minimally invasive methods such as FloTrac, ClearSight, LiDCO, and PiCCO can calculate cardiac output and help with fluid management. Esophageal Doppler monitoring is used to monitor hemodynamic changes. Transesophageal echocardiography (TEE) represents the gold standard for intraoperative hemodynamic monitoring. It provides recognition of conditions such as hypovolemia, right/left ventricular dysfunction, tamponade, and valvular regurgitation (Halvorsen et al., 2022; American Society of Anesthesiologists (ASA), n.d.).

Intraoperative Hemodynamics

Most anesthetic techniques reduce sympathetic tone, which decreases venous return, resulting in vasodilation and decreased blood pressure. Adequate organ perfusion is of key importance in patients with heart failure. According to the ESC 2022 guideline, it is recommended to prevent the mean arterial pressure from decreasing by more than 20% of the basal values or below 60-70 mmHg for more than 10 minutes in the intraoperative period to minimize postoperative organ dysfunction (Halvorsen et al., 2022).

There is insufficient evidence to determine an upper value for arterial blood pressure for patients undergoing noncardiac surgery. However, pressures above 160 mmHg are associated with myocardial damage and myocardial infarction. Intraoperative tachycardia negatively affects the oxygen balance of the myocardium and can lead to myocardial damage (Halvorsen et al., 2022).

Selection of an Anesthesia Method

It is necessary to create an anesthesia plan according to the type of surgery and the individual characteristics of the patient. Regional anesthesia is beneficial in patients with heart failure, as it reduces the risk of postoperative pneumonia and provides postoperative analgesia. Hypotension can develop due to suppression of the sympathetic system. Alpha-1 receptor antagonists (e.g., phenylephrine) or direct/indirect sympathomimetics (e.g., ephedrine) can be used in the case of hypotension. The development of hypotension must be avoided during the induction of general anesthesia. Intravenous induction agents can be used for the maintenance of anesthesia. Since inhalation anesthetics may have a myocardial depressant effect, they must be appropriately titrated. Postoperative cardiac events in noncardiac surgeries are not volatile or associated with the choice of intravenous anesthetic. Since opioid agents inhibit adrenergic activation, they may be beneficial in patients with heart failure (Halvorsen et al., 2022).

Fluid Therapy

It is recommended to regularly evaluate volume status and signs of organ perfusion in patients with heart failure. In minor surgeries, fluid replacement should be performed only as much as the maintenance fluid requirement. Restrictive transfusion management is preferred. However, blood transfusion should be considered in case the hemoglobin level drops to 8 or below. Fluid therapy must be carefully planned to prevent heart failure from decompensating and rapid practices should be avoided. It is necessary to utilize fluid heaters to prevent shivering due to hypothermia (Halvorsen et al., 2022; Hines & Jones, 2022a).

Anesthesia Management in Patients with Cardiac Implanted Electronic Devices

Patients with cardiac implanted electronic devices (CIEDs) must be checked preoperatively. Control must be performed within 12 months prior to pacemaker surgery and within 6 months for ICD. The device of all patients with CIED should be reprogrammed prior to surgery, checked again after the operation, and reprogrammed if necessary. In pacemaker-dependent patients, devices should be taken in the non-sensing or asynchronous pace mode to prevent device inhibition. This can be achieved by placing a magnet on the pacemaker in most pacemaker models. ICD devices must be turned off during surgery or a magnet should be placed on the device. Until the deactivated ICD is reactivated, the patient must be continuously monitored with the ECG and under the supervision of personnel who can intervene in case of arrhythmia (Halvorsen et al., 2022).

Anesthesia Management in Patients with Ventricular Assist Devices

It is recommended to establish a multidisciplinary team, involving a Ventricular Assist Device (VAD) specialist, in the perioperative management of patients receiving mechanical circulatory support. Anticoagulant therapy, rhythm monitoring, and antibiotic prophylaxis are essential in the anesthesia management of a patient with VAD. The use of electrocautery can lead to electromagnetic interference and impact the pump current. Therefore, bipolar cautery should be used if possible (Halvorsen et al., 2022).

The hemodynamic monitoring of patients with implantable non-pulsatile devices is a special subject. Because most of these patients have non-pulsatile flow, it is impossible to safely use non-invasive blood pressure monitoring and pulse oximetry. In a few patients, the blood is pumped intermittently from the ventricle, and oxygen saturation can be measured by pulse oximetry in these patients. Cerebral oximetry, which does not depend on pulsatile flow, can be utilized instead of pulse oximetry. The oxygenation status can be monitored by intermittent blood gas studies. An intraarterial catheter is necessary to monitor the mean arterial pressure. It can be challenging to insert a catheter into the non-pulsatile artery, so ultrasound-assisted placement is recommended. With TEE, ventricular function and volume status can be measured (Hines & Jones, 2022a).

Anesthesia Management of Patients with Heart Transplantation

Patients who have undergone heart transplantation and who will undergo a surgical procedure represent a special group. These patients receive long-term immunosuppressive therapy, which puts them at risk of infection. Aseptic techniques must be applied very strictly when invasive procedures are performed. The transplanted heart is denervated. Therefore, the heart rate can only be increased with direct-acting beta-adrenergic agonists such as isoproterenol and epinephrine. Likewise, heart rate does not change with atropine or pancuronium. The transplanted heart can increase output by increasing the volume of cardiac stroke. Therefore, these patients must be considered to be preload dependent. Ensuring adequate preload must be aimed at fluid applications; however, it should not be forgotten that the administration of excess fluid can cause pulmonary edema (Hines & Jones, 2022a).

Postoperative Management

Patients who develop heart failure during surgery must be followed up in the intensive care unit during the postoperative period. Adequate analgesia should be provided using appropriate methods, as pain and hemodynamic status may worsen. It is necessary to continue treatment in the postoperative period in patients using beta-blockers. In the postoperative period, it is recommended to evaluate patients with ECG, markers of myocardial damage, and echocardiography and to continue the specific treatment for the individual (Halvorsen et al., 2022).

The incidence of acute heart failure was found to be 1-2% within 30 days after surgery and 4-6% within 365 days in patients with known coronary artery disease, pulmonary artery disease, or over 65 years of age who underwent major non-cardiac surgery. Chronic or undiagnosed heart failure and volume overload constitute important factors. The general principles in the diagnosis and treatment of acute heart failure are also applied in postoperative acute heart failure (Halvorsen et al., 2022).

Peripheral Arterial Diseases

Peripheral arterial disease (PAD) represents a pathology that causes decreased blood flow to the limbs. Individuals with PAD usually have advanced atherosclerosis and a worse prognosis than those without PAD. The risk profile in peripheral arterial diseases varies depending on whether the surgery is vascular or non-vascular. Performing a cardiac evaluation and optimizing cardiac status are recommended before elective surgery in patients with limited functional capacity or cardiac risk factors (Halvorsen et al., 2022).

Chronic Arterial Insufficiency

Peripheral arterial insufficiency is diagnosed when the ankle-brachial index (ABI) is below 0.9. The ABI is calculated as the ratio of the systolic blood pressure at the ankle to the systolic blood pressure at the brachial artery. Peripheral atherosclerosis is similar to atherosclerosis in the aorta or coronary arteries. The prevalence of peripheral atherosclerosis increases with age and is over 70% in people over 75 years of age. Atherosclerosis is a systemic disease. Therefore, patients with peripheral arterial disease have a 3-5 times higher risk of developing cardiovascular ischemic events than the general population. Critical limb ischemia is associated with very high mid- to late-year morbidity and mortality. The risk of developing peripheral atherosclerosis is associated with the same factors as the risk of developing ischemic heart disease, which are advanced age, family history, diabetes mellitus, smoking, obesity, hypertension, and dyslipidemia (Selvin & Erlinger, 2004; Taylor Piliae et al., 2011).

Intermittent claudication and pain at rest are the main symptoms of peripheral arterial disease. A decreased pulse or non-palpable pulse is the most reliable sign of the disease. A murmur can be heard in the abdomen, pelvis, and inguinal region, and a decreased pulse in the femoral, popliteal, and posterior tibial regions may indicate the anatomical location of the arterial stenosis. Coldness, pallor, cyanosis, and hair loss are symptoms of chronic leg ischemia. Doppler ultrasonography, MRI (magnetic resonance imaging), and contrast angiography are used in the diagnosis. Transcutaneous oximetry can determine the severity of skin ischemia (Pollak et al., 2012; Hines & Jones, 2022b).

Treatment of peripheral arterial disease involves exercise programs and lifestyle and treatment changes for risk factors for atherosclerosis. Although exercise programs do not change ABI in such patients, they can ensure progress in walking capacity. The prognosis can be improved by quitting smoking. Lipid lowering therapies and the treatment of diabetes mellitus may slow the progression of microvascular disease. Treatment of accompanying hypertension, if present, reduces stroke and cardiovascular morbidity. Conditions such as disabling claudication, ischemic resting pain, and the risk of loss of the limb are indications for revascularization. It is possible to determine the prognosis of the limb by the dimension of the arterial disease, the severity of the ischemia in the limb and the speed of arterial circulation. Revascularization can be applied with surgical reconstruction and endovascular methods (Taylor Piliae et al., 2011; Hines & Jones, 2022b).

Anesthesia Management

Comorbidities in patients with chronic arterial insufficiency influence risk during the perioperative period. In the preanesthesia evaluation, it is essential to evaluate accompanying cardiovascular diseases, chronic obstructive pulmonary disease, diabetes, and renal failure in these patients.

Due to the high prevalence of coronary artery disease in patients with peripheral arterial diseases, the risk of perioperative MI and cardiac death increases. Mortality after revascularization surgery in patients with preoperative ischemic heart disease generally occurs as a result of MI. Because patients with claudication cannot participate in the exercise stress test, pharmacological stress test and echocardiography, nuclear imaging methods enable determining the presence or severity of ischemic heart disease in patients. Treatment of ischemic heart disease with interventional methods or coronary bypass graft operation can be considered prior to revascularization surgery in some cases (Hines & Jones, 2022b). It is necessary to check the creatinine value before beginning endovascular revascularization attempts. The risk of developing contrast-related nephropathy is high in patients with chronic renal failure (Asif & Epstein, 2004).

Perioperative heart rate control decreases the risk of myocardial ischemia in high-risk patients in vascular surgery. ACC / AHA guidelines recommend perioperative beta-blocker therapy in intermediate and high-risk patients undergoing vascular surgery. The acute discontinuation of beta-blocker use on the day of surgery and the beginning of high-dose beta-blocker therapy are associated with increased mortality (van der Meer et al., 2019).

Anesthesia techniques must be chosen individually. General anesthesia and regional anesthesia techniques have their advantages and disadvantages. The advantages of epidural and spinal anesthesia can be summarized as increased blood flow from the graft, less activation of the coagulation system, postoperative analgesia, and fewer postoperative respiratory complications. Intraoperative heparin administration is not a contraindication to epidural anesthesia; if an epidural intervention has been performed, at least 1 hour must pass between it and intraoperative heparinization. Furthermore, prior to intervention, if a blood tap occurs during epidural intervention, the surgical team should be informed and a joint decision should be taken on the need to postpone the operation. Combinations of femoral and sciatic nerve blocks can be used in patients with chronic limb-threatening ischemia and severe pain (Marcus et al., 2006). General anesthesia can be preferred in long operations or in cases where vein grafts must be taken from the upper limb. It has not been proven that one general anesthetic agent is superior to the other. Infrarenal cross-clamping during aortoiliac and aortofemoral surgery is associated with fewer hemodynamic side effects and there are fewer hemodynamic changes during unclamping. A central venous catheter can be placed in the said group of patients; unless there is symptomatic left ventricular dysfunction, placement of a pulmonary artery catheter is not preferred. Invasive arterial monitoring is applied in addition to the standard monitoring methods recommended by the ASA (American Society of Anesthesiologists (ASA), n.d.; Halvorsen et al., 2022; Hines & Jones, 2022b).

Heparin is generally administered before vascular cross-clamp placement to prevent thromboembolic complications in revascularization surgeries. The ACT (activated clotting time) test is applied. The targeted ACT value varies by centers; some clinics target a value between 200-250, while other clinics target a value twice the patient's baseline value. The patient is at risk of developing distal embolization despite administering heparin (Mabry et al., 1979; Goldhammer & Zimmerman, 2018).

A study conducted in the geriatric population found no difference in 30-day mortality between the general anesthesia group and the regional anesthesia group among patients who underwent revascularization surgery in the lower extremities. However, intraoperative dopamine and epinephrine use, postoperative oxygen therapy, and mechanical ventilation support were found to be higher in the general anesthesia group (Lim et al., 2022). No differences in 30-day mortality were detected between surgeries performed with peripheral block and spinal anesthesia in cases of amputation above the knee (Pisansky et al., 2018). In patients receiving antiplatelet, antithrombotic, or thrombolytic therapy, it should be remembered that discontinuation of this therapy may not be appropriate and spinal anesthesia may involve higher risk than general anesthesia.

Postoperative Management

It is essential to provide analgesia, regulate fluid-electrolyte balance, control heart rate and blood pressure, and maintain optimal oxygenation and ventilation with the aim of preventing myocardial ischemia and infarction in the postoperative period in patients with chronic PAD.

Acute Arterial Occlusion

Acute arterial occlusion occurs mainly as a result of cardiogenic embolism. Systemic embolism can originate from a thrombus in the left ventricle or from an atrial myxoma at the onset of atrial fibrillation. Noncardiac causes can be plaque rupture and hypercoagulability, as well as aortic dissection and trauma, which can lead to acute occlusion in the arteries with disruption of the vessel lumen structure.

In acute arterial occlusion in the limb, signs of ischemia, e.g., severe pain in the distal part of the arterial occlusion, paresthesia, and weakness in the limb, are observed. In the distal part of the occlusion, an undetectable peripheral pulse, cold skin, and skin discoloration with a demarcation line are observed. Surgical embolectomy can be applied in acute systemic embolism. Heparin anticoagulation is administered when the diagnosis of acute arterial embolism is confirmed. Intraarterial thrombolysis with urokinase or recombinant tPA can provide patency of the vessel. Clinical outcomes are associated with rapid implementation of revascularization. Some patients may need an amputation. Anesthesia management in surgeries performed in acute arterial occlusion is similar to that of chronic peripheral arterial disease (Iyem & Nesimi Eren, 2009; Hines & Jones, 2022b).

Peripheral Vein Diseases

Superficial thrombophlebitis, deep vein thrombosis (DVT), and chronic venous insufficiency are the most frequently observed diseases in surgical patients. Pulmonary embolism, an important cause of perioperative morbidity and mortality, is the most significant complication of DVT.

Deep Vein Thrombosis

DVT is commonly observed in surgical patients, but most of these resolve completely when mobilization begins. Deep and superficial vein thrombosis may coexist. However, isolated deep vein thrombosis can be differentiated from superficial venous thrombosis by examination and ultrasound findings. Superficial thrombophlebitis is rarely associated with pulmonary embolism. Superficial thrombophlebitis can lead to total venous occlusion. During examination, the vein can be palpated as a cord-like structure and erythema, increased temperature, and edema are observed around it. DVT is characterized by widespread pain, tenderness, and unilateral swelling of the affected limb. Doppler ultrasonography performed with vein compression is highly sensitive in the diagnosis of proximal vein (femoral or popliteal) thrombosis, but less sensitive in detecting thrombosis in the calf. Venography and impedance plethysmography represent other potential diagnostic methods (Di Nisio et al., 2010).

To prevent deep vein thrombosis, determining clinical risk factors is important for taking prophylactic measures. Minimal measures such as postoperative mobilization and compression stockings are sufficient in low-risk patients. Patients over 40 years of age who have undergone surgery lasting more than 1 hour, lower extremity orthopedic surgery, and pelvic and abdominal surgery are at higher risk. Thrombotic complications are also increased in cancer patients. External pneumatic compression devices and heparin administration reduce the risk of DVT (Hines & Jones, 2022b).

The incidence of postoperative DVT is lower in surgeries performed with regional anesthesia applications. Epidural or spinal anesthesia instead of general anesthesia in total knee and hip replacement surgeries reduces the risk of postoperative DVT by up to 50%. However, no significant differences were revealed in the incidence of DVT in patients who underwent chemical antithrombotic prophylaxis before the operation and were operated under general anesthesia. Possible reasons why regional anesthesia is beneficial are thought to be the development of vasolidation, increasing blood flow and allowing early mobilization by providing good postoperative analgesia (Hu et al., 2009; Johnson et al., 2016; Kang et al., 2022).

Anticoagulation is the primary treatment in patients diagnosed with DVT. Since it has a fast-onset effect, treatment is started with heparin. The advantages of low molecular weight heparin (LMWH) over unfractionated heparin are its longer half-life, the absence of need to look at the activated partial thromboplastin time, and fewer bleeding complications. Its disadvantages are its high cost and the lack of a rapid reversing agent (Holbrook et al., 2012).

Conclusion

Patients with heart failure and peripheral vascular disease are at risk of encountering various complications during the perioperative period. Hence, it is essential to take these patients to surgery with good preoperative preparation and closely follow them for complications that may develop in the perioperative and postoperative periods.

References

Asif, A., & Epstein, M. (2004). Prevention of radiocontrast-induced nephropathy. *American Journal of Kidney Diseases,* 44(1), 12–24. https://doi.org/10.1053/J.AJKD.2004.04.001.

Delicce, A. V., & Makaryus, A. N. (2022). Physiology, Frank Starling Law. *StatPearls.* Retrieved from https://www.ncbi.nlm.nih.gov/books/NBK470295/.

Di Nisio, M., Van Sluis, G. L., Bossuyt, P. M. M., Büller, H. R., Porreca, E., & Rutjes, A. W. S. (2010). Accuracy of diagnostic tests for clinically suspected upper extremity deep vein thrombosis: A systematic review. *Journal of Thrombosis and Haemostasis,* 8(4), 684–692. https://doi.org/10.1111/j.1538-7836.2010.03771.x.

Goldhammer, J. E., & Zimmerman, D. (2018). Pro: Activated Clotting Time Should Be Monitored During Heparinization For Vascular Surgery. *Journal of Cardiothoracic and Vascular Anesthesia*, 32(3), pp. 1494–1496. W. B. Saunders. https://doi.org/10.1053/j.jvca.2017.04.047.

Halvorsen, S., Mehilli, J., Cassese, S., Hall, T. S., Abdelhamid, M., Barbato, E., De Hert, S., de Laval, I., Geisler, T., Hinterbuchner, L., Ibanez, B., Lenarczyk, R., Mansmann, U. R., McGreavy, P., Mueller, C., Muneretto, C., Niessner, A., Potpara, T. S., Ristić, A., Sade, L. E, Schirmer, H., Schüpke, S., Sillesen, H., Skulstad, H., Torracca, L., Tutarel, O., Van Der Meer, P., Wojakowski, W., & Zacharowski, K. (2022). 2022 ESC Guidelines on cardiovascular assessment and management of patients undergoing non-cardiac surgery. *European Heart Journal,* 43(39), 3826–3924. https://doi.org/10.1093/eurheartj/ehac270.

Heidenreich, P. A., Bozkurt, B., Aguilar, D., Allen, L. A., Byun, J. J., Colvin, M. M., Deswal, A., Drazner, M. H., Dunlay, S. M., Evers, L. R., Fang, J. C., Fedson, S. E., Fonarow, G. C., Hayek, S. S., Hernandez, A. F., Khazanie, P., Kittleson, M. M., Lee, C. S., Link, M. S., Milano, C. A., Nnacheta, L. C., Sandhu, A. T., Stevenson, L. W., Vardeny, O., Vest, A. R. & Yancy, C. W. (2022). 2022 AHA/ACC/HFSA Guideline for the Management of Heart Failure: A Report of the American College of Cardiology/American Heart Association Joint Committee on Clinical Practice Guidelines. *Journal of the American College of Cardiology,* 79(17), e263–e421. https://doi.org/10.1016/j.jacc.2021.12.012.

Hines, R. L., & Jones, S. B. (2022a). Heart Failure and Cardiomyopathies. In *Stoeltıng's Anesthesıa And Co-Exıstıng Dısease* (8th Edıtıon, pp. 203–230). Elsevier.

Hines, R. L., & Jones, S. B. (2022b). Vascular Disease. In *Stoeltıng's Anesthesıa And Co-Exıstıng Dısease* (8th Edıtıon, pp. 245–272). Elsevier.

Holbrook, A., Schulman, S., Witt, D. M., Vandvik, P. O., Fish, J., Kovacs, M. J., Svensson, P. J., Veenstra, D. L., Crowther, M., & Guyatt, G. H. (2012). Evidence-based management of anticoagulant therapy. Antithrombotic therapy and prevention of thrombosis, 9th ed: American College of Chest Physicians evidence-based clinical practice guidelines. *Chest*, 141(2 SUPPL.), e152S-e184S. https://doi.org/10.1378/chest.11-2295.

Hu, S., Zhang, Z. Y., Hua, Y. Q., Li, J., Cai, Z. D., & Surgeon, O. (2009). A comparison of regional and general anaesthesia for total replacement of the hip or knee A META-ANALYSIS. *J Bone Joint Surg [Br],* 7, 91–935. https://doi.org/10.1302/0301-620X.91B7.

Iyem, H., & Nesimi Eren, M. (2009). Should embolectomy be performed in late acute lower extremity arterial occlusions? *Vascular Health and Risk Management,* 5, 621–626. https://www.dovepress.com/.

Johnson, R. L., Kopp, S. L., Burkle, C. M., Duncan, C. M., Jacob, A. K., Erwin, P. J., Murad, M. H., & Mantilla, C. B. (2016). Neuraxial vs general anaesthesia for total hip and total knee arthroplasty: A systematic review of comparative-effectiveness research. *British Journal of Anaesthesia*, 116(2), 163–176. Oxford University Press. https://doi.org/10.1093/bja/aev455.

Kang, J., Lin, W., Wang, H., Liang, Y., & Yu, Z. (2022). Effects of general anesthesia and epidural anesthesia on deep vein thrombosis and perioperative cognitive function of patients undergoing total knee arthroplasty. *Am J Transl Res,* 14(7), 4786–4794. www.ajtr.org.

Lim, J. A., Seo, Y., Choi, E. J., Kwak, S. G., Ryu, T., Lee, J. H., Park, K. H., & Roh, W. S. (2022). Impact of regional anesthesia on outcomes of geriatric patients undergoing lower extremity revascularization A propensity score-matched cohort study. *Medicine (United States),* 101(52). https://doi.org/10.1097/MD.0000000000032597.

Mabry, C. D., Thompson, B. W., & Read, R. C. (1979). Activated clotting time (ACT) monitoring of intraoperative heparinization in peripheral vascular surgery. *The American Journal of Surgery,* 138(6), 894–900. https://doi.org/10.1016/0002-9610(79)90318-0.

Marcus, A. J., Lotzof, K., Kamath, B. S. K., Shanthakumar, R. E., Munir, N., Loh, A., Bird, R., & Howard, A. (2006). A new approach: Regional nerve blockade for angioplasty of the lower limb. *CardioVascular and Interventional Radiology*, 29(2), 235–240. https://doi.org/10.1007/s00270-004-0084-7.

Masarone, D., Kittleson, M. M., Pollesello, P., Marini, M., Iacoviello, M., Oliva, F., Caiazzo, A., Petraio, A., & Pacileo, G. (2022). Use of Levosimendan in Patients with Advanced Heart Failure: An Update. *Journal of Clinical Medicine,* 11(21), 6408. https://doi.org/10.3390/jcm11216408.

Nehler, M. R., Duval, S., Diao, L., Annex, B. H., Hiatt, W. R., Rogers, K., Zakharyan, A., & Hirsch, A. T. (2014). Epidemiology of peripheral arterial disease and critical limb ischemia in an insured national population. *Journal of Vascular Surgery*, 60(3). https://doi.org/10.1016/j.jvs.2014.03.290.

Pisansky, A. J. B., Brovman, E. Y., Kuo, C., Kaye, A. D., & Urman, R. D. (2018). Perioperative Outcomes after Regional Versus General Anesthesia for Above the Knee Amputations. *Annals of Vascular Surgery,* 48, 53–66. https://doi.org/ https://doi.org/10.1016/j.avsg.2017.10.014.

Pollak, A. W., Norton, P. T., & Kramer, C. M. (2012). Multimodality imaging of lower extremity peripheral arterial disease current role and future directions. *Circulation: Cardiovascular Imaging,* 5(6), 797–807. https://doi.org/10.1161/CIRCIMAGING. 111.970814.

Raphael, C., Briscoe, C., Davies, J., Whinnett, Z. I., Manisty, C., Sutton, R., Mayet, J., & Francis, D. P. (2007). Limitations of the New York Heart Association functional classification system and self-reported walking distances in chronic heart failure. *Heart*, 93(4), 476–482. https://doi.org/10.1136/hrt.2006.089656.

Selvin, E., & Erlinger, T. P. (2004). Prevalence of and risk factors for peripheral arterial disease in the United States: Results from the National Health and Nutrition Examination Survey, 1999-2000. *Circulation*, 110(6), 738–743. https://doi.org/ 10.1161/01.CIR.0000137913.26087.F0.

American Society of Anesthesiologists (ASA). (n.d.). *Standards for Basic Anesthetic Monitoring*. Retrieved March 6, 2023, from https://www.asahq.org/standards-and-guidelines/standards-for-basic-anesthetic-monitoring.

Taylor Piliae, R. E., Fair, J. M., Varady, A. N., Hlatky, M. A., Norton, L. C., Iribarren, C., Go, A. S., & Fortmann, S. P. (2011). Ankle brachial index screening in asymptomatic older adults. *American Heart Journal,* 161(5), 979–985. https://doi.org/10.1016/j.ahj.2011.02.003.

van der Meer, P., Gaggin, H. K., & Dec, G. W. (2019). ACC/AHA Versus ESC Guidelines on Heart Failure: JACC Guideline Comparison. In *Journal of the American College of Cardiology,* 73(21), 2756–2768. Elsevier USA. https://doi.org/10.1016/j.jacc.2019.03.478.

Chapter 5

Respiratory Insufficiencies and Anesthesia

Başar Erdivanlı[1,*], MD
and Özlem Çelebi Erdivanlı[2], MD
[1]Department of Anesthesiology, Recep Tayyip Erdogan University, Rize, Turkiye
[2]Department of Otorhinolaryngology, Recep Tayyip Erdogan University, Rize, Turkiye

Abstract

This chapter discusses ways to adapt anesthetic techniques to the patient suffering from respiratory insufficiency. Traditionally, the word "respiratory" is associated with the lungs. However, the lungs are only as important as the bellows of an anesthesia workstation. The respiratory system is a complex consisting of several organs organized according to the metabolic needs of the body.

Therefore, this chapter starts with a concise review of respiratory physiology. Subsequently, pathologies related to both organs and control mechanisms are discussed. To avoid repeating things, acute pathologies are discussed first, so that comorbidities introduced due to long-standing diseases do not complicate the discussion. Pathologies are ordered from extrinsic to intrinsic as much as possible. With so many pathologies, it is difficult to summarize the text, let alone highlight the highlights. One thing to bring home though is that in many cases the treatment comes before the diagnosis. Once the patient is prevented from imminent death, treatment continues with a history and physical examination.

Anesthesia itself may cause respiratory failure. Therefore, a short section is dedicated to the mechanism, prevention, and management of crises in intraoperative and postoperative respiratory failure. Finally, some topics are suggested for future research.

* Corresponding Author's Email: basar.erdivanli@erdogan.edu.tr.

In: Organ Failure and Anesthesia Practices
Editors: Ahmet Şen and Basar Erdivanli
ISBN: 979-8-89113-486-7

Keywords: respiratory failure, anesthesia, hypoxemia, hypercarbia

Introduction

The reader will not benefit from this chapter without understanding the impact of respiratory insufficiencies on anesthesia. The respiratory system is thought to be primarily the lungs and upper airway, both of which are thought to be under the control of the anesthesiologist. That is an illusion. If the airways are under control, it means the patient is intubated or tracheotomized. If the lungs are under control, it means that the patient is not self-breathing but ventilated. None of these situations promote self-care and must be sacrificed if one wants the patient to return to his/her daily life.

Furthermore, positive pressure ventilation with any means, invasive or not, is prone to damage the lungs. So, it is not easy to maintain for a long time.

This illusion comes partly from the similarity of the lungs to the bellows of the anesthesia machine, and partly from not knowing how the lungs or a bellow works. This simplified view states that the lungs act as the primary site of gas exchange in the body, by simply inflating and deflating. This view negates the functions of the endothelium and the immune system functioning within the lungs.

Furthermore, the lungs are not an isolated organ, but rather an integral part of the respiratory system, including the airways, the diaphragm, the intercostal muscles, and the nervous system that controls respiration. These, in turn, are closely connected to other systems in the body, such as the cardiovascular system, which delivers oxygen and nutrients to the tissues and removes waste products. All of these components work together to ensure adequate gas exchange, regulation of the pH balance, and control of the temperature and fluid balance. Finally, the upper airways and lungs also act as a filter, protecting the body from harmful inhalational substances.

In summary, while the lungs may seem like simple bellows, they are in fact a complex and vital organ that plays a crucial role in overall health and functioning of the body.

Anatomy and Mechanical Aspects of Breathing

The anatomy or physiology of the lungs are vast topics beyond this chapter. This section will compare positive pressure ventilation (PPV), the dominant form of mechanical ventilation, with spontaneous breathing. At the end of this section, the reader should appreciate the unphysiological aspects and harms of positive pressure ventilation.

The vital structures involved in the mechanical aspects of breathing are the rib cage and the diaphragm, and the intercostal muscles. When we inhale, the diaphragm contracts and moves downward, increasing the volume of the chest cavity and creating negative pressure in the lungs. This negative pressure draws air into the lungs through the airways. The intercostal muscles are located between the ribs and help to expand and contract the chest cavity during breathing. When we inhale, the intercostal muscles contract, lifting the ribcage and further expanding the chest cavity. This increases the volume of the lungs and allows more air to enter.

Spontaneous ventilation is the natural process of breathing, in which the diaphragm and intercostal muscles contract and relax to draw air into and out of the lungs. During spontaneous inhalation, the diaphragm generates a negative pressure of approximately -3 mmHg to -5 mmHg in the thoracic cavity. This negative pressure helps to expand the lungs and draw air into the respiratory system. Pressure can vary depending on individual factors such as age, health status, and lung capacity.

In some respiratory conditions that limit airflow, such as chronic obstructive pulmonary disease (COPD), asthma, pneumonia, and fibrosis, the negative pressure needed to expand the chest wall may be increased, making it more difficult to breathe. Pulmonary fibrosis and chest wall diseases such as kyphosis or scoliosis can limit the volume of expansion regardless of the negative pressure generated.

In such conditions, the application of positive pressure to the airways can prevent the collapse of the airways (COPD), atelectasis (pneumonia), or simply reduce the patient's effort to inhale the same amount of air.

On the contrary, PPV is a mechanical process that involves insufflation of pressurized air into the lungs through a mask or endotracheal tube. This pressurized air helps to inflate the lungs and facilitate gas exchange, but requires much higher pressures. Please note that the positive pressure should be at least 10-15 mmHg to provide sufficient opening of the alveoli. Almost all side effects of PPV are due to the two- or three-fold increase in airway pressure.

PPV has four side effects (Tonetti et al., 2017). In historical order, the first is barotrauma, which is damage to the lungs or other organs caused by excessive pressure. Although it depends on the degree of pressure, the duration of exposure, the age of the patient, nutritional status, and several other factors, there are some empirical limits: the alveolar endothelium can easily accommodate pressures <20 mmHg for a few hours. If prolonged, such pressure will stretch the alveolar endothelium and cause increased metabolism and secretion. With pressures >20 mmHg, the endothelium begins to become inflamed. With pressures >30 mmHg, the endothelium will be damaged, which will heal depending on the general state of the patient. Patients with poor nutritional status or underlying infection will build scar tissue. Otherwise, the damage may heal better. With pressures >35 mmHg, there will be a time-dependent risk of pneumothorax or subcutaneous emphysema.

Observing these risks, the early ventilators switched from pressure generators to flow generators, which is theoretically the same but a completely different concept. With flow generation, or as more commonly known as volume-controlled ventilators, artificial breathing became more physiological. However, since the underlying principle is the same, namely lung expansion, the damage mechanism became volutrauma. Excessive stretching of the chest wall causes inhibitory signals that depress the regulatory centers and cause atrophy of the diaphragm and intercostal muscles. Especially if used for an extended period, respiratory muscle weakness can cause difficulty in weaning the patient off the ventilator and may require rehabilitation. Overstretching of the alveoli causes inflammation, which in turn causes edema and promotes bacterial growth and ruptures. Finally, overstretching is almost always heterogeneous, which means that it silently progresses if it is not checked rigorously.

Next, in order, comes atelectrauma, which is caused by the cyclic opening and closing of the alveoli. The most common reason is disruption of the extracellular matrix of the lung parenchyma.

Finally, ergotrauma is the latest observed cause of lung damage due to PPV. The main reason is the force delivered by a supranormal respiratory rate. It should be noted that although all these causes are intuitive, there is a reason why it took four decades to become aware of ergotrauma. Each type of trauma is the result of maneuvers used to evade the former type of trauma. That is, volutrauma may become inevitable if the peak airway pressure or the duration of maximal pressure need to be limited. Similarly, atelectrauma can become inevitable if lung volumes are reduced to extremes to accommodate all alveoli. And ergotrauma may be inevitable if one tries to avoid high pressures and high tidal volumes with the use of high respiratory rates and flows.

Ventilator-associated pneumonia is a type of pneumonia that can develop when bacteria enter the lungs through a ventilator tube. This has several causes, such as inadequate oral and bronchial hygiene, frequent tracheal aspirations, damage due to PPV, depression of the immune system, and poor nutritional status. Clearly, all these factors may be exacerbated if the endotracheal tube remains in place for an extended period. Two contrasting factors should be discussed in more detail. Using pressurized air or oxygen supplied by a gas cylinder will desiccate the alveolar endothelium over time, regardless of the fluid balance of the patient. Therefore, moisture-protecting filters or external humidification devices may be required. On the other hand, continuous humidification of the airways is one way to promote bacterial overgrowth. An unfortunate scenario may start with positive pressure ventilation in a patient with pneumonia, and external humidification may be used to promote the removal of thick mucus, but instead promote bacterial overgrowth. Another mishap may start with positive pressure ventilation, which can weaken the respiratory muscles, thus dragging the weaning and desiccating of the alveoli in time. Late treatment with an external humidification device may cause inflammation and edema in the already damaged endothelium due to hot water vapor.

The effects of spontaneous breathing and PPV differ significantly. Spontaneous breathing cyclically causes a negative intrathoracic pressure, which decreases the right atrial pressure, which increases the diastolic filling of the right ventricular, which increases the left ventricular afterload. The resulting decrease in stroke volume will eventually be limited within 1 to 2 beats due to the increase in left atrial and consequently left ventricular preload (Magder, 2018). PPV, in turn, cyclically increases intrathoracic pressure and causes reduced preload, which can decrease stroke volume in hypovolemic patients. However, its effects on stroke work are mixed and may differ between individuals. Basically, increased pulmonary vascular resistance increases stroke work, while decreased pressure gradient between intra- and extra-thoracic aortic pressure may decrease stroke work (Bubshait & Alabbasi, 2021).

Continuous or increased exposure to positive intrathoracic pressures may also limit lymphatic drainage and promote pleural effusion. Such effects should be considered when initiating, maintaining, and weaning PPV, or mobilizing a patient while on PPV. Diagnostic work, decision making, and interventions will be highlighted in the perioperative care and management section.

Noninvasive PPV can cause gastric distension and tracheal aspiration of the gastric contents and all forms of PPV can cause psychological distress and anxiety in some patients, especially if they are aware and aware of the mechanical ventilation.

Finally, it should be noted that the effects of PPV are not equal to the side effects of mechanical ventilation, which is more like a package. This consists of analgesia, sedation, and immobility that promote thrombosis, poor oral hygiene, and constant pressure on the tracheal mucosa.

Control of Breathing

The respiratory system is responsible for the removal of acids in the form of carbon dioxide (CO_2) and the supply of enough oxygen (O_2). Therefore, the depth and rate of respiration are strictly controlled by several chemical and mechanical sensors.

The control centers of respiration are in the brainstem, specifically in the medulla oblongata and pons. These control centers receive input from various sources, including chemoreceptors, mechanoreceptors, and central nervous system receptors.

The medulla oblongata contains the primary respiratory center, which is responsible for controlling the rhythm and depth of breathing. The neurons in this center generate rhythmic signals that drive the contraction of the respiratory muscles. The medulla also contains chemoreceptors that are sensitive to changes in the levels of carbon dioxide, oxygen, and pH in the blood. When the levels of carbon dioxide in the blood increase, the medulla responds by increasing the respiratory rate and depth to eliminate excess carbon dioxide.

The pons contains additional respiratory centers that work together with the medulla to modulate the respiratory rhythm and maintain the balance of oxygen and carbon dioxide in the body. The pons also contains mechanoreceptors that are sensitive to changes in lung volume and work to adjust respiratory rate and depth accordingly.

Disorders that affect respiratory control centers can lead to respiratory failure or insufficiency. For example, neurological disorders that affect the medulla or pons, such as strokes or tumors, can disrupt the normal functioning of the respiratory centers and lead to breathing problems. Additionally, drugs or toxins that affect the central nervous system can also interfere with the normal functioning of respiratory control centers and lead to respiratory depression or failure.

Both the medulla oblongata and the pons are important for the control of respiration. The medulla oblongata contains the primary respiratory center that generates the rhythmic signals that drive breathing, while the pons contains additional respiratory centers that modulate the respiratory rhythm and adjust the respiratory rate and depth (Lumb, 2017). The medulla is considered the most important of the two centers for the generation of the basic respiratory rhythm. If the medulla is depressed, the patient may experience respiratory failure or arrest. However, the pons can still provide some respiratory force in the absence of medullary activity. In some cases, the pons may be able to take over respiratory drive and support ventilation in the absence of medullary function. However, this is only possible if the pons is intact and functioning properly.

Overall, it is important to note that the medulla oblongata and the pons work together in the control of respiration, and disruptions in either center can lead to respiratory failure or failure. But they serve different functions. The medulla is responsible for vital functions such as breathing, heart rate, and blood pressure, while the pons is involved in functions such as sleep, arousal, and facial movements. This share of responsibilities allows for differential diagnosis.

Some examples where the medulla is depressed but the pons is still functioning are opioid overdose. Opioid drugs such as morphine and fentanyl can depress the medulla, leading to respiratory depression and potentially fatal consequences. However, the pons may still be functioning, as the person may still be able to respond to stimuli and have some level of consciousness. Such a patient will be apneic, but will breath when tactile stimuli is applied. Repetitive tactile stimuli can allow for adequate ventilation. Although it may seem cumbersome, this may be desirable in certain situations. If an opioid overdose is reversed with an antagonist such as naloxone, the patient may rigorously inhale against a closed glottis. This may result in negative pressure lung edema. Prevention could be as simple as jaw thrust maneuver or application of an airway, whereas treatment may require prolonged use of invasive or noninvasive mechanical ventilation, which may cause tracheal aspiration or similar complications. A postoperative patient, who received excessive doses of opioids for analgesia, may experience an abrupt return of pain and the consequences of hypertension and tachycardia, which can be as severe as myocardial infarction or ventricular tachycardia.

A stroke that affects the medulla can cause symptoms such as difficulty breathing, changes in heart rate, and loss of consciousness. However, if the pons is not affected, the person may still be able to move their limbs and respond to stimuli. The combination of a patient looking intelligently but not breathing or coughing may confuse the examiner and postpone definitive interventions such as tracheostomy or percutaneous enterogastrostomy by futile trials such as amantadine, etc.

Some examples where the pons is depressed but the medulla is still functioning are Locked-in syndrome, which is a condition in which the pons is damaged, leading to complete paralysis of all voluntary muscles except those that control eye movement. However, the medulla is still functioning, so that the person can breathe and maintain his heart rate. This may confuse the examiner and cause an early tracheostomy due to a low Glasgow coma scale score.

Barbiturates, which are also found in certain sleeping pills, can depress the pons, leading to symptoms such as slowed breathing and decreased heart rate. However, the medulla may still function, so the person may still be able to breathe and maintain their blood pressure.

It is important to note that these examples are simplified and that in reality, the effects of brainstem damage can vary widely depending on the extent and location of the damage. Finally, stretch receptors located in the pleura limit lung overextension, while chemical receptors that detect arterial blood pressure of O_2 and CO_2 promote sighs. All of these receptors are prone to inhibition by anesthetic drugs and overstimulation by prolonged or excessive PPV.

In the context of anesthesia, it is important for anesthesiologists to be aware of respiratory control centers and their regulation of breathing. Anesthetic agents can depress respiratory centers, leading to respiratory depression and potentially respiratory failure. Therefore, monitoring respiratory function during anesthesia is crucial to ensure patient safety.

Carbon Dioxide Removal, Oxygen Transport and Delivery

The respiratory depth and rate are regulated according to ventilation requirements (to keep $PaCO_2 < 50$ mmHg and pH > 7.3), oxygen requirements (to keep $PaO_2 > 60$ mmHg), and metabolic requirements (to match DO_2 to VO_2 and CO_2 to pH). This regulation may not achieve the expected result due to two reasons:

It is understandable that the depth and rate of respiration will increase if any of the above-mentioned requirements will increase. But without a proportional increase in cardiac output, this will not increase the transport of O_2 and CO_2 between tissues and the lungs. Taking into account the effects of PPV on cardiac output, it should be understandable that although PPV may improve exposure to the alveoli and surrounding capillaries, gas exchange may not always improve if cardiac output deteriorates due to hypovolemia or worsening of cardiac mechanics. As mentioned above, if the injury is only pulmonary, PPV and mechanical ventilation will probably improve the patient's condition. In mixed pathologies, individual components of PPV should be titrated accordingly. In short, the lungs are not the only organs that can interact if one needs to improve gas exchange. The good side is that the gas exchange can improve without overstretching the lungs. The bad side is that gas exchange can worsen if mechanical ventilation or weaning can negatively affect the cardiovascular system.

Another problem is that the lungs do not exchange respiratory gases homogeneously throughout the parenchyma. Apart from variations in tissue properties, interactions with the diaphragm and the heart, and gravitational effects do prevail. Despite all this heterogeneity, a healthy lung fulfills its required gas exchange role very well. And the lungs can tolerate a considerable amount of structural deterioration before an individual becomes symptomatic due to poor gas exchange. Before we examine which disease causes what kind of deterioration, we now have the question of how to assess lung function.

Other Functions of the Respiratory System

The lungs act as a natural filter. Smoking-related chemicals can lead to COPD, lung cancer, and other respiratory diseases. Exposure to second-hand smoke can also damage the lungs and increase the risk of respiratory infections, asthma, and COPD. Exposure to pollutants such as particulate matter, ozone, nitrogen dioxide, and sulfur dioxide can damage the lungs and increase the risk of respiratory infections, asthma, and COPD. Occupational exposure to asbestos, silica, and coal dust, which can damage the lungs and cause occupational lung diseases such as pneumoconiosis and lung cancer. Radon is a naturally occurring radioactive gas that can seep into homes and buildings. Prolonged exposure to high levels of radon can increase the risk of lung cancer.

The lungs play a role in regulating body temperature by altering the amount of heat and water that is lost during breathing. When we exhale, we lose heat and water from our bodies, and the lungs can help regulate the amount of heat and water lost by adjusting the rate and depth of breathing. If the lungs do not regulate body temperature properly, it can lead to overheating or hypothermia. There are several conditions in which the role of the lungs in temperature regulation may be impaired.

People with COPD may have difficulty regulating body temperature, particularly in extreme heat or cold. Respiratory infections, such as pneumonia and influenza, can cause inflammation in the lungs and impair their ability to regulate body temperature. Trauma to the lungs, such as from a chest injury or surgery, can affect lung function and affect their ability to regulate body temperature. Certain medications, such as beta-blockers and antidepressants, can affect the ability of the lungs to regulate body temperature.

In summary, the lungs play a role in regulating body temperature by adjusting the amount of heat and water lost during breathing. However, certain conditions and medications can affect this function, leading to overheating or hypothermia.

The lungs play an important role in maintaining fluid balance in the body by regulating the exchange of water and electrolytes during breathing. When we inhale, the lungs humidify and warm the air, helping to prevent excessive fluid loss from the body. When we exhale, we remove carbon dioxide and excess water from the body. Respiratory insufficiencies can lead to various electrolyte imbalances in the body, including sodium and potassium disorders.

Hyponatremia is a common electrolyte abnormality in patients with pneumonia. Pneumonia can cause an inflammatory response in the body, leading to the release of certain hormones and chemicals that affect the balance of fluid and electrolytes. Additionally, pneumonia can cause fever, sweating, and an increased respiratory rate, which can lead to increased fluid loss from the body and a dilution of sodium levels in the blood.

Other respiratory insufficiencies, such as COPD, can also lead to electrolyte imbalances. For example, COPD can cause chronic respiratory acidosis, which can lead to retention of bicarbonate ions in the body and a subsequent decrease in chloride levels, resulting in hypochloremic metabolic alkalosis. COPD can also cause hypoxemia, which can lead to increased erythropoietin production and subsequent polycythemia. This can lead to increased blood viscosity and decreased renal blood flow, which can contribute to the development of electrolyte imbalances such as hyponatremia, hypocalcemia, and hyperkalemia (Schiavo et al., 2016).

In summary, respiratory insufficiencies such as pneumonia and COPD can lead to electrolyte imbalances in the body, with hyponatremia being a common electrolyte abnormality in patients with pneumonia. Proper management and treatment of these conditions, including appropriate replacement of fluids and electrolytes, can help mitigate these risks and prevent further complications.

Assessment of Lung Function and Respiratory Status

Since all respiratory failures will end with intubation, the logical next step after medical history and physical examination is to assess the airways for difficult airway. Certain characteristics and comorbidities of the patient, such as obesity, neck stiffness, a history of sleep apnea, or a difficult airway in a previous procedure, should raise suspicion of a potentially difficult airway. The use of a scoring system will help ensure an overall assessment (Phero et al., 2012; Stojanovic, 2017). Some commonly used scoring systems are the following:

- *Mallampati score:* This is a simple, noninvasive assessment of pharyngeal structures that can predict difficult intubation. The score ranges from I to IV, with higher scores indicating greater difficulty in visualizing the larynx.
- *Cormack-Lehane score*: This is a classification system that describes the degree of visualization of the larynx during direct laryngoscopy. The score ranges from I to IV, with higher scores indicating greater difficulty with intubation.
- *Wilson score*: This scoring system incorporates several factors related to the airways, such as mouth opening, neck movement, and upper lip bite test, to predict difficult intubation.
- *LEMON score*: This mnemonic stands for: Externally, evaluate 3-3-2, Mallampati score, obstruction, and neck mobility. Each of these factors is scored, and the total score can help predict difficult intubation.
- *MACOCHA score*: This scoring system incorporates several factors, including Mallampati score, airway obstruction, body mass index, neck circumference, and age, to predict difficult intubation in patients undergoing general anesthesia.

The important point is that the evaluation should be on par with the skill of the practitioner and available tools such as a video laryngoscope or supraglottic airway devices.

Respiratory insufficiency refers to a condition in which the lungs cannot exchange oxygen and carbon dioxide adequately with the environment, leading to a decrease in oxygen levels and an increase in carbon dioxide levels in the blood. There are various conditions that can lead to respiratory failure, and these can be broadly categorized as extrinsic or intrinsic factors.

Another classification is hypoxemic versus hypercapnic respiratory failure. In hypoxemic respiratory failure, the lungs may not adequately humidify and warm the air, leading to excessive loss of fluid from the body. This can result in dehydration and hypovolemia, which can lead to decreased blood pressure, decreased urine output, and other signs of fluid depletion.

In hypercapnic respiratory failure, the lungs may retain excess carbon dioxide in the body, leading to increased blood acidity. This can lead to fluid retention and hypervolemia, as the body tries to compensate for acidosis by retaining fluids.

In both types of respiratory failure, the patient may be at risk of developing imbalances in fluid and electrolyte levels, which can lead to further complications such as electrolyte abnormalities, kidney failure, and cardiac arrhythmias.

In summary, respiratory failure can have implications for fluid balance in the body, and hypoxemic and hypercapnic respiratory failure can put the patient at risk of developing imbalances in fluid and electrolyte levels. Proper management of respiratory failure, including appropriate oxygenation and ventilation strategies, can help mitigate these risks and prevent further complications.

Given the common overlap between these two classifications and other classifications, this section will outline the steps to assess lung function in acute respiratory failure. Chronic respiratory failure will not be mentioned, as the only difference is the availability of more time for medical history and physical examination. In acute failures, treatment of the most prominent symptoms of distress should start first, then follow by obtaining medical history as the patient's condition allows.

Some general approaches for assessing lung function in various examples of acute respiratory failure are given below:

In cases of trauma, it is important to assess potential chest injuries, such as pneumothorax, flail chest, hemothorax, or pulmonary contusion, which can result in decreased lung function and respiratory failure. Patients with chest trauma should be closely monitored for signs of respiratory distress, such as increased breathing work, hypoxemia, and decreased tidal volume. Adequate pain control and mechanical ventilation may be necessary to support lung function.

Spinal trauma patients may be at risk for respiratory failure due to impaired respiratory muscle function. Patients with spinal cord injuries above the level of C4 may need mechanical ventilation to support breathing. Additionally, patients with spinal cord injuries may be at risk for pulmonary complications such as pneumonia and atelectasis.

Patients with burns or inhalational injuries may develop airway edema, which can obstruct the airway and cause respiratory failure. Early intubation and mechanical ventilation may be necessary to maintain adequate oxygenation and prevent further damage to the lungs.

In cases of poisoning, the patient should be evaluated immediately for respiratory rate, oxygen saturation, and level of consciousness. Toxicology screens and blood gas analysis may help identify the specific toxin involved and guide treatment. In all cases, the determination of the basal vital signs and laboratory values of organ functions should be made. The possibility of the removal of the toxin or an antidote should be actively sought, and the response should be closely monitored.

Patients with neuromuscular disorders such as myasthenia gravis or amyotrophic lateral sclerosis may develop respiratory failure due to impaired respiratory muscle function. It is important to monitor for signs of respiratory distress and consider mechanical ventilation, if necessary. Succinylcholine can further damage the abnormal muscle membrane in patients with muscular dystrophies. In addition, such patients may have an abnormal heat dissipation mechanism and need central temperature monitoring (Bauman & Tobin, 2012).

Patients with acute respiratory distress syndrome can develop severe respiratory failure due to alveolar damage and pulmonary edema. It is important to monitor signs of respiratory distress, such as tachypnea, dyspnea, and hypoxemia. Treatment may involve mechanical ventilation with positive end-expiratory pressure and other supportive measures.

In patients with suspected pulmonary embolism, it is important to assess signs of respiratory distress, such as tachypnea, dyspnea, and hypoxemia. Patients with aspiration pneumonia can develop respiratory failure due to lung inflammation and infection. It is important to assess signs of respiratory distress, such as tachypnea, dyspnea, and hypoxemia. Treatment may involve antibiotics and supportive measures such as oxygen therapy.

In acute exacerbations of COPD, it is important to assess signs of respiratory distress, such as increased work of breathing and hypoxemia. Treatment may involve bronchodilators, steroids, and oxygen therapy.

Patients with interstitial lung disease may experience acute exacerbations characterized by worsening dyspnea, cough, and hypoxemia. Treatment may involve high-dose steroids and oxygen therapy. Neuromuscular diseases such as muscular dystrophy, myasthenia gravis, or amyotrophic lateral sclerosis can cause respiratory muscle weakness and respiratory failure due to the decreased ability to adequately ventilate the lungs. Similarly, patients with chest wall abnormalities such as scoliosis or kyphosis, pectus excavatum, or pectus carinatum may be at increased risk for acute respiratory failure due to decreased lung volumes and impaired respiratory muscle function. Treatment may involve mechanical ventilation and supportive measures such as oxygen therapy and pain control. Sarcoidosis is a systemic inflammatory disease that can affect the lungs, leading to granulomatous inflammation and fibrosis, which can cause restrictive lung disease and respiratory failure. Idiopathic pulmonary fibrosis is a progressive chronic lung disease that can cause fibrosis and scarring of the lung tissue, leading to decreased lung function and respiratory failure during acute exacerbations. Radiation pneumonitis is a lung inflammation that can occur as a side effect of radiation therapy for lung cancer, breast cancer, or lymphoma, leading to restrictive lung disease and respiratory failure.

It is important to correctly assess the survival of a patient. This can be complex and depends on many factors such as the underlying cause of the disease, the severity of the lung disease, comorbidities, age, and overall health status of the patient. This is especially important in patients with restrictive lung disease, but also with chronic obstructive lung disease, as some of these patients are not expected to survive, whereas some may be potentially saved with lung transplantation, and should be treated accordingly.

Prognostic factors should be sought. For example, in idiopathic pulmonary fibrosis, the presence of certain factors such as older age, male sex, low forced vital capacity, low carbon monoxide diffusion capacity of the lung, and the extent of fibrosis on high-resolution computed tomography can be associated with poorer survival. Oxygenation status is an important predictor of survival. In general, patients with severe hypoxemia or hypercapnia are at increased risk of mortality. However, it is important to consider the overall clinical picture, as some patients with chronic respiratory failure may have adapted to their baseline oxygenation level and may not require aggressive intervention. In acute exacerbations, response to treatment may be an important predictor of survival. Patients who respond well to medical therapy, such as corticosteroids or immunosuppressants, may have better results compared to those who do not respond. However, the frequency of exacerbations and the trend of increase or decrease are equally important predictors. Quality of life is an important consideration in determining whether a patient may be a candidate for lung transplantation. Patients who have significant impairment in their activities of daily living, despite medical therapy, can be considered for lung transplantation if they are suitable candidates. Finally, comorbidities such as cardiovascular disease, diabetes, or chronic kidney disease can affect survival, frequency, and severity of exacerbations, and quality of life. All these factors should be taken into account when deciding to receive palliative care or aggressive treatment.

Anesthetic Considerations for Patients with Respiratory Insufficiencies

In patients with respiratory insufficiency due to any pathology, it is important for anesthesiologists to carefully monitor and manage their breathing during anesthesia to ensure that the balance of oxygen and carbon dioxide is maintained within safe levels. This section will discuss general considerations for anesthesia in patients with respiratory insufficiencies, choice of anesthesia technique (e.g., regional vs. general anesthesia), and preoperative optimization of respiratory function (e.g., bronchodilators, mucolytics). Please note that, in accordance with the section "CO_2 removal, transport and delivery," the anesthesiologist cannot confine his attention to the airways and the lungs. The positioning of the patient, the cardiovascular system, and the expectation of worsening or improvement after the intervention affect the management. Various anesthetic techniques can be used for patients with respiratory insufficiency, depending on the severity and cause of the condition. Understanding anesthesia can be a challenge for those not familiar with the field. By breaking it down into the four parts that make up its package - hypnosis, amnesia, analgesia and prevention of muscular and autonomic reflexes - it becomes easier to comprehend.

Hypnosis refers to the induction and maintenance of a state of unconsciousness, during which the patient is unaware of his surroundings and does not respond to external stimuli. The goal is to ensure that the patient is completely unaware of the surgical procedure, which helps minimize pain and reduce psychological trauma.

Amnesia refers to the prevention of the formation and retention of new memories during the anesthesia period. This helps to reduce the psychological stress associated with surgery and prevent the patient from remembering the traumatic experience.

Analgesia refers to the prevention or reduction of pain during the surgical procedure. This is typically achieved through the administration of opioids or other pain reliever medications. The goal of analgesia is to ensure that the patient is pain-free during the procedure and during the recovery period.

Prevention of reflex activity is commonly understood as the suppression of movement or reflexes that may occur during the surgical procedure, such as coughing or movement. This is typically achieved with muscle relaxants or other medications that suppress the autonomic nervous system. However, prevention of autonomic reflexes such as hypertension or hypotension is equally important. With the availability of ultrasound devices and several local anesthetic medications with varying effective duration, the use of regional anesthesia is widespread. It is increasingly used as it allows for more rational use of the operating room, earlier mobilization and discharge, and the opportunity to interact with the patient during the procedure. With so many advantages, it may seem contradictory that sedation may be used to facilitate some nerve blocks on the scalp or face. However, such blocks may induce dangerous hypotension.

Another misconception is that the patient should be pain-free if he/she does not move. This is apparent in common talk, and unfortunately, many physicians are prone to this misconception, although the complexity of several physical signs had long been difficult for over seven decades, beginning with the Guedel's four stages of anesthesia (Atkinson et al., 1977), and the "Curare cleft" experiment which preceded that. This experiment was conducted by a team of researchers at the University of Oxford in England in the late 1940s and is considered a landmark study in the history of anesthesia. It involved administering a muscle relaxant called curare to an anesthesiologist, who had a sleeve on one of his arms, which prevented the curare from affecting that limb. The curare rendered him paralyzed and unable to speak or move. However, he was still conscious and able to understand what was happening around him. This experiment demonstrated that curare does not have hypnotic or amnestic action, which means that it does not affect the patient's level of consciousness or the ability to remember what happened during anesthesia.

Finally, the main anesthetic drugs provide hypnosis at a much lower serum concentration compared to amnesis. Like analgesia, this is commonly interpreted as hypnosis is present if the patient does not move, which is understandably wrong. Furthermore, it should be noted that if a patient becomes aware of the surrounding, amnesis is certainly lost.

The highlight of the preceding paragraphs is that each component of anesthesia should be evaluated separately. Hopefully, monitoring each of these components is possible, albeit with some pitfalls, which require expertise.

As it should be clear by now that any anesthetic technique may be used in isolation and in combination with the others, here are a few examples for the nonanesthesiologist:

Regional anesthesia involves numbing only a specific part of the body, such as an arm or a leg, without affecting the patient's ability to breathe on their own. This can be a good option for patients with mild to moderate respiratory insufficiency who can tolerate lying flat. Please note that this is an oversimplification. Spinal anesthesia is associated with acute exacerbation of multiple sclerosis, where the mechanism is unclear, but speculated to be related to increased sensitivity of demyelinated areas of the spinal cord to local anesthetics (Bauman & Tobin, 2012).

Sedation involves the use of medications to help the patient relax and reduce anxiety while still maintaining their ability to breathe on their own. This can be a good option for patients with mild respiratory insufficiency who are able to maintain their airways and breathing without assistance.

Inhalational anesthesia involves the delivery of anesthetic gases through a mask or a breathing tube to induce and maintain general anesthesia. This can be a good option for patients with moderate to severe respiratory failure who require help with breathing.

Total intravenous anesthesia involves the delivery of anesthesia medications through an intravenous catheter, rather than using inhalational gases. This can be a good option for patients with respiratory failure who may be more sensitive to the effects of inhalational gases. Additionally, it will be safer to induce and maintain anesthesia in patients with damaged lungs, as the inhalational route of anesthetic drug administration is inhibited and shared with the route of O2.

It is important to note that the choice of anesthetic technique for a patient with respiratory insufficiency will depend on a variety of factors, including the severity and cause of the condition, the patient's overall health and medical history, and the type of surgery or procedure being performed. Anesthesiologists are trained to evaluate each patient individually and develop a personalized anesthetic plan that takes all of these factors into account.

Perioperative Care and Management

Complications and the management of respiratory insufficiencies during anesthesia are critical topics that all anesthesiologists must be aware of. Respiratory insufficiencies can occur during anesthesia due to a variety of factors, including pre-existing respiratory conditions, drug interactions, and physiological changes induced by the anesthesia itself.

Some of the most common complications associated with respiratory failure during anesthesia include hypoxemia, hypoventilation, hypercapnia and respiratory acidosis, airway obstruction, bronchospasm, aspiration, pulmonary edema, and pneumothorax. These complications can lead to serious adverse events such as brain damage, cardiac arrest, and death. As almost all of these complications can occur and are commonly seen during the induction of anesthesia and the securing of the airway, laryngeal intubation and tracheotomy will be discussed separately.

To manage respiratory failures during anesthesia, anesthesiologists must be familiar with a variety of techniques and interventions. These may include adjusting the dose of anesthesia, administering oxygen or other respiratory support, performing endotracheal intubation, and using positive pressure ventilation.

In some cases, it may be necessary to interrupt anesthesia and reverse its effects using reversal agents such as naloxone or flumazenil. In addition, careful monitoring of the patient's vital signs, including blood pressure, heart rate, and oxygen saturation, is essential to ensure timely intervention in the event of respiratory complications.

Anesthesiologists must be familiar with a range of techniques and interventions to manage these complications, including adjusting the dose of anesthesia, administering oxygen or other respiratory support, performing endotracheal intubation, and using positive pressure ventilation. Careful monitoring of the patient's vital signs and a thorough preoperative evaluation of respiratory status can also help minimize the risk of respiratory complications during anesthesia.

Emergent Interventions and Crisis Management

In general, emergent interventions and crisis management require prompt recognition of respiratory distress and a rapid response. Rapid response should include calling for help if necessary and appropriate interventions such as airway management, oxygenation, fluid management, and pharmacological interventions. Close monitoring and frequent reassessment of the patient's respiratory status are essential, as is collaboration with other members of the anesthesia team and other medical professionals when necessary. The importance of correctly identifying the need for help cannot be overemphasized. In cases of severe respiratory distress, calling for the help of other members of the anesthesia team, as well as other medical professionals, to provide additional support and expertise may determine the outcome.

Some emergency situations are discussed in the following:

Hypoxemia can be caused by a decreased fraction of inspired O_2 (FiO_2), decreased alveolar ventilation, or shunt physiology. Predictive factors are obesity, preexisting lung disease, higher age, duration of anesthesia. It may be prevented by monitoring oxygen saturation, using additional oxygen. Treatment includes increasing FiO_2, positive pressure ventilation, and correcting underlying causes. The potential long-term lung damage and the need for postoperative oxygen therapy should be evaluated.

Hypoventilation can be caused by respiratory depressants, neuromuscular blockade, or inadequate ventilation. Predictive factors are opioid use, preexisting respiratory disease, obesity, sedation level. It can be prevented by monitoring the respiratory rate and depth, avoiding excessive opioid use. Treatment involves increasing ventilation, reversing neuromuscular blockade, and correcting the underlying causes. The potential for postoperative respiratory failure or pneumonia should be evaluated.

Airway obstruction can be caused by laryngospasm, bronchospasm, foreign body aspiration, or upper airway edema. Predictive factors are preexisting airway disease, history of difficult airway management, surgery involving airway manipulation. It may be prevented by proper management of the airways, the use of prophylactic bronchodilators, or steroids in at-risk patients. Treatment involves positive pressure ventilation, administering bronchodilators, removing foreign bodies, or addressing edema. The potential for prolonged mechanical ventilation or tracheostomy should be evaluated.

Bronchospasm can be caused by irritants, allergens, or hyperresponsiveness of the airways. Predictive factors are preexisting asthma or COPD, history of bronchospasm with anesthesia or surgery. It may be prevented by using prophylactic bronchodilators or steroids in at-risk patients. Treatment involves administering bronchodilators, increasing FiO_2, positive pressure ventilation. The potential for prolonged mechanical ventilation or tracheostomy should be evaluated.

Pneumothorax can be caused by trauma, barotrauma, or lung disease. Predictive factors are preexisting lung disease, history of pneumothorax, and certain surgical procedures. It may be prevented by careful monitoring during surgery, avoiding excessive positive pressure ventilation. Treatment involves the insertion of the chest tube and the adjustment of mechanical ventilation.

The potential for prolonged hospitalization or the development of chronic lung disease should be evaluated.

Tracheal aspiration of gastric contents can be caused by inadequate fasting, delayed gastric emptying, or altered protective reflexes of the airways. Predictive factors are obesity, history of gastroesophageal reflux disease or esophageal dysfunction, and certain surgical procedures. It can be prevented by proper fasting guidelines, although even fasting times in excess of 12 hours are associated with a full stomach. Additional preventive measures include the prophylactic use of proton pump inhibitors in at-risk patients to decrease the probability of lung damage. Treatment involves antibiotics and mechanical ventilation, if necessary. The potential for prolonged mechanical ventilation or the development of chronic lung disease should be evaluated.

Pulmonary edema during anesthesia can occur for several reasons, including fluid overload, heart failure, increased vascular permeability, and impaired lymphatic drainage. Predictive factors are a history of heart failure, renal failure, or COPD. The incidence of pulmonary edema during anesthesia varies depending on the underlying patient population, ranging from less than 1% to 30%. Prevention strategies for pulmonary edema during anesthesia include optimizing fluid management, avoiding excessive administration of intravenous fluids, and ensuring adequate oxygenation and ventilation. Treatment involves addressing the underlying cause, such as administering diuretics, optimizing heart function, or providing positive end-expiratory pressure ventilation. Supplemental oxygen and inotropic agents may also be necessary. Patients who develop pulmonary edema during anesthesia should be closely monitored in the postoperative period for signs of respiratory distress and hemodynamic instability. Further management may involve adjustment of fluid and medication management, as well as further investigation and treatment of underlying cardiovascular or pulmonary pathology.

Endotracheal Intubation and Other Ways to Secure the Airway

In the case of a patient with respiratory failure, the list of necessary equipment is massively expanded to include additional personnel to help with positioning, intubation, or suction. Video laryngoscope or fiberoptic bronchoscope to visualize airways, supraglottic airways, and several masks of different sizes and types should be prepared. The use of trays, pre-packaged kits, or crash carts is encouraged to ensure teaching, standardization, and preparedness.

Preoxygenation is applied to fill the dead anatomic space, including the oropharynx and conducting airways, and the functional residual capacity with oxygen. To maximize benefit, 100% O_2 is used to denitrogenate the space. It should be noted that the anatomic dead space is 2 ml/kg, whereas the functional residual capacity is almost 3 liters in an average adult. However, it may become smaller due to thoracic conditions such as thoracic cage deformities (scoliosis, kyphosis, pectus carinatum), lung damage (tumors, pneumo or hemothorax, pleural effusion), a hypertrophied heart or pericardial effusion, abdominal conditions such as tumors, fetus, ascites, diaphragmatic herniation of the stomach or intestines, or ileus. Smaller individuals have smaller functional residual capacity, which is the reason why a newborn can never tolerate apnea for 5-10 seconds, regardless of how long it had been pre-oxygenated (Hopkins & Sharma, 2022).

In practice, concentrations <100% are preferred in elective conditions to prevent hyperoxia-related harms, such as increased atelectasis or mortality in critically ill patients (Branson & Robinson, 2011; Duggan & Kavanagh, 2007; Pelletier et al., 2021). However, such a practice cannot be safely advised without the use of appropriate equipment to monitor the oxygen reserve of the patient (Yoshida et al., 2020). Even then, it should be noted that hemoglobin saturation of oxygen is not the primary determinant of tissue oxygenation. For this, there should be enough oxygen content in the blood, the circulation of blood should be adequate, the mean arterial blood pressure should be adequate to perfuse the organ, the capillary network should be adequate, and finally the amount of oxygen served should match the requirements of the tissue.

One way to ensure this match is to sedate the patient. The patient may receive sedative medications to relax and reduce anxiety and muscle relaxants to paralyze the vocal cords and facilitate intubation.

Overall, endotracheal intubation is a complex procedure that requires skill and experience. It is typically performed by an anesthesiologist or other trained healthcare professional in a hospital or clinical setting. The complexity is due to the high risks involved in each step and the fact that almost all steps may be modified or canceled in experienced hands. On the contrary, an inexperienced physician may find it safest to completely sedate and paralyze the patient and quickly try to intubate the patient. Such a practice requires careful patient selection and is otherwise not safe.

Another point that requires careful patient selection is the use of video laryngoscopes. Their use is increasing because of their availability. The results with inexperienced users are conflicting. Some studies report increased success but increased time-to-intubation or vice versa (Hansel et al., 2022; Tung & Griesdale, 2013; van Schuppen et al., 2022). The Difficult Airway Society recently emphasized the use of video laryngoscopes in difficult airways during the first attempt, which may be interpreted differently (*DAS Guidelines for Management of Unanticipated Difficult Intubation in Adults 2015 | Difficult Airway Society*, n.d.; Frerk et al., 2015). The short advice is that video laryngoscopes are tools that improve the success of the first intubation attempt, but they are not a tool to negate the effect of experience.

The guidelines also emphasize the use of supraglottic devices to facilitate preoxygenation, intubation, and ventilation in case of "unable to intubate" situations. Therefore, the period of induction of anesthesia and laryngeal intubation should be well planned, with all the necessary tools in mind.

Tracheostomy

Tracheostomy is a surgical procedure that involves making a small incision between the second and third rings and inserting a tracheostomy tube into the trachea to create an open airway. A higher incision will risk fracture of the cricoid cartilage and subglottic stenosis (Cooper, 2018; Shinn et al., 2019). A lower incision will risk a tracheoinnominate fistula, which is a life-threatening condition (Reger et al., 2018; Shamji et al., 2018). The surgeon will carefully separate the muscles and tissues around the incision site to expose the trachea and may use retractors to separate the tissues and provide a clear view of the trachea.

The correct placement will be confirmed by suctioning to feel the tugging or clicking of the trachea, listening to breath sounds, monitoring the rise and fall of the chest, and checking carbon dioxide levels in exhaled air using a capnography device. Although widely used as part of the removal of secretions and blood from the trachea, note that while tracheal tug is a normal finding during suction, it can also indicate that the suction catheter is in contact with the tracheal wall, which can cause irritation or injury. Therefore, it is important for the operator to be gentle and use caution when suctioning the trachea to avoid causing any damage to the airway.

Overall, tracheostomy is a complex surgical procedure that requires skill and experience. It is typically performed by a surgeon in a hospital or clinical setting. Tracheotomy may be performed as a temporary or permanent procedure, depending on the patient's condition and needs.

Percutaneous tracheotomy involves using the Seldinger technique to introduce the tracheotomy tube. Percutaneous tracheotomy is generally considered less invasive and faster than open tracheostomy, but it may be associated with a higher risk of complications, such as bleeding or tube displacement. On the contrary, open tracheotomy is generally considered a more invasive and complex procedure, but it provides better visualization and control of the airway.

Also, it should be emphasized that the open technique frequently involves creating a u-shaped flap called the tracheal or mucosal flap. The flap is then bent upward and sutured to the skin edges, creating a seal around the tracheostomy tube and preventing air or fluid from escaping around the tracheostomy tube, which could lead to obstruction of the airways, infection, or other complications. By creating a seal between the tracheal wall and the skin edges, it helps direct air and secretions through the tracheostomy tube and prevent leakage around the tube. It also helps to anchor the tracheostomy tube in place, reducing the risk of accidental dislodgement or displacement. Furthermore, the flap provides some protection to the tracheal mucosa, which can be vulnerable to irritation or damage due to the presence of the tracheostomy tube.

Postoperative Care and Management

It is important to classify the patient's condition before and after the operation to properly discuss postoperative care and management. Different types of respiratory failure require different interventions and management strategies.

For example, a patient who developed respiratory failure during the operation due to a variety of reasons, such as anesthesia-induced respiratory depression, gastric contents aspiration, or an allergic reaction, may need immediate intervention, such as intubation and mechanical ventilation, while the underlying cause of respiratory failure is being identified and treated. In contrast, a patient who had respiratory failure before the operation and is not expected to recover postoperatively may require long-term mechanical ventilation or other respiratory support measures.

A patient who is undergoing surgery to resolve the cause of respiratory failure, such as COPD, who undergoes lung transplant surgery to improve their respiratory function, may require close monitoring of respiratory function during and after the operation, while a patient with multiple organ failure, including respiratory failure, may require a more comprehensive approach to management, including fluid management, nutritional support, and intensive care.

Third, a patient with severe respiratory failure along with other organ failures, such as renal or cardiac failure, that require intensive care management may require a comprehensive approach to managing multiple organ systems, including mechanical ventilation, hemodynamic support, and renal replacement therapy during postoperative care. For example, a patient with sepsis and acute respiratory distress syndrome may require postoperative mechanical ventilation and renal replacement therapy to manage multiple organ failures.

In general, a proper classification of the patient's condition allows for a more targeted and effective postoperative care and management plan, taking into account the specific needs and challenges of each patient.

Complications in the post-anesthesia care unit were and are still common, which is a consequence of caring for high-risk postoperative patients. Airway obstruction due to tongue displacement, laryngeal edema or laryngospasm, paralysis of the vocal cord, or trachea due to external compression can be seen. Delayed emergence from general anesthesia and inadequate reversal of neuromuscular blockade can require prolonged intubation, promoting hemodynamic instability such as hypotension, cardiac dysrhythmias, or hypertension. Urinary retention and oliguria are also frequent due to hypovolemia or response to surgical stress (Bittner et al., 2012).

Two other aspects deserve some in-depth discussion: pain management and its impact on respiratory function, and early mobilization and respiratory therapy.

Pain Management and Its Impact on Respiratory Function

Effective pain management is an essential component of patient care, and its impact on respiratory function should be carefully considered, particularly in patients with preexisting respiratory impairment or those undergoing surgery or other invasive procedures. Pain can affect respiratory function by reducing tidal volume, functional residual capacity, and respiratory rate, leading to hypoxemia, hypercapnia, and other complications.

The use of opioid analgesics is still a common approach to pain management, but the advantage of these drugs is mostly offset due to the need to monitor early (with synthetic opioids) or late (with morphine) respiratory depression, delayed discharge due to sedation, constipation, and similar complications (Lee et al., 2015). Alternative pain management strategies, such as regional anesthesia, non-steroidal anti-inflammatory drugs, or more commonly a combination of all (multimodal analgesia) should be considered in all appropriate cases.

Early Mobilization and Respiratory Therapy

Early mobilization and respiratory therapy are two important components of postoperative care, particularly in patients with respiratory compromise or those undergoing cardiothoracic surgery. Early mobilization can help improve lung function, prevent complications such as pneumonia and atelectasis, and reduce the duration of mechanical ventilation and the length of hospital stay. Respiratory therapy, including techniques such as incentive spirometry, deep breathing exercises, and chest physiotherapy, can also help improve respiratory function and prevent complications (Zhang et al., 2018).

Conclusion

In conclusion, administering anesthetic to a patient with respiratory failure begins with addressing the life-threatening issue. This is then supplemented with a review of the patient's medical history and correlating it with their physical examination results.

It is important to differentiate between a patient not expected to survive, a patient who may be rescued from respiratory failure, and a patient who will continue to have respiratory failure postoperatively.

Positive pressure ventilation, the dominant form of mechanical ventilation, decreases the patient's work of breathing and rescues a fatigued patient from hypoxemia and respiratory acidosis. However, extra thoracic effects should be considered when initiating, titrating, or weaning artificial ventilation.

Ergo trauma is the latest acknowledged form of damage due to positive pressure ventilation. Since invasive mechanical ventilation comes with an additional burden of sedation, immobilization, and continuous pressure on the tracheal mucosa, weaning from invasive forms of mechanical ventilation should begin with the onset.

Knowledge about the control centers of breathing is necessary for a complete neurological examination and objective evaluation of lung functions.

The less known functions of the lungs, such as filtering, thermoregulation, and regulation of fluid balance, are quickly deteriorated with mechanical ventilation and should be replaced as soon as possible to improve patient comfort and effort.

The anesthesiologic plan should include a detailed plan for induction and airway security. Postoperative care should also be planned, but since the intraoperative period is prone to so many complications, it is best to prevent them rather than account for them.

References

Atkinson, R. S., Rushman, G. B., & Lee, J. A. (1977). *A synopsis of anaesthesia*. Butterworth-Heinemann.

Bauman, L. A., & Tobin, J. R. (2012). Evaluation of the Patient with Neuromuscular, Skeletal, or Motion Disorders. In D. E. Longnecker, D. L. Brown, M. F. Newman, & Zapol W. M. (Eds.), *Anesthesiology* (2nd ed.). McGraw Hill. https:/ accessanesthesiology.mhmedical.com/content.aspx?bookid=490&sectionid=40114694.

Bittner, E. A., Grecu, L., & George, E. (2012). Postoperative Complications. In D. E. Longnecker, D. L. Brown, M. F. Newman, & W. M. Zapol (Eds.), *Anesthesiology* (2nd ed.). McGraw Hill. https://accessanesthesiology.mhmedical.com/content.aspx?bookid=490&sectionid=40114761.

Branson, R. D., & Robinson, B. R. H. (2011). Oxygen: When is more the enemy of good? *Intensive Care Medicine*, *37*(1), 1–3. https://doi.org/10.1007/S00134-010-2034-Y/METRICS.

Bubshait, K., & Alabbasi, Y. (2021). Influence of Spontaneous and Mechanical Ventilation on Frequency-Based Measures of Heart Rate Variability. *Critical Care Research and Practice*, *2021*. https://doi.org/10.1155/2021/8709262.

Cooper, J. D. (2018). Tracheal Injuries Complicating Prolonged Intubation and Tracheostomy. *Thoracic Surgery Clinics*, *28*(2), 139–144. https://doi.org/10.1016/J.THORSURG.2018.01.001.

DAS guidelines for management of unanticipated difficult intubation in adults 2015 | Difficult Airway Society. (n.d.). Retrieved March 31, 2023, from https://das.uk.com/guidelines/das_intubation_guidelines.

Duggan, M., & Kavanagh, B. P. (2007). Atelectasis in the perioperative patient. *Current Opinion in Anaesthesiology*, *20*(1), 37–42. https://doi.org/10.1097/ACO.0B013E328011D7E5.

Frerk, C., Mitchell, V. S., McNarry, A. F., Mendonca, C., Bhagrath, R., Patel, A., O'Sullivan, E. P., Woodall, N. M., Ahmad, I. & Difficult Airway Society intubation guidelines working group (2015). Difficult Airway Society 2015 guidelines for management of unanticipated difficult intubation in adults. *BJA: British Journal of Anaesthesia*, *115*(6), 827–848. https://doi.org/10.1093/BJA/AEV371.

Hansel, J., Rogers, A. M., Lewis, S. R., Cook, T. M., & Smith, A. F. (2022). Videolaryngoscopy versus direct laryngoscopy for adults undergoing tracheal intubation. *The Cochrane Database of Systematic Reviews*, *4*(4). https://doi.org/10.1002/14651858.CD011136.PUB3.

Hopkins, E., & Sharma, S. (2022). Physiology, Functional Residual Capacity. *StatPearls*. https://www.ncbi.nlm.nih.gov/books/NBK500007/.

Lee, L. A., Caplan, R. A., Stephens, L. S., Posner, K. L., Terman, G. W., Voepel-Lewis, T., & Domino, K. B. (2015). Postoperative opioid-induced respiratory depression: a closed claims analysis. *Anesthesiology*, *122*(3), 659–665. https://doi.org/10.1097/ALN.0000000000000564.

Lumb, A. B. (2017). Control of Breathing. In *Nunn's Applied Respiratory Physiology* (pp. 51-72.e2). Elsevier. https://doi.org/10.1016/B978-0-7020-6294-0.00004-6.

Magder, S. (2018). Heart-Lung interaction in spontaneous breathing subjects: the basics. *Annals of Translational Medicine*, *6*(18), 348–348. https://doi.org/10.21037/ATM.2018.06.19.

Pelletier, J. H., Ramgopal, S., & Horvat, C. M. (2021). Hyperoxemia Is Associated with Mortality in Critically Ill Children. *Frontiers in Medicine*, *8*, 723. https://doi.org/10.3389/FMED.2021.675293/BIBTEX.

Phero, J. C., Patil, Y. J., & Hurford, W. E. (2012). Evaluation of the Patient with a Difficult Airway. In D. E. Longnecker, D. L. Brown, M. F. Newman, & W. M. Zapol (Eds.), *Anesthesiology* (2nd ed.). McGraw Hill. https://accessanesthesiology.mhmedical.com/content.aspx?bookid=490&sectionid=40114692.

Reger, B., Neu, R., Hofmann, H. S., & Ried, M. (2018). High mortality in patients with tracheoarterial fistulas: clinical experience and treatment recommendations. *Interactive Cardiovascular and Thoracic Surgery*, *26*(1), 12–17. https://doi.org/10.1093/ICVTS/IVX249.

Schiavo, A., Renis, M., Polverino, M., Iannuzzi, A., & Polverino, F. (2016). Acid-base balance, serum electrolytes and need for non-invasive ventilation in patients with hypercapnic acute exacerbation of chronic obstructive pulmonary disease admitted to an internal medicine ward. *Multidisciplinary Respiratory Medicine*, *11*(1). https://doi.org/10.1186/S40248-016-0063-2.

Shamji, F. M., Deslauriers, J., & Nelems, B. (2018). Recognition and Management of Life-Threatening Tracheovascular Fistulae and How to Prevent Them. *Thoracic Surgery Clinics*, *28*(3), 403–413. https://doi.org/10.1016/J.THORSURG.2018.05.005.

Shinn, J. R., Kimura, K. S., Campbell, B. R., Sun Lowery, A., Wootten, C. T., Garrett, C. G., Francis, D. O., Hillel, A. T., Du, L., Casey, J. D., Ely, E. W., & Gelbard, A. (2019). Incidence and Outcomes of Acute Laryngeal Injury After Prolonged Mechanical Ventilation. *Critical Care Medicine*, *47*(12), 1699–1706. https://doi.org/10.1097/CCM.0000000000004015.

Stojanovic, D. (2017). Difficult Endotracheal Intubation-Scales and Causes. *Journal of Pharmacy and Pharmacology*, *5*, 775–786. https://doi.org/10.17265/2328-2150/2017.010.012.

Tonetti, T., Vasques, F., Rapetti, F., Maiolo, G., Collino, F., Romitti, F., Camporota, L., Cressoni, M., Cadringher, P., Quintel, M., & Gattinoni, L. (2017). Driving pressure and mechanical power: new targets for VILI prevention. *Annals of Translational Medicine*, *5*(14). https://doi.org/10.21037/ATM.2017.07.08.

Tung, A., & Griesdale, D. E. G. (2013). Comparing the novel GlideScope Groove videolaryngoscope with conventional videolaryngoscopy: a randomized mannequin study of novice providers. *Journal of Clinical Anesthesia*, *25*(8), 644–650. https://doi.org/10.1016/J.JCLINANE.2013.07.005.

van Schuppen, H., Wojciechowicz, K., Hollmann, M. W., & Preckel, B. (2022). Tracheal Intubation during Advanced Life Support Using Direct Laryngoscopy versus Glidescope® Videolaryngoscopy by Clinicians with Limited Intubation Experience: A Systematic Review and Meta-Analysis. *Journal of Clinical Medicine*, *11*(21). https://doi.org/10.3390/JCM11216291.

Yoshida, K., Isosu, T., Noji, Y., Ebana, H., Honda, J., Sanbe, N., Obara, S., & Murakawa, M. (2020). Adjustment of oxygen reserve index (ORi^{TM}) to avoid excessive hyperoxia during general anesthesia. *Journal of Clinical Monitoring and Computing*, *34*(3), 509–514. https://doi.org/10.1007/S10877-019-00341-9.

Zhang, G., Zhang, K., Cui, W., Hong, Y., & Zhang, Z. (2018). The effect of early mobilization for critical ill patients requiring mechanical ventilation: a systematic review and meta-analysis. *Journal of Emergency and Critical Care Medicine*, *2*(1), 9–9. https://doi.org/10.21037/JECCM.2018.01.04.

Chapter 6

Anesthesia Considerations in Liver Failure

Süheyla Karadağ Erkoç*
and Neslihan Alkış
Department of Anesthesiology and Reanimation, Ankara University Faculty of Medicine, Ankara, Turkiye

Abstract

Chronic liver disease (CLD) is a progressive deterioration of liver functions for more than 6 months, including protein synthesis, detoxification of harmful metabolic products, and excretion of bile. The most common causes of chronic liver diseases are chronic viral hepatitis, alcoholic liver disease, and nonalcoholic steatohepatitis. CLD causes portal hypertension that can cause complications such as ascites, gastrointestinal bleeding, encephalopathy, hepatorenal syndrome, hepatopulmonary syndrome, portopulmonary syndrome, cardiomyopathy, and coagulopathy. The reported mortality rates in patients with cirrhosis undergoing various surgical procedures range from 8.3% to 25%. This wide range of mortality rates depends on severity of liver disease, type of surgery, comorbidities, expertise of the surgical, anesthesia, and intensive care unit team (Millwala et al., 2007). Predictors of perioperative mortality are the severity of hepatic dysfunction, the degree of portal hypertension, the urgency of surgery, and the severity of complications. The Child-Turcotte-Pugh (CTP) and end-stage liver disease model (MELD) can be used to assess the severity of liver disease and determine the risk of perioperative morbidity and mortality. The main course of anesthetic evaluation is optimizing the patient prior to surgery. Perioperative management in patients with

---

* Corresponding Author's Email: suheylakaradag@hotmail.com.

In: Organ Failure and Anesthesia Practices
Editors: Ahmet Şen and Basar Erdivanli
ISBN: 979-8-89113-486-7

chronic liver disease should be individualized by assessing the severity of cirrhosis and the presence of accompanying complications.

Keywords: anesthesia, perioperative management, liver failure, cirrhosis

Introduction

Acute liver failure is defined as the loss of liver function in a short period, such as days or weeks, without any previous liver disease. Chronic liver disease "CLD" is a progressive loss of liver functions for more than six months. It is a continuous and progressive process that leads to fibrosis and cirrhosis due to inflammation, destruction, and regeneration of the liver parenchyma. Most patients with cirrhosis remain asymptomatic, as no obvious symptoms or signs appear in the early stage. The most common causes of CLD are nonalcoholic fatty liver disease, viral hepatitis (hepatitis B, or hepatitis C), and alcoholic liver disease. Chronic liver disease (CLD) affects approximately 1.5 billion people worldwide and approximately 2 million people die each year as a result of CLD (Zhang et al., 2022). Recently, nontransplant surgical procedures have been planned more frequently in patients with liver failure, and anesthesia management involves many difficulties due to accompanying complications.

This chapter summarizes the anatomy, physiology, pathophysiological changes in chronic liver disease, and anesthetic management during the perioperative period.

Anatomy and Physiology of the Liver

The liver is located below the diaphragm in the right upper quadrant. It is approximately 1.5 kg, accounting for approximately 2%-3% of average body weight. The falciform ligament separates the liver into the right and left lobes. The right lobe is larger than the left lobe with two more lobes on the posterior inferior surface named caudate and quadrate lobes (Chernobylsky et al., 2021).

The total amount of blood supply to the liver at rest is 20-25% of the total cardiac output. It has dual blood supply. The first is the hepatic artery which contributes 25% of the blood and 50%-70% of the liver's oxygen requirements. The second is the portal vein, which is responsible for the remaining 75% of the blood supply and the remaining 30%-50% of the liver oxygen needs (Chernobylsky et al., 2021). The arterial and portal blood mix within the hepatic sinusoids. The common hepatic artery originates from the celiac trunk together with the left gastric and splenic arteries, and then the hepatic artery divides into the left and right hepatic arteries to feed the hepatic lobes. The portal vein is formed by the superior mesenteric vein and the splenic vein. Venous drainage of the liver is through the intrahepatic veins that join into three hepatic veins that finally drain into the inferior vena cava.

Sympathetic and parasympathetic innervation of the liver is supplied by the sympathetic nerve fibers of T6-T11, the parasympathetic fibers of the right and left vagal nerve, and the fibers of the right phrenic nerve. Sympathetic activation results in vasoconstriction that decreases hepatic blood flow. β-adrenergic stimulation vasodilates the hepatic artery.

The normal portal venous pressure is approximately 7-10 mmHg. Small changes in hepatic venous tone and hepatic venous pressure can result in large changes in hepatic blood volume. This causes the liver to act as a blood reservoir. The increase in central venous pressure is transmitted to the hepatic veins and causes liver congestion (Ramsay, 2018).

There are many enzymatic reactions in the liver. Liver plays a key role in the metabolism of carbohydrates, fats, proteins, drugs, and other substances, including bile production, plasma protein synthesis (e.g., clotting factors), drug metabolism, and vitamin, mineral, and glucose storage. The liver maintains glucose homoeostasis through several mechanisms. Glucose, fructose, and galactose are the end products of carbohydrate digestion. In addition, conversion of fats and proteins to glucose by gluconeogenesis, glucogenesis, and glucose release from glycogen by glycogenolysis are enzymatic reactions that occur in the liver.

When carbohydrate stores are saturated or exceeded, excess glucose is converted into fat. Average glucose consumption is 150 g/d and after 24 hours of fasting, hepatic glycogen stores are normally depleted. The liver is capable of high rates of fatty acid oxidation and forms acetoacetic acid from excess acetyl-CoA. Acetyl-CoA is also used by the liver to produce cholesterol and phospholipids (Ramsay, 2018).

The liver plays a critical role in protein metabolism, such as amino acid metabolism, urea formation, protein production such as albumin, α1-antitrypsin, and other proteases/elastases, and coagulation factors.

Many exogenous substances, mainly drugs, are metabolized in the liver (biotransformation). The end products of these reactions are usually inactive or converted to water-soluble substances that can be readily excreted from bile or urine. This biotransformation occurs through two types of reaction: in phase I reaction; modification occurs through cytochrome P-450 enzyme systems, resulting in oxidation, reduction, deamination, dealkylation, or methylation. Phase II reactions consist of conjugation of metabolites with glucuronide, sulfate, taurine, or glycine to be excreted by urine or bile.

The liver also plays an important role in the metabolism of many hormones, vitamins, and minerals. The main storage sites for retinoic acid (vit A), cobalamin (B12), E, D, and K are also liver.

Anesthesia Management in Liver Disease

The prevalence of liver disorders is increasing all over the world. End-stage liver disease (ESLD) has a general population incidence of up to 5% in autopsy series (Csikesz et al., 2009). Cirrhosis, as a result of ESLD, viral hepatitis, and hepatocellular carcinoma and their complications are estimated to cause approximately 2 million deaths worldwide per year (Endale Simegn et al., 2012). Chronic liver disease is becoming more common due to the increased prevalence of hepatitis C (HCV), hepatitis B (HBV), alcohol and nonalcoholic fatty liver disease (NAFLD). Ten percent of patients with ESLD experience surgical procedures during the last 2 years of their life. As the liver has a remarkable functional reserve, this masks the clinical manifestations and signs of hepatic disease until the liver is extensively damaged. When elective surgery is planned for these patients, anesthesia and the surgical procedure itself could precipitate hepatic decompensation and hepatic failure, significantly increasing morbidity and mortality.

Preoperative Evaluation

The preoperative evaluation of patients with ESLD should include a detailed medical history, physical examination, and laboratory tests, current complications, medications used, and the existence of other complications.

Patients with ESLD who plan to undergo nonhepatic surgery have a high risk of transfusion requirements, infection, cardiac compromise, prolonged hospital stay, and operative morbidity and mortality. Various scoring systems for liver failure, such as Child-Turcotte-Pugh (CTP), or the model for end-stage liver disease (MELD), should be evaluated, patient-specific risk factors, and surgical risk factors should be defined and optimized before surgery to decrease the rate of complications and mortality (Table 1) (Kamath et al., 2001).

It is important to assess the presence and severity of liver disease. Decompensating symptoms such as coagulopathy, ascites, renal dysfunction, jaundice, electrolyte disturbances, and encephalopathy should be evaluated. Preoperative optimization should be individualized and a multidisciplinary team approach should be established.

Table 1. Perioperative risk factors associated with complications and mortality

Scoring system
– Modified Child–Turcotte–Pugh (CTP)
– Model for end-stage liver disease (MELD)
– ASA-PS IV or V
Patient-specific risk factors
– Male gender
– Age > 70 years
– Preoperative infection
– Elevated creatinine
– Chronic obstructive pulmonary disease
– Intraoperative hypotension
– Upper gastrointestinal bleeding
– Cirrhosis other than primary biliary cirrhosis
– Ascites
High-risk surgeries
– Emergency surgery
– Trauma laparotomy
– Abdominal surgery
– Open cholecystectomy
– Cardiothoracic surgery
– Esophageal surgery

Central Nervous System Complications

The most important manifestation of the central nervous system (CNS) in patients with liver failure is hepatic encephalopathy (HE), which is characterized by changes in behavior, cognitive function, consciousness, and neuromuscular function. Depending on the severity of the condition, HE is classified as covert HE (CHE) and overt HE (OHE). CHE is characterized by minimal hepatic encephalopathy or grade I encephalopathy, and diagnosis is made with psychometric and electrophysiological tests. On the other hand,

OHE is characterized by grade II-IV encephalopathy accompanied by precipitating factors. In both forms of HE, quality of life is decreased, hospital admissions are increased, and the risk of death is increased. Hyperammonemia is the most important factor in the pathogenesis of HE; however, additional factors such as inhibition of neurotransmission through CNS gamma-aminobutyric acid (GABA) receptors and changes in other levels of CNS neurotransmitters and circulating amino acids also play a role in pathogenesis (Hoilat et al., 2022). The exact prevalence and incidence of HE is unknown because different factors play a role in the etiology of the disease, the severity of the disease differs in each patient and there are difficulties in the diagnosis of minimal or subclinical HE. However, HE has been detected in up to 40% of cirrhotic patients (López-Franco et al., 2021). HE is generally triggered by a precipitating factor such as gastrointestinal bleeding, sepsis, alterations in gut flora, neuroinflammation, presence of spontaneous or iatrogenic portosystemic shunt, hypokalemia, hyponatremia and use of sedatives and is rarely caused by liver failure (Hoilat et al., 2022). Many of these triggering factors could be prevented or treated during the early period in patients with HE. Inactivity, lack of cooperation during nursing procedures, and HE-caused aspiration pneumonia in the postoperative period and unnecessary investigations could have negative effects on the clinical state of the patient in the postoperative period (Millwala et al., 2007). Following transplantation surgery, neurological complications increase in patients with HE. Postoperative cognitive dysfunction (POCD) in cirrhotic patients is described as a 'more than expected' decline in cognitive function. Specific preventive measures to reduce the risk of additional neurocognitive decline could be beneficial in patients with preoperative HE. Adequate monitoring of depth of anesthesia intraoperatively, selection of appropriate anesthetic agents, and opioid-sparing techniques have been shown to demonstrate favorable results in terms of POCD (Ingustu et al., 2023).

Cardiovascular Complications

Cardiovascular complications are commonly seen in patients with liver disease and are major risk factors for postoperative mortality and morbidity. Cirrhosis patients typically have a hyperdynamic circulation that mimics hyperdynamic circulatory changes in patients with sepsis. Both are characterized by tachycardia, elevated cardiac output, low arterial pressure, and low systemic vascular resistance. Cirrhotic cardiomyopathy is described as a condition of normal to increased cardiac output and contractility at rest, but a blunted response to pharmacologic, physiological, or pathologic stress that can result in overt heart failure. Perioperative intravenous fluids should be carefully managed to avoid volume overload. Cirrhotic cardiomyopathy is often reversible and inotropic and diuretic support is necessary to prevent increased central venous pressure and hepatic congestion, prior to surgery and anesthesia to prevent complications (Rahman & Mallett, 2015).

Coronary artery disease (CAD) risk factors, including hypertension, hyperlipidemia, diabetes, obesity, smoking, malnutrition, sedentary lifestyle, age, sex, family history of CAD, should be evaluated in cirrhotic patients. Dobutamine stress echocardiography (DSE) can be used to detect myocardial ischemia.

Pulmonary Complications

The manifestations of the pulmonary system in patients with hepatic insufficiency include hepatic hydrothorax (HH), hepatic pulmonary syndrome (HPS), and portopulmonary hypertension.

Hepatic hydrothorax (HH) is a rare disease and can be found in 5-10% of patients with ESLD. Pleural effusion of 500 ml and above is defined as hepatic hydrothorax (HH) in patients with ESLD, in the absence of cardiopulmonary and pleural diseases. Pleural effusion is generally localized on the right side (85% of cases) (Garbuzenko & Arefyev, 2017). Small defects located on the right hemidiaphragm allow for the passage of ascitic fluid from the peritoneal cavity into the pleural cavity due to negative intrathoracic pressure. Patients with liver hydrothorax have dyspnea, nonproductive cough, pleuritic chest pain, and fatigue. HH can be detected on a chest radiograph. Treatment of HH involves a sodium restricted diet and diuretics. In the presence of refractory ascites, therapeutic thoracentesis could be repeated every 2-3 weeks and this procedure should be accompanied by albumin infusion and diuretic administration in patients who have a urine sodium concentration > 30 mEq/dl (Solà et al., 2016). Chest tubes should not be placed for the treatment of hepatic hydrothorax due to the risk of electrolyte imbalance, infection, renal dysfunction, and bleeding.

Hepatic pulmonary syndrome (HPS) is a clinical state of hypoxemia resulting from vascular dilatations within pulmonary tissue and shunts in the presence of portal hypertension. The diagnostic criteria for HPS is the degree of hypoxemia, and the prevalence of HPS in patients with liver disease ranges from 4% to 45% (Fauconnet et al., 2013). Patients with HPS have symptoms such as cyanosis, dyspnea, platypnea, orthodeoxia, digital clubbing spider nevus, and peripheral arterial oxygen saturation <96%. Orthodeoxia is defined as a decrease in PaO_2 of more than 5% or more than 4 mm Hg during movement from a supine position to an upright position. Platypnea is defined as a dyspnea that worsens during movement from a supine to an upright position. (Ho, 2008). Pulmonary angiography is a previously used invasive diagnostic method in patients with HPS. Type I lesions are diffuse pulmonary vascular dilations at the precapillary level close to the normal gas exchange units of the lung and supplemental oxygen provides improvement. Type II lesions are large arteriovenous communications away from gas exchange units, and these lesions do not improve with supplemental oxygen (Krowka & Cortese, 1990). Arterial blood gas analysis should be performed sitting upright in room air in patients with clinical symptoms and with a pulse oximetry <96%. Hypoxemia is defined as a partial pressure of oxygen (PaO_2) <80 mm Hg or an alveolar-arterial oxygen gradient ($A\text{-}aO_2$) $\geq$ 15 mm. In patients $\geq$65 years of age, PaO_2 <70 mmHg or $A\text{-}aO_2$ $\geq$20 mmHg can be considered hypoxemia. Contrast-enhanced echocardiography with agitated saline could be a useful diagnostic test for pulmonary vascular dilation. Preparation before liver transplantation is necessary in patients with severe or very severe HPS, while those with mild to moderate disease are regularly monitored. The presence of HPS should be evaluated in the preoperative period in patients with hepatic insufficiency. HPS should be considered in patients who develop intraoperative respiratory failure and intraoperative transesophageal contrast echocardiography should be performed to confirm diagnosis. Mechanical ventilatory support can be performed in the supine position to prevent orthodeoxia (Mandell et al., 2007).

Portopulmonary hypertension (PoPH) is defined as pulmonary arterial hypertension (mean pulmonary artery pressure >25 mmHg) in the presence of portal hypertension with or without hepatic disease. The prevalence of PoPH in liver transplant patients ranges from approximately 5% to 8.5% (Rodríguez-Roisin et al., 2004). PoPH should be investigated in patients with portal hypertension with symptoms and signs that include exertion dyspnea, fatigue, weakness, orthopnea, atypical chest pain, syncope, increased jugular venous pressure, and leg edema. Symptomatic patients with chronic liver disease should be evaluated for PH by transthoracic echocardiography (TTE). All patients who are scheduled to undergo liver transplantation and with right ventricular systolic pressure (RVSP) $\geq$45 mmHg on transthoracic echocardiography should be evaluated with right heart catheterization. In patients with mPAP >35 mmHg, liver transplantation can be planned if mPAP decreases to 35 mmHg by medical therapy (Martin et al., 2014). During preoperative evaluation of patients with established pulmonary hypertension, a risk assessment should be taken into account evaluating the functional state, severity of the disease, and type of surgery planned. Before laryngoscopy and tracheal intubation, we should be sure that an adequate depth of anesthesia is established. Otherwise, sympathetic stimulation at this stage could have deleterious effects on right ventricular afterload. We should also avoid acidosis, hypercarbia, hypothermia, elevated PEEP levels, and inspiratory pressures. By invasive arterial monitoring before anesthetic induction, it is possible to recognize hemodynamic instability immediately and take intermittent arterial blood gas sampling. All patients with severe PH or mild to moderate PH with existing right-sided heart failure require intraoperative transoesophageal echocardiography (TOE) and / or pulmonary artery catheter monitoring (Pilkington et al., 2015).

These patients are at risk for right heart failure, and, as in other patients with pulmonary hypertension, the risk of perioperative morbidity and mortality is high in these patients, so anesthesia management should aim to control hypoxia, hypercarbia, acidosis, pain, and hypothermia and thus prevent increased pulmonary vascular resistance. Patients with ascites can develop shortness of breath, ventilation/perfusion mismatch, pleural effusion, and decreased lung capacity, mainly due to compressive atelectasis. Patients with massive ascites do not tolerate lying supine for induction of anesthesia or during procedures performed under monitored anesthesia care or regional anesthesia. Compressive atelectasis reduces functional residual capacity and decreases the time to oxygen desaturation. During anesthesia, lung recruitment maneuvers and pleural fluid drainage can improve pulmonary mechanics.

Electrolyte Imbalance and Metabolic Disorders

Hyponatremia, hypomagnesemia, and hypocalcemia are common metabolic disorders observed in this group of patients. Patients are at risk for central pontine myelinolysis perioperatively, and this hyponatremia should be corrected slowly. Total serum calcium is low due to low serum albumin with reduced calcium binding. Patients with chronic liver disease and cirrhosis demonstrate multifactorial glucose metabolism disorders, including the inflammatory response to surgery, steroid administration, liver dysfunction, altered glycogen stores, and insulin resistance.

Renal Dysfunction

Many varieties such as diuretics, nephrotoxic drugs, infections, large volume paracentesis, gastrointestinal bleeding, or hepatorenal syndrome (HRS) might result in renal failure in patients with advanced liver disease (Millwala et al., 2007). Vasodilation induced by general anesthesia may cause renal hypoperfusion and the end result may be prerenal renal failure. Postoperative hemodialysis may be required in the presence of hepatorenal failure and is associated with a poor prognosis.

In patients with cirrhosis, plasma creatinine >1.5 mg/dl is defined as HRS despite discontinuation of the diuretic for 2 days and volume expansion with albumin. Diagnosis requires the absence of previous kidney disease, nephrotoxic drug use, and hemodynamic alterations leading to renal hypoperfusion. A progressive increase in cardiac output and a reduction in systemic vascular resistance develops due to the severity of the actual disease. This causes activation of renin-angiotensin resulting in renal hypoperfusion. Secondary hyperaldosteronism leads to water retention and hyponatremia, resulting in the formation of ascites.

Type I HRS is defined as the doubling of baseline plasma creatinine to a level greater than >2.5 mg/dL or a 50% reduction in creatinine clearance at 24 hours to <20 ml/min in less than 2 weeks. The prognosis of type 1 HRS is poor, with a mortality rate exceeding 50% after one month (Arroyo et al., 2002). Large-volume paracentesis without adequate albumin administration, gastrointestinal hemorrhage, bacterial infections, massive diuretic use are the main precipitating factors causing Type 1 HRS. Type 2 HRS is defined as an increase in serum creatinine level to >133 μmol/L (1.5 mg/dL) or a creatinine clearance of less than 40 mL/min, and urine sodium < 10 μmol/L. In Type 2 HRS, renal dysfunction and diuretic-resistant ascites develop characteristically slowly. Survival time for these patients is longer than Type 1. The definitive therapy for HRS is liver transplantation (Ng et al., 2007).

Coagulation Disorders

The decreased liver function has procoagulant and anticoagulant effects. Patients with liver disease frequently have abnormalities in routine coagulation tests and the balance between coagulation and anticoagulation changes, including prolongations of the PT, INR, and activated partial thromboplastin time, thrombocytopenia, and elevated D-dimer. Prolongation of the INR may reflect instability of the hemostatic balance, but not hypocoagulability or hypercoagulability in cirrhosis. In patients with a risk of bleeding due to percutaneous procedures or surgery, platelet transfusion both preoperatively and intraoperatively should be administered to achieve a platelet count ≥50,000/μl, and cryoprecipitate to maintain fibrinogen levels ≥200 mg/dl should be given, whereas routine administration of fresh frozen plasma is not suggested to correct INR. Viscoelastic tests (thromboelastography (TEG)) are very useful in guiding preoperative correction of coagulation disorders during surgery in patients with liver disease (De Pietri et al., 2016).

Despite coagulation disorder, thrombotic events, including DVT and PE, are common in liver failure, despite irregular standard coagulation tests. Therefore, LWMH thromboprophylaxis should be prescribed in patients with liver cirrhosis who are at high risk for thrombotic complications. If there are significant risk factors for bleeding, compression stockings or intermittent pneumatic compression should be considered to prevent deep venous thrombosis (Senzolo et al., 2009).

Laboratory

Preoperative laboratory tests for patients with liver disease should include full blood count, coagulation profile, serum electrolytes, creatinine, glucose, blood urea nitrogen, transaminase levels (alanine aminotransferase, aspartate aminotransferase), bilirubin and albumin. Other blood tests may be indicated, depending on the co-morbidities of the patient. Physician-led preoperative evaluation also consists of baseline blood tests, ECG, chest radiograph, ECHO, and cardiopulmonary exercise monitoring (Endale Simegn et al., 2022).

Risk Stratification

Child-Turcotte-Pugh (CTP) and the end-stage liver disease (MELD) model scores can be used to determine the severity of the disease (Wiesner et al., 2001; Pugh et al., 1973) (Table 2). The CTP and MELD scores should be considered together to provide a more precise measure of liver dysfunction and decompensation. Child A patients are acceptable for elective procedures with special intraoperative care. Child B patients should be optimized before surgery to be converted to Child A, while the risk of anesthesia is increased in Child C patients or patients with a MELD score greater than 20, and surgery should be postponed (Endale Simegn et al., 2022).

The MELD score was developed to predict short-term survival in patients who are candidate and awaiting liver transplant. This objective score is calculated from serum bilirubin, serum creatinine, INR, and the etiology of liver disease. The MELD score ranges between 6 and 40 and a MELD score of 10 to 15 confers increased perioperative risk, and patients with MELD scores >15 should not undergo elective surgery. In 2016, the MELD score was modified to include serum sodium concentration and recognize hyponatremia as an independent prognostic factor (Nagai et al., 2018). The MELD score is increasingly used in other settings, including prediction of perioperative mortality in patients with cirrhosis who undergo nontransplant surgery in combination with CTP.

Table 2. Child-Turcotte-Pugh (CTP) score

Classification			
Clinical parameter	1 point	2 points	3 Points
Total bilirubin (mg/dL)	<2	2-3	>3
Serum albumin (g/dL)	>3.5	2.9-3.5	<2.8
INR	<1.7	1.7-2.3	>2.3
Ascites	None	Mild	Moderate to severe
Hepatic encephalopathy	None	Grade I-II	Grade III-IV
Interpretation			
Points	Class		Mortality
5-6	A		10%
7-10	B		30%
10-15	C		76-82%

Anesthesia Management

Perioperative evaluation and anesthesia management of patients with liver disease aim to preserve hepatic blood flow and oxygen supply and minimize hepatotoxic drug exposure. All drugs, anesthetic techniques, intraoperative fluid management, monitoring tools, or even pain management after surgery should be chosen based on this principle. The selection of drugs and dose adjustments depend on the severity of liver disease. Patients with mild liver disease could usually be treated with a similar choice of drugs as healthy patients (Imani et al., 2014). The incidence of gastroparesis is increased in patients with cirrhosis, and these patients frequently have postprandial abdominal pain, nausea, and vomiting (Verne et al., 2004). Patients who have abdominal distention due to massive ascites or patients with nausea and vomiting require a well-planned induction that includes preoxygenation and rapid-sequence induction/intubation with cricoid pressure. Even awake intubation or rapid sequence induction with high-dose rocuronium is suggested for unstable patients or patients with active bleeding.

Besides standard ASA monitorization (ECG, pulse oximetry, capnography, temperature, urine output, noninvasive blood pressure), continuous invasive arterial pressure monitoring is often used for high-risk patients because of hemodynamic instability. One of the minimally invasive hemodynamic monitorization techniques can be preferred to monitor hemodynamic instability via cardiac output, systemic vascular resistance, pleth variability index, or even TEE can be considered. Due to cardiovascular instability, invasive monitors should be used in the perioperative period, especially in major surgeries. Beat-to-beat arterial pressure is monitored and blood is frequently sampled through a radial artery catheter. Pulse pressure variation evaluates fluid responsiveness, and it is calculated from invasive arterial monitoring. Peripheral arterial pressure measurements can be unreliable in patients with severe vasoconstriction or vasodilation. Central venous access is also necessary to measure right atrial pressure and to administer high-volume fluids, rapid infusion, or drugs. It is difficult to optimize intravascular volume status and goal-directed hemodynamic and fluid therapy using esophageal Doppler, arterial waveform analysis, or TEE will guide to maintain stability.

The choice of anesthetic technique for patients with liver disease should be based on the surgical procedure and factors of the patient. Neuraxial anesthesia, general anesthesia, and monitored anesthesia care may be options depending on the preoperative status of the patients.

All anesthetic agents and opioids are well tolerated in patients with compensatory liver disease. However, they should be used with caution in patients with decompensatory hepatic dysfunction. Anesthesia induction decreases hepatic blood flow by up to 40% in patients without liver disease. If there is evident hepatic dysfunction, especially in cases of cirrhosis, compensation for reduced portal blood flow is affected during anesthesia. This may worsen hepatic dysfunction and lead to difficulty in anesthesia management (Rahimzadeh et al., 2014).

Sedation with benzodiazepines, especially with repeated doses, may cause a prolonged duration of action, so a dose reduction for midazolam should be considered or should be titrated.

Regional anesthesia may be a choice of anesthesia in ESLD. Neuraxial anesthesia (ie, spinal or epidural) should be considered in patients with liver failure. Even this technique can cause systemic hypotension and reduced hepatic blood flow as a result of induced sympathectomy, and is also contraindicated in patients with severe coagulopathy and/or thrombocytopenia due to the increased risk of spinal epidural hematoma, lower drug dosages are used and locally administered drugs have less systemic effects.

Propofol induction followed by isoflurane, sevoflurane, or desflurane with an oxygen - air mixture is commonly used for general anesthesia in many situations. Currently and frequently used volatile anesthetics (i.e, isoflurane, sevoflurane, and desflurane) may reduce liver blood flow but are not associated with hepatic toxicity. Isoflurane and sevoflurane decrease hepatic blood flow very little at 1 minimum alveolar concentration, but desflurane can decrease by up to 30% at 1 MAC. This decrease is dose-dependent. As isoflurane and desflurane undergo less metabolism to trifluoroacetyl chloride (TFA), which is thought to be involved in hepatic toxicity, hepatic injury due to volatile agents is extremely low. Sevoflurane does not undergo metabolism to TFA, but produces fluoride and hexa-fluoro-iso-propanol (HFIP) which are conjugated by the liver and excreted by the kidney (Frink, 1995). There is no evidence that these metabolites, or compound A, cause hepatic damage. Nitrous oxide, NO is not known to cause liver injury, although it may decrease hepatic blood flow primarily through sympathetic stimulation. Therefore, it is not a choice during inhalation anesthesia for patients with liver failure (Obata et al., 2000).

Intravenous anesthetics (e.g., propofol, thiopental, etomidate, midazolam), when used for induction of anesthesia or for short procedures, or even for the maintenance of anesthesia like propofol, do not appear to affect liver function, as long as stable cardiac output and blood pressure are maintained.

In clinical practice, the clearance of standard induction doses of propofol, thiopental, etomidate and ketamine are similar in patients with liver disease and healthy patients. Patients with liver disease are more sensitive to the pharmacodynamic effects of induction agents. Dose adjustment should be made according to the severity of the disease. In addition, the clinical recovery duration can be prolonged after discontinuation of propofol infusions, when used for maintenance (Servin et al., 1998). The depth of anesthesia monitoring with bispectral index (BIS) during both total intravenous anesthesia (TIVA) and inhalation techniques guides the titration of anesthetic agents and can reduce intraoperative awareness (Brezeanu et al., 2020).

Liver disease affects the onset, metabolism, and duration of action of neuromuscular blocking agents (NMBAs). NMBAs should be titrated to effect, and preferably administration should be guided by monitoring with TOF monitors. The drug metabolism of rocuronium and vecuronium (clearance, elimination, and duration of action) that is dependent on liver function is prolonged in liver disease (Magorian et al., 1995). But atracurium and cis-atracurium undergo organ-independent elimination, and their elimination half-life and duration of action are not affected. The reversal agent sugammadex is excreted in the urine unchanged.

Opioids, especially remifentanil infusion, reduce the dose of the volatile agent required, but as the metabolism of opioids is reduced in patients with liver disease, the half-lives of opioids are often significantly prolonged, which can cause postoperative respiratory depression. Long-acting opioids such as morphine should be avoided, but shorter-acting opioids such as fentanyl or remifentanil are well tolerated when given in small doses or titrated as infusion. Morphological clearance is up to 35 to 60% in patients with liver disease. If morphine is needed, the intervals between doses should be increased to prevent accumulation (Potosek et al., 2014). Elimination of a bolus dose of fentanyl is not appreciably altered in patients with cirrhosis, though with repeat administration or infusion prolonged effects can occur. Remifentanil is rapidly hydrolyzed by esterase of blood and tissue esterase. Clearance and elimination and recovery from the effects of remifentanil are unchanged in patients with severe liver disease (Vaja et al., 2010).

Conclusion

Perioperative complications in patients with chronic liver disease scheduled for nonhepatic surgery are increased and even leading to death. Preoperative evaluation and optimization efforts should aim to modify the patient's preoperative Child's class or MELD score before an elective operation, if possible. In these patients, anesthesia and surgery may worsen liver functions or patient status; therefore, choosing anesthetics and anesthesia technique will determine the outcome. The cirrhotic liver depends on hepatic arterial perfusion due to portal hypertension. Therefore, the objective of anesthesia management should focus on preservation of hepatic arterial blood flow and avoidance of agents with potentially adverse effects on hepatic function during induction and maintenance.

References

Arroyo, V., Guevara, M., & Ginès, P. (2002). Hepatorenal syndrome in cirrhosis: pathogenesis and treatment. *Gastroenterology*, *122*(6), 1658–1676. https://doi.org/10.1053/gast.2002.33575.

Brezeanu, L. N., Brezeanu, R. C., Diculescu, M., & Droc, G. (2020). Anaesthesia for Liver Transplantation: An Update. *Journal of critical care medicine (Universitatea de Medicina si Farmacie din Targu-Mures), 6(2), 91–100.* https://doi.org/10.2478/jccm-2020-0011.

Chernobylsky D. J., & Kaye A. D., & Fuller M. C., & Hall S. M. (2021). Hepatic and biliary physiology. In Levitzky, M., & McDonough, K., & Kaye, A., & Hall S. (Eds.), *Clinical Physiology in Anesthetic Practice.* McGraw Hill. https://accessanesthesiology.mhmedical.com/content.aspx?bookid=2979&sectionid=249590985.

Csikesz, N. G., Nguyen, L. N., Tseng, J. F., & Shah, S. A. (2009). Nationwide volume and mortality after elective surgery in cirrhotic patients. *Journal of the American College of Surgeons*, *208*(1), 96–103. https://doi.org/10.1016/j.jamcollsurg.2008.09.006.

De Pietri, L., Bianchini, M., Montalti, R., De Maria, N., Di Maira, T., Begliomini, B., Gerunda, G. E., di Benedetto, F., Garcia-Tsao, G., & Villa, E. (2016). Thrombelastography-guided blood product use before invasive procedures in cirrhosis with severe coagulopathy: A randomized, controlled trial. *Hepatology (Baltimore, Md.)*, *63*(2), 566–573. https://doi.org/10.1002/hep.28148.

Endale Simegn, A., Yaregal Melesse, D., Belay Bizuneh, Y., & Mekonnen Alemu, W. (2022). Perioperative management of patients with liver disease for non-hepatic surgery: A systematic review. *Annals of medicine and surgery (2012)*, *75*, 103397. https://doi.org/10.1016/j.amsu.2022.103397.

Fauconnet, P., Klopfenstein, C. E., & Schiffer, E. (2013). Hepatopulmonary syndrome: the anaesthetic considerations. *European journal of anaesthesiology*, *30*(12), 721–730. https://doi.org/10.1097/EJA.0b013e328365bb6f.

Frink, E. J., Jr (1995). The hepatic effects of sevoflurane. *Anesthesia and analgesia*, *81*(6 Suppl), S46–S50. https://doi.org/10.1097/00000539-199512001-00007.

Garbuzenko, D. V., & Arefyev, N. O. (2017). Hepatic hydrothorax: An update and review of the literature. *World journal of hepatology*, *9*(31), 1197–1204. https://doi.org/10.4254/wjh.v9.i31.1197.

Ho, V. (2008). Current concepts in the management of hepatopulmonary syndrome. *Vascular health and risk management*, *4*(5), 1035–1041. https://doi.org/10.2147/vhrm.s3608.

Hoilat, G. J., Suhail, F. K., Adhami, T., & John, S. (2022). Evidence-based approach to management of hepatic encephalopathy in adults. *World journal of hepatology*, *14*(4), 670–681. https://doi.org/10.4254/wjh.v14.i4.670.

Imani, F., Motavaf, M., Safari, S., & Alavian, S. M. (2014). The therapeutic use of analgesics in patients with liver cirrhosis: a literature review and evidence-based recommendations. *Hepatitis monthly*, *14*(10), e23539. https://doi.org/10.5812/hepatmon.23539.

Ingustu, D. G., Pavel, B., Paltineanu, S. I., Mihai, D. I., Cotorogea-Simion, M., Martac, C., Florescu, M. M., Cobilinschi, C., Isac, S., & Droc, G. (2023). The Management of Postoperative Cognitive Dysfunction in Cirrhotic Patients: An Overview of the Literature. *Medicina*, *59*(3), 465. https://doi.org/10.3390/medicina59030465.

Kamath, P. S., Wiesner, R. H., Malinchoc, M., Kremers, W., Therneau, T. M., Kosberg, C. L., D'Amico, G., Dickson, E. R., & Kim, W. R. (2001). A model to predict survival in patients with end-stage liver disease. *Hepatology (Baltimore, Md.)*, *33*(2), 464–470. https://doi.org/10.1053/jhep.2001.22172.

Krowka, M. J., & Cortese, D. A. (1990). Hepatopulmonary syndrome: an evolving perspective in the era of liver transplantation. *Hepatology (Baltimore, Md.)*, *11*(1), 138–142. https://doi.org/10.1002/hep.1840110123.

López-Franco, Ó., Morin, J. P., Cortés-Sol, A., Molina-Jiménez, T., Del Moral, D. I., Flores-Muñoz, M., Roldán-Roldán, G., Juárez-Portilla, C., & Zepeda, R. C. (2021). Cognitive Impairment After Resolution of Hepatic Encephalopathy: A Systematic Review and Meta-Analysis. *Frontiers in neuroscience*, *15*, 579263. https://doi.org/10.3389/fnins.2021.579263.

Magorian, T., Wood, P., Caldwell, J., Fisher, D., Segredo, V., Szenohradszky, J., Sharma, M., Gruenke, L., & Miller, R. (1995). The pharmacokinetics and neuromuscular effects of rocuronium bromide in patients with liver disease. *Anesthesia and analgesia*, *80*(4), 754–759. https://doi.org/10.1097/00000539-199504000-00018.

Mandell, M. S., Stoner, T. J., Barnett, R., Shaked, A., Bellamy, M., Biancofiore, G., Niemann, C., Walia, A., Vater, Y., Tran, Z. V., & Kam, I. (2007). A multicenter evaluation of safety of early extubation in liver transplant recipients. *Liver transplantation : official publication of the American Association for the Study of Liver Diseases and the International Liver Transplantation Society*, *13*(11), 1557–1563. https://doi.org/10.1002/lt.21263.

Martin, P., DiMartini, A., Feng, S., Brown, R., Jr, & Fallon, M. (2014). Evaluation for liver transplantation in adults: 2013 practice guideline by the American Association for the Study of Liver Diseases and the American Society of Transplantation. *Hepatology (Baltimore, Md.)*, *59*(3), 1144–1165. https://doi.org/10.1002/hep.26972.

Millwala, F., Nguyen, G. C., & Thuluvath, P. J. (2007). Outcomes of patients with cirrhosis undergoing non-hepatic surgery: risk assessment and management. *World journal of gastroenterology*, *13*(30), 4056–4063. https://doi.org/10.3748/wjg.v13.i30.4056.

Nagai, S., Chau, L. C., Schilke, R. E., Safwan, M., Rizzari, M., Collins, K., Yoshida, A., Abouljoud, M. S., & Moonka, D. (2018). Effects of Allocating Livers for Transplantation Based on Model for End-Stage Liver Disease-Sodium Scores on

Patient Outcomes. *Gastroenterology*, *155*(5), 1451–1462.e3. https://doi.org/10.1053/j.gastro.2018.07.025.

Ng, C. K., Chan, M. H., Tai, M. H., & Lam, C. W. (2007). Hepatorenal syndrome. *The Clinical biochemist. Reviews*, *28*(1), 11–17.

Obata, R., Bito, H., Ohmura, M., Moriwaki, G., Ikeuchi, Y., Katoh, T., & Sato, S. (2000). The effects of prolonged low-flow sevoflurane anesthesia on renal and hepatic function. *Anesthesia and analgesia*, *91*(5), 1262–1268. https://doi.org/10.1097/00000539-200011000-00039.

Pilkington, S. A., Taboada, D., & Martinez, G. (2015). Pulmonary hypertension and its management in patients undergoing non-cardiac surgery. *Anaesthesia*, *70*(1), 56–70. https://doi.org/10.1111/anae.12831.

Potosek, J., Curry, M., Buss, M., & Chittenden, E. (2014). Integration of palliative care in end-stage liver disease and liver transplantation. *Journal of palliative medicine*, *17*(11), 1271–1277. https://doi.org/10.1089/jpm.2013.0167.

Pugh, R. N., Murray-Lyon, I. M., Dawson, J. L., Pietroni, M. C., & Williams, R. (1973). Transection of the oesophagus for bleeding oesophageal varices. *The British journal of surgery*, *60*(8), 646–649. https://doi.org/10.1002/bjs.1800600817.

Rahimzadeh, P., Safari, S., Faiz, S. H., & Alavian, S. M. (2014). Anesthesia for patients with liver disease. *Hepatitis monthly*, *14*(7), e19881. https://doi.org/10.5812/hepatmon.19881.

Rahman, S., & Mallett, S. V. (2015). Cirrhotic cardiomyopathy: Implications for the perioperative management of liver transplant patients. *World journal of hepatology*, *7*(3), 507–520. https://doi.org/10.4254/wjh.v7.i3.507.

Ramsay, M. (2018). Hepatic physiology & anesthesia. Butterworth IV, J. F., & Mackey, D. C., & Wasnick J. D. (Eds.), *Morgan & Mikhail's Clinical Anesthesiology, 6e*. McGraw Hill. https://accessmedicine.mhmedical.com/Content.aspx?bookid=2444&sectionid=193561933.

Rodríguez-Roisin, R., Krowka, M. J., Hervé, P., Fallon, M. B., & ERS Task Force Pulmonary-Hepatic Vascular Disorders (PHD) Scientific Committee (2004). Pulmonary-Hepatic vascular Disorders (PHD). *The European respiratory journal*, *24*(5), 861–880. https://doi.org/10.1183/09031936.04.00010904.

Senzolo, M., Sartori, M. T., & Lisman, T. (2009). Should we give thromboprophylaxis to patients with liver cirrhosis and coagulopathy? *HPB: the official journal of the International Hepato Pancreato Biliary Association*, *11*(6), 459–464. https://doi.org/10.1111/j.1477-2574.2009.00079.x.

Servin, F., Desmonts, J. M., Haberer, J. P., Cockshott, I. D., Plummer, G. F., & Farinotti, R. (1988). Pharmacokinetics and protein binding of propofol in patients with cirrhosis. *Anesthesiology*, *69*(6), 887–891. https://doi.org/10.1097/00000542-198812000-00014.

Solà, E., Solé, C., & Ginès, P. (2016). Management of uninfected and infected ascites in cirrhosis. *Liver international : official journal of the International Association for the Study of the Liver*, *36 Suppl 1*, 109–115. https://doi.org/10.1111/liv.13015.

Vaja, R., McNicol, L., & Sisley, I. (2010). Anaesthesia for patients with liver disease. *Continuing Education in Anaesthesia Critical Care & Pain*, 10(1), 15–19. https://doi.org/10.1093/bjaceaccp/mkp040.

Verne, G. N., Soldevia-Pico, C., Robinson, M. E., Spicer, K. M., & Reuben, A. (2004). Autonomic dysfunction and gastroparesis in cirrhosis. *Journal of clinical gastroenterology*, *38*(1), 72–76. https://doi.org/10.1097/00004836-200401000-00015.

Wiesner, R. H., McDiarmid, S. V., Kamath, P. S., Edwards, E. B., Malinchoc, M., Kremers, W. K., Krom, R. A., & Kim, W. R. (2001). MELD and PELD: application of survival models to liver allocation. *Liver transplantation: official publication of the American Association for the Study of Liver Diseases and the International Liver Transplantation Society*, *7*(7), 567–580. https://doi.org/10.1053/jlts.2001.25879.

Zhang, Y. Y., & Meng, Z. J. (2022). Definition and classification of acute-on-chronic liver diseases. *World journal of clinical cases*, *10*(15), 4717–4725. https://doi.org/10.12998/wjcc.v10.i15.4717.

Chapter 7

Anesthesia During Renal Failure

Lerzan Doğan, MD
Bülent Güçyetmez*, MD
and Fevzi Toraman, MD
Department of Anesthesiology and Reanimation, Acibadem University, Istanbul, Turkiye

Abstract

Patients with renal failure undergoing surgery pose significant challenges, given their increased vulnerability to increased morbidity and mortality. Their pre-existing medical condition and the planned surgical procedure require special consideration. Electrolyte imbalances, fluid overload, and acid-base abnormalities are among the potential medical problems these patients may face, all of which can interfere with their reactions to anesthesia and perioperative stress. Given that many anesthetics depend to some extent on renal excretion, patients with renal failure are at increased risk of experiencing adverse events due to physiologic changes associated with their condition, including reduced metabolism and elimination. Consequently, some anesthetics must be administered with caution or entirely avoided, as they can accumulate in the body or exacerbate kidney injury. Anesthetics are mainly metabolized and eliminated by the liver, so it may be preferred since the liver is able to clear them even with a low glomerular filtration rate. Therefore, it is of paramount importance to implement controlled fluid management, maintain normovolemia, optimize renal blood flow and renal perfusion, avoid hypotension, and abstain from nephrotoxic substances to prevent further renal injury. Maintenance of residual renal function should be the

* Corresponding Author's Email: bulentgucyetmez@gmail.com.

In: Organ Failure and Anesthesia Practices
Editors: Ahmet Şen and Basar Erdivanli
ISBN: 979-8-89113-486-7

main goal during anesthesia, rather than the selection of anesthetic agents and techniques.

Keywords: decreased clearance, fluid overload, maintenance of normovolemia

Introduction

Renal failure is a pathological condition that results from the inability of the kidneys to maintain fluid and electrolyte balance, eliminate metabolic waste products, and regulate vascular tone (Wagener & Brentjens, 2006). Glomerular filtration rate (GFR), assessed by creatinine clearance, provides an indicator of kidney filtering capacity. Patients may remain asymptomatic even with a GFR decrease of 120 to 60 ml/min, and only have mild renal impairment when the decrease is gradual, between 40-60 ml/min (Hartmann et al., 2010). Moderate renal failure is defined as a decrease in creatinine clearance of less than 40 ml/min, while failure is characterized by a decrease of less than 25 ml/min (Hartmann et al., 2010). Dialysis dependency develops when creatinine clearance is less than 10 ml/min. Patients are asymptomatic as long as at least 40% of their nephrons are operating; Insufficiency is seen when just 10% to 40% of the patient's nephrons are functioning, and this places the patient at risk of failure because there is essentially no renal reserve. Renal failure occurs when more than 90% of functioning nephrons are lost, and survival requires the initiation of renal replacement therapy (RRT) (Table 1) (Wagener & Brentjens, 2006).

Table 1. The severity of renal insufficiency and stages of chronic kidney disease

CKD stage	GFR (ml/min)	Renal insufficiency
1	120-90	none
2	90-60	mild
3	60-30	intermediate
4	30-15	severe
5	15-0	Preterminal requires dialysis

Modified from "Drug Therapy in Patients with Chronic Renal Failure" (Hartmann et al., 2010).

Renal failure can be classified into two main types: acute and chronic. Acute renal failure (ARF) is characterized by a rapid and reversible deterioration of renal function, which can occur over a period of hours or days and is commonly caused by acute tubular necrosis, prerenal azotemia, acute interstitial nephritis, acute glomerular and vasculitic renal diseases, acute postrenal obstructive nephropathy, or a combination of these factors (Koza, 2016). The decline in renal function results in the accumulation of metabolic waste products, leading to extensive organ dysfunction and increases postoperative morbidity by three times and mortality by five times (Kheterpal et al., 2009). Chronic renal failure (CRF) is a persistent and progressive condition characterized by irreversible renal damage that requires dialysis or kidney transplantation. The main mechanisms underlying CRF are glomerular dysfunction, tubular dysfunction, and urinary tract obstruction, caused by intravascular volume depletion, sepsis, obstructive jaundice, crush injuries, and exposure to nephrotoxic agents such as radiocontrast agents, certain antibiotics, angiotensin converting enzyme inhibitors, and non-steroidal anti-inflammatory drugs. Among these etiologies, hypovolemia and reduced renal perfusion are the most significant factors contributing to the decline in renal function, underscoring the importance of proper perioperative patient management. To prevent the progression of CRF, it is imperative to prevent further renal insults and support compromised physiological systems (Wagener & Brentjens, 2010; Blantz, 1998).

The diagnosis of ARF is based primarily on changes in urine output and serum creatinine levels. The three most commonly used staging systems are the Acute Dialysis Quality Initiative RIFLE criteria, the Acute Kidney Injury Network (AKIN) (Bellomo et al., 2004; Lin & Chen, 2012), and Kidney Disease Improving Global Outcomes (KDIGO) (Table 2) (Shin et al., 2016). The RIFLE criteria contain 5 elements including risk, injury, failure, loss, and end-stage kidney disease (Bellomo et al., 2004). The Acute Kidney Injury Network is based on a change in serum creatinine level greater than 0.3 mg/dL within 48 hours after injury (Mehta et al., 2007). Furthermore, novel plasma and urine biomarkers, such as cystatin C, neutrophil gelatinase-associated lipocalin, interleukin-18, and kidney injury molecule-1, are currently under extensive investigation. Biomarkers are expected to take center stage in the diagnosis, staging, and prognostic evaluation of renal failure in the near future (Srisawat & Kellum, 2020).

Table 2. Comparison of RIFLE, AKIN, and KDIGO classifications

RIFLE Criteria: Creatinin definition	AKIN Criteria: Creatinin definition	KDIGO Criteria: Creatinin definition	Urine Output
Risk ≥1.5-fold increase from baseline SCr or decrease in GFR ≥25%	Stage 1 ≥0.3 mg/dL increase or ≥1.5-fold increase from baseline within 48 h	Stage 1 ≥0.3 mg/dL increase within 48 hrs or 1.5-1.9 times baseline within 7 days	<0.5 mL/kg/h for >6h
Injury ≥2-fold increase from baseline SCr or decrease in GFR ≥50%	Stage 2 ≥2-fold increase from baseline Scr	Stage 2 2.0-2.9 times from baseline within 7 days	<0.5 mL/kg/h for 12 hours
Failure ≥3-fold increase from baseline SCr or increase to ≥4mg/dl or decrease in GFR ≥75%	Stage 3 ≥3-fold increase from baseline SCr or increase to ≥4.0 mg/dl with an acute increase of >0.5 mg/dl or initiation of RRT	Stage 3 ≥3 times from baseline within 7 days or increase to ≥4.0 mg/dl with an acute increase of >0.5 mg/dl or initiation of RRT	<0.3 ml/kg/h for 24 hours or anuria for >12 hours

Modified from "Prediction and Prevention of Acute Kidney Injury after Cardiac Surgery." (Shin et al., 2016).

Patients with renal failure can exhibit a wide range of metabolic disturbances, including metabolic acidosis, hyperkalemia, hyperphosphatemia, hypocalcemia, and uremia. Administration of depolarizing muscle relaxants, such as succinylcholine, can exacerbate hyperkalemia and therefore should be avoided until serum potassium levels have been determined (Wagener & Brentjens, 2010). Furthermore, rapid transfusion of multiple units of packed red blood cells can significantly elevate potassium levels. The co-occurrence of hyperkalemia and metabolic acidosis, frequently observed in individuals with renal failure, can lead to potentially fatal cardiac arrhythmias and cardiac arrest (Smith et al., 2008). Treatment of hyperkalemia requires the elimination of potassium overload while providing interim measures to alleviate the condition. If previous interventions have not succeeded in controlling hyperkalemia, urgent initiation of hemodialysis is warranted (Wagener & Brentjens, 2010). Furthermore, in cases of acute renal failure, in addition to hyperkalemia, acidosis is also frequent. It is imperative to perform regular point-of-care monitoring of electrolytes and arterial blood gases to facilitate the prompt identification and correction of these disturbances. In spontaneously breathing patients, the maintenance of adequate minute ventilation to normalize pH levels is often compromised. However, mechanically ventilated patients can achieve hyperventilation to restore homeostasis. Consequently, extubation should be delayed until metabolic imbalances have been rectified (Elapavaluru & Kellum, 2007). Failure to address the uncorrected manifestations of renal failure can result in cardiac dysrhythmias and respiratory failure due to increased breathing effort, leading to cardiorespiratory collapse. Therefore, extubation in precarious situations should not be rushed. Moreover, fluid overload and anemia, common occurrences in renal failure, are associated with left ventricular hypertrophy and are autonomous risk factors for cardiovascular abnormalities and premature mortality (Foley et al., 1996). Furthermore, complications related to uremia cover a variety of issues, such as reduced levels of von Willebrand factor, impaired platelet aggregation and adhesion, and leukocyte dysfunction (Wagener & Brentjens, 2006). To treat uremic coagulopathy before or during surgery, desmopressin may be used (Galbusera et al., 2009).

Anesthetic Effects on Renal Function

The renal excretion of numerous drugs typically used in anesthesia is significant and this must be taken into account when administering anesthesia to patients with renal dysfunction (Liu & Gropper, 2003). Such drugs may be suboptimal for use in these cases as they may have prolonged effects due to the delayed elimination of active metabolites. Furthermore, it should be noted that anesthesia can exert an indirect effect on the kidneys by altering systemic hemodynamics and inducing hypotension. Reduced systemic vascular resistance or cardiac output can cause decreased renal perfusion (Herd, 1991).

Patients with renal failure are more susceptible to the effects of benzodiazepines and barbiturates due to reduced protein binding. Hence, a dose reduction of midazolam is recommended due to its abbreviated onset of action and prolonged duration (Maddern, 1983). On the contrary, patients with renal failure generally respond to ketamine and in some animal models it has been shown to maintain or increase renal perfusion (Priano, 1982). When administering opioids to patients with renal failure, it is crucial to take into account the potential for drug accumulation and prolonged activity due to the presence of active metabolites. Morphine and meperidine, for example, should be used with caution due to their active metabolites (Wagener & Brentjens, 2006). Morphine is metabolized to morphine-3-glucuronide (M3G), morphine-6-glucuronide (M6G), and normorphine, all of which are excreted by the kidneys (Hasselström & Säwe, 1993). There is a case report of respiratory arrest linked to the metabolite morphine-6-glucuronide (Talbott et al., 1997). In particular, M6G can cross the blood-brain barrier and continue to have effects on the central nervous system even after the medication has been discontinued or dialysis has been performed to remove the metabolite (Angst et al., 2000). Furthermore, the accumulation of these metabolites between dialysis sessions can exacerbate their effects. Dialysis can remove both the parent substance and its metabolites; however, morphine should be avoided whenever possible and alternative options should be considered (Angst et al., 2000). Fentanyl, on the other hand, is metabolized in the liver and does not accumulate significantly in renal failure, making it a safer option for patients with renal dysfunction (Mercadante et al., 1997), and is also dialyzable, which is a beneficial attribute (Joh et al., 1998). Other synthetic opioids like sufentanil and remifentanil are not significantly affected by renal failure; decreased clearance has been observed in patients with severe uremia, necessitating close monitoring for signs of gradual accumulation (Koehntop & Rodman, 1997; Dean, 2004).

Nondepolarizing neuromuscular agents (NMDAs) are subject to renal elimination for inactivation, leading to a prolonged duration of action in patients with renal dysfunction (Craig & Hunter, 2009). Historically, longer-acting NMDAs, such as pancuronium and d-tubocurarine, have been associated with delayed recovery due to reduced renal clearance and increased volume of distribution. However, the degradation pathways of newer NMDAs, such as atracurium, cisatracurium, and mivacurium, are independent of kidney function ("Neuromuscular Blocking Agents", n.d.). Atracurium may be the NMDA of choice for these patients, as it has a low rate of renal excretion, with only 10% excreted in urine in 24 hours even after repeated doses. Rocuronium has a longer duration of action and reduced clearance in patients with renal failure (Robertson et al., 2005). Its renal excretion profile is dose-dependent, with 12-22% of the dose excreted in urine at 0.6 mg/kg and about 33% excreted at 1 mg/kg in patients with normal renal function (Wierda et al., 1991). Therefore, caution is recommended when using rocuronium, particularly when combined with neuromuscular monitoring and sugammadex administration if possible (Seidl & Eberle, 2015). Succinylcholine can be used but should be avoided when potassium levels are unclear. In contrast, cisatracurium and atracurium are nondepolarizing muscle relaxants that are metabolized through ester hydrolysis and Hoffmann elimination, not dependent on renal activity for clearance.

Volatile anesthetics, including isoflurane and sevoflurane, have been shown to reduce GFR by reducing renal perfusion pressure through a decrease in cardiac output and systemic vascular resistance (e.g., halothane), with this effect being further exaggerated by hypovolemia (Kusudo et al., 2004). Enflurane is no longer commonly used in clinical practice due to its association with renal damage, whereas desflurane and isoflurane are generally considered safe for individuals with renal injury (Wagener & Brentjens, 2006). Sevoflurane is metabolized to produce inorganic fluoride, which has the potential to be a tubular nephrotoxin. However, clinical studies have not shown a significant adverse effect in practice (Herd, 1991). Sevoflurane has been shown to have a similar effect on serum creatinine levels as control anesthetics (Mazze et al., 2000), and the effects of low-flow anesthesia on renal function are not significantly different from those of isoflurane (Higuchi et al., 2001). Although sevoflurane is generally considered safe, some studies have indicated that total intravenous anesthesia (TIVA) with propofol may be safer than inhalational anesthesia in terms of postoperative AKI (Kim et al., 2021). Propofol is mainly metabolized through hepatic pathways (Hiraoka, 2004) and has minimal urinary excretion of unchanged propofol (Simons et al., 1988). The pharmacokinetics of propofol are similar in patients with and without renal failure (Ickx et al., 1998; Kirvelä et al., 1992; Ickx et al., 1998), but its metabolites can be detected in urine during the anhepatic phase (Veroli et al., 1992). Propofol has been shown to be safe and effective for individuals undergoing kidney transplants.

In renal failure, anticholinergics may be used at the standard dose, as their pharmacokinetics are not affected by GFR or urine flow. However, caution should be exercised when using adjuvant therapy, such as duloxetine, venlafaxine, gabapentin, and pregabalin, as they have the potential to increase the risk of adverse effects on the central nervous system and can require dose adjustments (Owsiany et al., 2019). Since nonsteroidal anti-inflammatory agents can exacerbate renal damage, they should be avoided (Wagener & Brentjens, 2010). Angiotensin-converting enzyme (ACE) inhibitors and beta-blockers should also be avoided; instead, calcium channel blockers may be preferred due to their nephroprotective effect (Olivero, 2015).

Preoperative Management

The preoperative management of patients with renal failure is determined by the severity of renal function and the type of surgery. Personalized preoperative care strategies must be developed in collaboration with the nephrologist and surgical team to ensure perioperative safety. A thorough evaluation of the systemic implications of renal failure, advanced age, and significant comorbidities is necessary. In general, some considerations for the preoperative management of a patient with renal failure include the following:

1. *Optimizing kidney function:* This includes agents to improve renal blood flow, diuretics to decrease fluid retention, and, if required, dialysis on the day of surgery or the day before (Byrick, 1999). When a patient is not hemodynamically stable, continuous renal replacement therapy (CRRT) is a better choice. Dialysis adequacy can be assessed with the measurement of electrolytes and renal markers. Hypovolemia or fluid overload can occur, depending on the presence of dialysis or residual renal function. Comparing the patient's current weight to pre- and post-dialysis weights in the past may be useful.
2. *Metabolic optimization:* Electrolyte imbalances and uremia should be corrected before the operation. Sodium abnormalities, if not too extreme, should be corrected more gradually. In emergency cases, electrolyte correction is implemented without postponing life-saving surgery, and dialysis is indicated if there are relevant electrolyte imbalances.

3. *Venous line:* Special attention must be paid to the presence and functionality of preexisting arteriovenous fistulas, hemodialysis catheters, or access to peritoneal dialysis. The placement of venous lines can be difficult due to several previous surgeries, preexisting fistulas, unsuccessful cannulation attempts, hematoma, venous collapse following hemodialysis, limited alternatives, and a long preparation time. To lower the complication rate, venous line insertion can be inserted guided by ultrasound (www.ahrq.gov 2001; www.nice.org.uk 2002). Furthermore, in order to reduce the risk of bloodstream infection associated with central venous catheterization, comprehensive barrier precautions (mask, cap, scrubbing, sterile gown and gloves, handling of sterile equipment handling) are required.
4. *Managing comorbidities:* Consultation should be requested from the required branches according to the severity of the additional diseases.
5. *Perioperative antibiotics:* Prophylactic antibiotics can be advised before and after surgery to reduce their increased risk of infection. The choice, timing, and administration of the drug must be clear. A single shot of antibiotic prophylaxis is not adapted to renal clearance, but in longer use, doses will need adaptation.
6. *ICU reservation:* If required, postoperative hemodialysis, intermediate, or intensive care should be scheduled.
7. *Drugs:* It is essential to conduct a detailed review of medications, paying particular attention to those with significant renal elimination (Table 3). The avoidance of such medications is recommended to minimize the risk of drug toxicity. When feasible, dosage adjustments and blood level monitoring should be implemented to further reduce this risk. Anticoagulant therapy must also be carefully managed to avoid interferering with scheduled surgery and prevent thromboembolic complications (Gogarten et al., 2010). Proper cessation, bridge, or timing directives must be established. Antihypertensive medications should continue until the time of surgery. Smoking cessation is recommended for at least 24 hours prior to surgery to improve tracheal clearance. Additionally, for insulin-dependent diabetics, blood glucose management can be complicated by presurgical fasting and potential delays in the OR schedule. Therefore, close control of blood glucose and insulin is necessary for these patients.

8. *Premedication:* In patients who are alert, stable, and scheduled for an overnight hospital stay, the use of benzodiazepines or opioids can be optimized by employing reduced doses. Alternatively, clonidine or haloperidol may be administered orally as a premedication. However, it should be noted that preoperative sedatives are not typically administered to ambulatory patients (Seidl & Eberle, 2015).
9. *Gastric emptying:* In patients with chronic renal failure, gastric emptying is often delayed (Hubalewska et al., 2004), which can increase the risk of regurgitation and aspiration during induction of anesthesia or deep sedation. To prevent aspiration, H2 blockers or proton pump inhibitors should be used as prophylactic measures. In addition, metoclopramide can help reduce the risk of aspiration and promote gastric emptying in patients with nausea and vomiting. It is also recommended that appropriate precautions be taken for rapid airway control in such patients.
10. *Anemia:* In patients with renal failure who are scheduled for elective surgery, it is vital to adequately address any anemia. Recombinant erythropoietin therapy combined with concurrent iron supplementation may be used as a hematopoietic stimulant to mitigate or prevent the need for perioperative blood transfusions. Typically, preoperative erythrocyte transfusions are reserved for patients with severe anemia. This is especially critical for those awaiting renal transplantation. (Seidl & Eberle, 2015).

Table 3. Drugs that do and do not depend on renal function

Class	Dependent on renal function	Independent of renal function
Opioids	Morphine, pethidine	Fentanyl, levomethadone
Antiarrhythmic drugs	Sotalol	Amiodarone
Antibiotics	Ciprofloxacin, Levofloxacin	Moxifloxacin
Antidiabetic drugs	Glibenclamide, Glimepiride Nateglinide Sitagliptine	Gliquidone, Gliclacide Pioglitazone
Anticonvulsants	Gabapentine, pregabalin, Lamotrigine, Levetiracetam	Carbamazepine, Phenytoin, Valproate
Antihypertensive drugs	Atenolol	Bisoprolol, Carvedilol Metoprolol, Propranolol
Cholesterol-lowering drugs	Bezafibrate, Fenofibrate	Simvastatin, Niacin

Class	Dependent on renal function	Independent of renal function
Drugs for gout and other rheumatological conditions	Methotrexate	Colchicine, Hydroxychloroquine, Leflunomide
Cardiovascular drugs	Digoxin	Digitoxin
Psychoactive drugs	Lithium, Mirtazapine	Amitriptyline, Citalopram, Haloperidol, Risperidone
Antiviral drugs	Acyclovir	Brivudine
Cytostatic drugs	Actinomycin D, Bleomycin, Capecitabine, Carboplatin, Cisplatin, Cyclophosphamide, Doxorubicin, Epirubicin, Etoposide, Gemcitabine, Ifosfamide, Irinotecan, Melphalan, Methotrexate, Oxaliplatin, Topotecan	Anastrozole, Docetaxel, Doxorubicin-peg-liposomal, Erlotinib, Fluorouracil, Gefitinib, Leuprorelin, Megestrol, Paclitaxel, Tamoxifen, Terozol, Vincristine, Trastuzumab

From 'Drug Therapy in Patients with Chronic Renal Failure' (Hartmann et al., 2010).

The Selection of Anesthetic Techniques

The selection of anesthesia techniques should not be made solely at the discretion of the anesthesiologist, but rather based on the patient's individual characteristics and the nature of the surgical procedure. Current clinical evidence does not suggest that any specific anesthesia technique is superior to others in terms of renal function and protection (Zacharias et al., 2008; Wagener & Brentjens, 2006). However, it is essential to maintain normovolemia and normotension during the administration of the chosen anesthesia technique (Wagener & Brentjens, 2010). When planning regional anesthesia techniques, the coagulation system must be carefully considered, as compromised coagulation is associated with a higher incidence of neurological complications than general anesthesia (Weinberg, 2012). However, if regional anesthesia is necessary, the use of ultrasound guidance is strongly recommended (Buhre & Rossaint, 2003). Additionally, epidural anesthesia does not affect renal blood flow when normotension and isovolemia are maintained in healthy volunteers (Guay, 2006); (Suleiman et al., 1997). Sympathetic blockade of levels from T4 to T10 may lead to blocking of sympathetic innervation of the kidneys. However, subsequent sympathetic blockage can reduce catecholamine-induced renal vasoconstriction if systemic vascular resistance and cardiac output are preserved throughout anesthesia

(Wagener & Brentjens, 2006). National Surgical Quality Improvement data indicate that for new arteriovenous fistulas, 85% of the patients underwent general anesthesia, 3% underwent local anesthesia and only 12% underwent regional anesthesia (Siracuse et al., 2014).

In patients with renal failure, general anesthesia has been associated with an increased risk of cardiorespiratory complications (Gao et al., 2020). Positive pressure ventilation can reduce cardiac output, renal blood flow, and GFR, with these effects further enhanced when high positive end-expiratory pressure is used. The decrease in renal blood flow is due to a reduction in cardiac output, which also triggers the release of catecholamines, renin, and angiotensin II, as well as activation of the sympathoadrenal system. Similar effects on renal blood flow and GFR are observed during laparoscopic surgery when the abdomen is insufflated. Furthermore, increased intra-abdominal pressure during laparoscopic surgery is immediately transmitted to the kidney, resulting in a further decrease in renal blood flow (Wagener & Brentjens, 2006).

Intraoperative Management

Monitoring

In the perioperative period, patients with renal failure require extensive follow-up due to their increased risk. It is crucial to avoid placing blood pressure cuffs, pulse oximeters, tourniquets, or peripheral venous cannulas on an arm with an arteriovenous fistula to prevent thrombosis. Similarly, a central line should not be placed in the same extremity as the arteriovenous access (Olivero, 2015). While basic monitoring standards may be acceptable for surgeries with minimal fluid loss and minimal risk, closer monitoring is necessary for intermediate or major surgeries. Patients with poorly controlled comorbidities should receive continuous intraarterial blood pressure monitoring, regardless of the type of surgery. Furthermore, it is recommended to maintain a urine output of at least 0.5 ml/kg/h in patients with preserved urinary output, although this is not a guarantee of the preservation of renal function.

Induction

During anesthetic induction, maintaining normotension and adequate oxygenation is of utmost importance. Preoxygenation is necessary, especially when anemia, reduced cardiorespiratory reserve, or a rapid induction sequence is anticipated (Maddern, 1983). Patients with end-stage renal disease undergoing hemodialysis may arrive at the operating room hypovolemic, putting them at an increased risk of postinduction hypotension (Byrick, 1999). Strategies to mitigate this risk include the judicious selection and dose reduction of anesthetics (Owsiany et al., 2019), and the careful titration of vasopressor drugs. Anesthetic dose adjustments are necessary due to changes in blood volume, protein binding, and pharmacodynamics, with a suggested dose reduction of 25-50%. More important is to ensure adequate intravascular volume than the choice of an induction agent, because post-induction hypotension occurs mostly in hypovolemic patients and typically resolves after intubation or surgical stimulation, rarely short-acting vasopressor usage. Once post-induction hypotension occurs, sympathetic or pharmacological mechanisms can cause renal vasoconstriction, which could exacerbate weakened renal perfusion. If hypotension persists, decreased renal perfusion can result in postoperative renal failure or impairment. And also tight blood pressure control and safe induction may be done using target-controlled infusion (TCI) systems (Guarracino et al., 2005). However, the use of TCI in patients with renal failure remains inconclusive, as sufficient data is lacking.

Maintenance

In the context of maintaining anesthesia, the primary objective should be to maintain normotension and cardiac output, regardless of the particular anesthetic used for maintenance purposes. Various anesthetic agents, such as remifentanil, propofol, fentanyl, sufentanil, and volatile anesthetics, can be employed with confidence for maintenance. However, nitrous oxide administration should be performed with caution in individuals with weak ventricular function or severe anemia to facilitate 100% oxygen delivery. In particular, total intravenous anesthesia (TIVA) has been found to produce more hypotension in patients with renal failure, necessitating a higher requirement for ephedrine, despite the use of lower concentrations of remifentanil (Byrick, 1999). Another important point is that inadequate spontaneous breathing under general anesthesia, combined with increased hypercarbia, poses a significant risk of respiratory acidosis. This condition can exacerbate preexisting acidemia, lead to severe circulatory depression, and dangerously elevate potassium levels. On the contrary, respiratory alkalosis can also be harmful by causing a shift to the left in the hemoglobin dissociation curve, worsening preexisting hypocalcemia, and potentially altering cerebral blood flow. Although vasoconstrictors can help maintain renal blood flow until hypotension is corrected, high doses, particularly α-adrenergic vasopressors, can have detrimental effects. It is essential to carefully manage the balance of the acid base and electrolyte during anesthesia to prevent potential complications (Olivero, 2015).

Fluid Therapy

In order to effectively treat patients with reduced renal function, it is crucial to ensure adequate fluid therapy. Treatment of negative effects caused by fluid overload, such as pulmonary congestion or edema, is much simpler compared to the management of renal injury by itself. However, rational fluid administration and appropriate monitoring can effectively prevent fluid overload. In stable clinical settings, the replacement of only insensible fluid losses during minimally invasive procedures or a minimal amount, i.e., not more than 1 ml/kg, is adequate (Olivero, 2015). Alternating one liter of each fluid may be employed during prolonged surgical procedures requiring large volumes. The optimal choice of intravenous solution can be made considering serum electrolyte levels. When administering large volumes of fluids, balanced solutions should be used instead of saline. For example, using lactated ringer solution, which contains only 4 mEq/L of potassium, is a safe alternative (O'Malley et al., 2002). Crystalloid solutions are commonly used for intravenous fluid therapy, but their volumetric effects are only temporary, and fluid overload can lead to unfavorable outcomes (Doherty & Buggy, 2012). Normal saline is usually preferred as crystalloid because it contains no potassium, but it can result in hyperchloremic metabolic acidosis, which has been associated with increased morbidity and mortality (Chowdhury et al., 2013). The use of chloride-poor or chloride-physiological fluids is associated with better renal outcomes (Yunos et al., 2012). Uremic patients require glucose-free solutions due to their glucose intolerance. Furthermore, artificial colloid solutions must be avoided as they are eliminated by the kidney (Bellomo & Hodgson, 2016). Hypotonic solutions pose a risk of severe hyponatremia in these patients (Olivero, 2015). When transfusion is necessary, careful monitoring of electrolytes and blood gases is necessary, along with consideration of volume burden and potassium load. Particular attention should be paid to hyperkalemia, which can be managed intraoperatively with calcium, insulin, and glucose, and metabolic acidosis can be improved by hyperventilation (Wagener & Brentjens, 2006). In cases of severe electrolyte abnormalities, urgent postoperative dialysis must be organized.

Postoperative Care

Patients with renal failure are at higher risk of developing postoperative complications. Various preventive strategies have been suggested in the literature; some general considerations include monitoring and improving cardiac output and stroke volume in patients with heart disease, adjusting blood pressure management goals in hypertensive patients, and using noradrenaline as the preferred vasopressor agent when necessary. Hydration is crucial without excessive fluid administration. For patients with known diabetes, it is recommended to target blood glucose levels between 7.8 and 11.1 mmol/l (Qaseem, 2011). Early mobilization is also recommended due to the higher risk of thromboembolism. Patients who have experienced an episode of acute renal failure are more likely to develop chronic kidney disease, and renal function should be evaluated at 6 months (Bellomo & Hodgson, 2016).

Conclusion

Intraoperative renal function deterioration may occur as a consequence of various factors, including surgical stress, anesthetic-induced effects, hormonal fluctuations, or obstacles to venous return due to positive pressure ventilation. Prophylaxis against these effects can be achieved by ensuring adequate intravascular volume through the administration of appropriate intravenous fluids. In addition, it is imperative to have a comprehensive understanding of the potential complications that can ensue, such as infections, hemorrhage, or renal injury, and to promptly manage them to avoid adverse outcomes.

References

Angst, M. S., Bührer, M., & Lötsch, J. (2000). Insidious intoxication after morphine treatment in renal failure: delayed onset of morphine-6-glucuronide action. *Anesthesiology,* 92(5), 1473–1476. https://doi.org/10.1097/00000542-200005000-00038.

Bellomo, R., & Hodgson, C. L. (2016). Improving the care of critically ill and postoperative patients with acute kidney injury. *Anaesthesia, Critical Care & Pain Medicine,* 35(2), 79–80. https://doi.org/10.1016/j.accpm.2016.02.002.

Bellomo, R., Ronco, C., Kellum, J. A., Mehta, R. L., Palevsky, P., & Acute Dialysis Quality Initiative workgroup. (2004). Acute renal failure - definition, outcome measures, animal models, fluid therapy and information technology needs: the Second International Consensus Conference of the Acute Dialysis Quality Initiative (ADQI) Group. *Critical Care/the Society of Critical Care Medicine,* 8(4), R204–R212. https://doi.org/10.1186/cc2872.

Blantz, R. C. (1998). Pathophysiology of pre-renal azotemia. *Kidney International*, 53(2), 512–523.

Buhre, W., & Rossaint, R. (2003). Perioperative management and monitoring in anaesthesia. *The Lancet*, 362(9398), 1839–1846. https://doi.org/10.1016/s0140-6736(03)14905-7.

Byrick, R. J. (1999). Anesthesia and end stage renal failure: is TIVA an advance? *Canadian Journal of Anesthesia/Journal canadien d'anesthésie,* 46(7), 621–625. https://doi.org/10.1007/bf03013948.

Chowdhury, A. H., Cox, E. F., Francis, S. T., & Lobo, D. N. (2013). A randomized, controlled, double-blind crossover study on the effects of 2-L infusions of 0.9% saline and plasma-lyte(R) 148 on renal blood flow velocity and renal cortical tissue perfusion in healthy volunteers. *Annals of Surgery* 258(6), 1118). https://doi.org/ 10.1097/sla.0000000000000346.

Craig, R. G., & Hunter, J. M. (2009). Neuromuscular blocking drugs and their antagonists in patients with organ disease. *Anaesthesia*, 64, 55–65. https://doi.org/10.1111/ j.1365-2044.2008.05871.x.

Dean, M. (2004). Opioids in renal failure and dialysis patients. *Journal of Pain and Symptom Management* 28(5), 497–504. https://doi.org/10.1016/j.jpainsymman. 2004.02.021.

Doherty, M., & Buggy, D. J. (2012). Intraoperative fluids: how much is too much? *British Journal of Anaesthesia*, 109(1), 69–79. https://doi.org/10.1093/bja/aes171.

Elapavaluru, S., & Kellum, J. A. (2007). Why Do Patients Die of Acute Kidney Injury? *Acta Clinica Belgica*, 62(sup2), 326–331. https://doi.org/10.1179/acb.2007.074.

Foley, R. N., Parfrey, P. S., Harnett, J. D., Kent, G. M., Murray, D. C., & Barre, P. E. (1996). The impact of anemia on cardiomyopathy, morbidity, and mortality in end-stage renal disease. *American Journal of Kidney Diseases,* 28(1), 53–61. https://doi.org/10.1016/s0272-6386(96)90130-4.

Galbusera, M., Remuzzi, G., & Boccardo, P. (2009). Treatment of Bleeding in Dialysis Patients. *Seminars in Dialysis,* 22(3), 279–286. https://doi.org/10.1111/j.1525-139x.2008.00556.x.

Gao, C., Weng, C., He, C., Xu, J., & Yu, L. (2020). Comparison of regional and local anesthesia for arteriovenous fistula creation in end-stage renal disease: a systematic review and meta-analysis. *BMC Anesthesiology,* 20(1), 219. https://doi.org/10.1186/s12871-020-01136-1.

Gogarten, W., Vandermeulen, E., Van Aken, H., Kozek, S., Llau, J. V., Samama, C. M., & European Scoeity of Anaesthesiology. (2010). Regional anaesthesia and antithrombotic agents: recommendations of the European Society of Anaesthesiology. *European Journal of Anaesthesiology*, 27(12), 999–1015. https://doi.org/10.1097/EJA.0b013e32833f6f6f.

Guarracino, F., Lapolla, F., Cariello, C., Danella, A., Doroni, L., Baldassarri, R., Boldrini, A., & Volpe, M. L. (2005). Target controlled infusion: TCI. *Minerva Anestesiologica*, 71(6), 335–337.

Guay, J. (2006). The benefits of adding epidural analgesia to general anesthesia: a metaanalysis. *Journal of Anesthesia,* 20(4), 335–340. https://doi.org/10.1007/s00540-006-0423-8.

Hartmann, B., Czock, D., & Keller, F. (2010). Drug Therapy in Patients with Chronic Renal Failure. *Deutsches Ärzteblatt international.* https://doi.org/10.3238/arztebl.2010.0647.

Hasselström, J., & Säwe, J. (1993). Morphine Pharmacokinetics and Metabolism in Humans. In *Clinical Pharmacokinetics*, 24(4), 344–354). https://doi.org/10.2165/00003088-199324040-00007.

Herd, J. A. (1991). Cardiovascular response to stress. *Physiological Reviews*, 71(1), 305–330. https://doi.org/10.1152/physrev.1991.71.1.305.

Higuchi, H., Adachi, Y., Wada, H., Kanno, M., & Satoh, T. (2001). The effects of low-flow sevoflurane and isoflurane anesthesia on renal function in patients with stable moderate renal insufficiency. *Anesthesia and Analgesia,* 92(3), 650–655. https://doi.org/10.1097/00000539-200103000-00019.

Hiraoka, H. (2004). Changes in drug plasma concentrations of an extensively bound and highly extracted drug, propofol, in response to altered plasma binding. *Clinical Pharmacology & Therapeutics*, 75(4), 324–330. https://doi.org/10.1016/j.clpt.2003.12.004.

Hubalewska, A., Stompór, T., Płaczkiewicz, E., Staszczak, A., Huszno, B., Sułowicz, W., & Szybiński, Z. (2004). Evaluation of gastric emptying in patients with chronic renal failure on continuous ambulatory peritoneal dialysis using 99mTc-solid meal. *Nuclear Medicine Review. Central & Eastern Europe*, 7(1), 27–30.

Ickx, B., Cockshott, I. D., Barvais, L., Byttebier, G., De Pauw, L., Vandesteene, A., & D'Hollander, A. A. (1998). Propofol infusion for induction and maintenance of anaesthesia in patients with end-stage renal disease. *British Journal of Anaesthesia*, 81(6), 854–860. https://doi.org/10.1093/bja/81.6.854.

Joh, J., Sila, M. K., & Bastani, B. (1998). Nondialyzability of fentanyl with high-efficiency and high-flux membranes. *Anesthesia and Analgesia*, 86(2), 447. https://doi.org/10.1097/00000539-199802000-00049.

Kheterpal, S., Tremper, K. K., Heung, M., Rosenberg, A. L., Englesbe, M., Shanks, A. M., & Campbell, D. A. (2009). Development and Validation of an Acute Kidney Injury

Risk Index for Patients Undergoing General Surgery. *Anesthesiology*, 110(3), 505–515. https://doi.org/10.1097/aln.0b013e3181979440.

Kim, B. R., Yoon, S., Song, G. Y., Lee, S., Bahk, J. H., & Nam, K. (2021). The impact of total intravenous anesthesia versus inhalation anesthesia on acute kidney injury after major abdominal surgery: a propensity score analysis. *Journal of Anesthesia*, 35(1), 112–121. https://doi.org/10.1007/s00540-020-02882-9.

Kirvelä, M., Olkkola, K. T., Rosenberg, P. H., Yli-Hankala, A., Salmela, K., & Lindgren, L. (1992). Pharmacokinetics of Propofol and Haemodynamic Changes During Induction of Anaesthesia in Uraemic Patients. *British Journal of Anaesthesia*, 68(2), 178–182. https://doi.org/10.1093/bja/68.2.178.

Koehntop, D. E., & Rodman, J. H. (1997). Fentanyl pharmacokinetics in patients undergoing renal transplantation. *Pharmacotherapy*, 17(4), 746–752.

Koza, Y. (2016). Acute kidney injury: current concepts and new insights. *Journal of Injury & Violence Research,* 8(1), 58–62.

Kusudo, K., Ishii, K., Rahman, M., Aki, Y., Miyatake, A., Kosaka, H., Kimura, S., Komatsu, T., Yokoyama, M., Morita, K., Abe, Y., & Nishiyama, A. (2004). Blood flow-dependent changes in intrarenal nitric oxide levels during anesthesia with halothane or sevoflurane. *European Journal of Pharmacology*, 498(1-3), 267–273. https://doi.org/10.1016/j.ejphar.2004.07.109.

Lin, C. Y., & Chen, Y. C. (2012). Acute kidney injury classification: AKIN and RIFLE criteria in critical patients. *Pediatric Critical Care Medicine: A Journal of the Society of Critical Care Medicine and the World Federation of Pediatric Intensive and Critical Care Societies,* 1(2), 40–45. https://doi.org/10.5492/wjccm.v1.i2.40.

Liu, L. L., & Gropper, M. A. (2003). Postoperative Analgesia and Sedation in the Adult Intensive Care Unit. *Drugs*, 63(8), 755–767. https://doi.org/10.2165/00003495-200363080-00003.

Maddern, P. J. (1983). Anaesthesia for the Patient with Impaired Renal Function. *Anaesthesia and Intensive Care,* 11(4), 321–332. https://doi.org/10.1177/0310057x8301100403.

Mazze, R. I., Callan, C. M., Galvez, S. T., Delgado-Herrera, L., & Mayer, D. B. (2000). The Effects of Sevoflurane on Serum Creatinine and Blood Urea Nitrogen Concentrations: A Retrospective, Twenty-Two–Center, Comparative Evaluation of Renal Function in Adult Surgical Patients. *Anesthesia & Analgesia,* 90(3), 683–688. https://doi.org/10.1097/00000539-200003000-00032.

Mehta, R. L., Kellum, J. A., Shah, S. V., Molitoris, B. A., Ronco, C., Warnock, D. G., Levin, A., & Acute Kidney Injury Network. (2007). Acute Kidney Injury Network: report of an initiative to improve outcomes in acute kidney injury. *Critical Care / the Society of Critical Care Medicine*, 11(2), R31. https://doi.org/10.1186/cc5713.

Mercadante, S., Caligara, M., Sapio, M., Serretta, R., & Lodi, F. (1997). Subcutaneous fentanyl infusion in a patient with bowel obstruction and renal failure. *Journal of Pain and Symptom Management*, 13(4), 241–244. https://doi.org/10.1016/s0885-3924(97)00076-6.

Neuromuscular blocking agents. (2018). *Morgan & Mikhail's Clinical Anesthesiology* (6th Ed., 348). McGraw Hill. https://accessmedicine.mhmedical.com/content.aspx?bookid=2444&sectionid=189636290.

Olivero, J. J., Sr. (2015). Administration of Anesthesia to Patients with Renal Failure. *Methodist DeBakey Cardiovascular Journal,* 11(3), 197. https://doi.org/10.14797/mdcj-11-3-197.

O'Malley, C. M. N., Frumento, R. J., & Bennett-Guerrero, E. (2002). Intravenous fluid therapy in renal transplant recipients: results of a US survey. *Transplantation Proceedings*, 34(8), 3142–3145. https://doi.org/10.1016/s0041-1345(02)03593-5.

Owsiany, M. T., Hawley, C. E., Triantafylidis, L. K., & Paik, J. M. (2019). Opioid Management in Older Adults with Chronic Kidney Disease: A Review. *The American Journal of Medicine*, 132(12), 1386–1393. https://doi.org/10.1016/j.amjmed.2019.06.014.

Priano, L. L. (1982). Comparative Renal Vascular Effects of Thiopental, Diazepam, Ketamine and Halothane. *Anesthesiology* 57(3), A34–A34. https://doi.org/10.1097/00000542-198209001-00034.

Qaseem, A. (2011). Use of Intensive Insulin Therapy for the Management of Glycemic Control in Hospitalized Patients: A Clinical Practice Guideline From the American College of Physicians. *Annals of Internal Medicine*, 154(4), 260. https://doi.org/10.7326/0003-4819-154-4-201102150-00007.

Robertson, E. N., Driessen, J. J., & Booij, L. H. D. J. (2005). Pharmacokinetics and pharmacodynamics of rocuronium in patients with and without renal failure. *European Journal of Anaesthesiology*, 22(1), 4–10. https://doi.org/10.1017/s0265021505000025.

Seidl, C., & Eberle, B. (2015). How to perform safe anesthesia in patients with end-stage renal disease. *Contributions to Nephrology*, 184, 107–122. https://doi.org/10.1159/000367905.

Shin, S. R., Kim, W. H., Kim, D. J., Shin, I. W., & Sohn, J. T. (2016). Prediction and Prevention of Acute Kidney Injury after Cardiac Surgery. *BioMed Research International*, 2016, 2985148. https://doi.org/10.1155/2016/2985148.

Simons, P. J., Cockshott, I. D., Douglas, E. J., Gordon, E. A., Hopkins, K., & Rowland, M. (1988). Disposition in male volunteers of a subanaesthetic intravenous dose of an oil in water emulsion of14C-propofol. *Xenobiotica*, 18(4), 429–440). https://doi.org/10.3109/00498258809041679.

Siracuse, J. J., Gill, H. L., Parrack, I., Huang, Z. S., Schneider, D. B., Connolly, P. H., & Meltzer, A. J. (2014). Variability in Anesthetic Considerations for Arteriovenous Fistula Creation. *The Journal of Vascular Access,* 15(5), 364–369. https://doi.org/10.5301/jva.5000215.

Smith, H. M., Farrow, S. J., Ackerman, J. D., Stubbs, J. R., & Sprung, J. (2008). Cardiac arrests associated with hyperkalemia during red blood cell transfusion: a case series. *Anesthesia and Analgesia*, 106(4), 1062–1069. https://doi.org/10.1213/ane.0b013e318164f03d.

Srisawat, N., & Kellum, J. A. (2020). The Role of Biomarkers in Acute Kidney Injury. *Critical Care Clinics,* 36(1), 125–140. https://doi.org/10.1016/j.ccc.2019.08.010.

Suleiman, M. Y., Passannante, A. N., Onder, R. L., Greene-Helms, W. F., & Perretta, S. G. (1997). Alteration of Renal Blood Flow During Epidural Anesthesia in Normal Subjects. *Anesthesia & Analgesia,* 84(5), 1076–1080. https://doi.org/10.1097/00000539-199705000-00022.

Talbott, G. A., Lynn, A. M., Levy, F. H., & Zelikovic, I. (1997). Respiratory Arrest Precipitated by Codeine in a Child with Chronic Renal Failure. *Clinical Pediatrics,* 36(3), 171–173. https://doi.org/10.1177/000992289703600308.

Veroli, P., O'Kelly, B., Bertrand, F., Trouvin, J. H., Farinotti, R., & Ecoffey, C. (1992). Extrahepatic metabolism of propofol in man during the anhepatic phase of orthotopic liver transplantation. *British Journal of Anaesthesia,* 68(2), 183–186. https://doi.org/10.1093/bja/68.2.183.

Wagener, G., & Brentjens, T. E. (2006). Renal Disease: The Anesthesiologist's Perspective. *Anesthesiology Clinics of North America,* 24(3), 523–547. https://doi.org/10.1016/j.atc.2006.04.001.

Wagener, G., & Brentjens, T. E. (2010). Anesthetic Concerns in Patients Presenting with Renal Failure. *Anesthesiology Clinics,* 28(1), 39–54. https://doi.org/10.1016/j.anclin.2010.01.006.

Weinberg, G. L. (2012). Lipid emulsion infusion: resuscitation for local anesthetic and other drug overdose. *Anesthesiology*, 117(1), 180–187. https://doi.org/10.1097/ALN.0b013e31825ad8de.

Wierda, J. M. K. H., Wierda, J. M. K., Kleef, U. W., Lambalk, L. M., Kloppenburg, W. D., & Agoston, S. (1991). The pharmacodynamics and pharmacokinetics of Org 9426, a new non-depolarizing neuromuscular blocking agent, in patients anaesthetized with nitrous oxide, halothane and fentanyl. *Canadian Journal of Anaesthesia,* 38(4), 430–435. https://doi.org/10.1007/bf03007578.

Yunos, N. M., Bellomo, R., Hegarty, C., Story, D., Ho, L., & Bailey, M. (2012). Association Between a Chloride-Liberal vs Chloride-Restrictive Intravenous Fluid Administration Strategy and Kidney Injury in Critically Ill Adults. *JAMA*, 308(15), 1566. https://doi.org/10.1001/jama.2012.13356.

Zacharias, M., Conlon, N. P., Herbison, G. P., Sivalingam, P., Walker, R. J., & Hovhannisyan, K. (2008). Interventions for protecting renal function in the perioperative period. *Cochrane Database of Systematic Reviews, 4,* CD003590. https://doi.org/10.1002/14651858.CD003590.pub3.

Chapter 8

Anesthesia for Endocrine Diseases

Selin Erel*, MD
and Ömer Kurtipek, MD
Department of Anesthesiology and Reanimation, Gazi University, Faculty of Medicine, Ankara, Turkey

Abstract

Dysfunctional endocrine organs can cause several anesthetic problems. The management of patients undergoing surgery who have primary or concomitant disease in one or more endocrine organs is discussed in this chapter. Pancreas-diabetes mellitus is the most common endocrine cause of main and secondary organ dysfunctions that affect anesthetic care. Adrenocortical hormone levels that are excessive or insufficient might lead to adrenal cortex dysfunction. Although phaeochromocytoma is uncommon, it may pose challenges during anesthesia. In the operating room, anesthesiologists may also encounter pathologies of the pituitary gland and disorders of the thyroid and parathyroid glands.

Keywords: endocrine diseases, anesthesia, perioperative management, hormones

* Corresponding Author's Email: selinerel@yahoo.com.

In: Organ Failure and Anesthesia Practices
Editors: Ahmet Şen and Basar Erdivanli
ISBN: 979-8-89113-486-7

Introduction

Hormones are substances that are secreted into the circulation in very small amounts to produce a physiological effect on distant target organs or cells. These hormones are secreted from several peripheral organs by the endocrine system, which is controlled by the hypothalamus and pituitary gland. In patients with endocrine abnormalities, care of the endocrine condition is equally crucial as the more typical characteristics of anesthetic management. Due to the complex relationships between the glands and their intended targets, this requires understanding the physiology and pathophysiology of endocrine function, which might be challenging.

The improved results seen in both endocrine surgery and the treatment of patients with endocrine disorders have been significantly attributed to advances in perioperative management. Greater knowledge of the perioperative outcomes of endocrine disorders and improved surgical methods have both contributed to these better outcomes. This chapter covers frequent endocrine diseases that an anaesthesiologist might encounter in the anaesthesia management and a summary of the most recent information on their best treatment options.

Diabetes Mellitus

Diabetes mellitus is the most common endocrine disease and is caused by inadequate insulin and/or inadequate tissue response to insulin. This leads to an increase in circulating glucose levels with eventual microvascular and macrovascular complications. There are two types of diabetes: Type 1 and Type 2 (American Diabetes Association, 2009).

Type 1 Diabetes

It accounts for 10% of all diabetes cases. One of the most prevalent chronic childhood diseases, it is typically diagnosed before the age of 40. Viruses, dietary proteins, drugs, and chemicals are just a few examples of environmental triggers that can start the autoimmune process in type 1a diabetes, although the exact cause is unknown. In most patients, a prolonged preclinical phase marked by the production of antibodies against cell antigens and loss of cell function occurs before the onset of clinical diabetes. At least 80% of β cell function must be lost before hyperglycemia occurs. Immune cells invade the pancreatic islets as the autoimmune attack first appears as islet inflammation. Circulating antibodies indicate islet cell damage. The disease typically begins abruptly and severely as a result of the loss of vital cell mass. Fatigue, weight loss, polyuria, polydipsia, impaired vision, episodes of hyperglycemia are common symptoms of diabetes. Ketoacidosis indicates severe insulin insufficiency and uncontrolled lipolysis (Cely et al., 2004).

Type 2 Diabetes

Type 2 diabetes is responsible for more than 90% of all diabetes mellitus cases around the world. By 2030, approximately. 600 million adults will have diabetes. Patients with type 2 diabetes are frequently overweight and tend to be in the middle or older age range (Galicia-Garcia et al., 2020).

Since it takes time to develop symptoms of type 2 diabetes, this condition is still underdiagnosed. Insulin resistance and relative cell failure are the defining features of the disease. In order to maintain normal plasma glucose levels, insulin secretion is increased due to the insensitivity of peripheral tissues to insulin. Insulin levels drop as the disease worsens and pancreatic cell function declines; this leads to hyperglycemia (Taniguchi et al., 2006; Herman & Kahn, 2006). Despite the importance of relative cell failure, type 2 is recognized by insulin resistance in the liver, adipose tissue, and skeletal muscle. While obesity and a sedentary lifestyle are acquired risk factors, insulin resistance appears to be a genetic factor of type 2 diabetes (American Diabetes Association, 2009).

Diagnosis and Treatment

The measurement of fasting plasma glucose levels is the recommended screening test for diabetes mellitus. Prediabetes can be detected in people using the same tests. In type 2 diabetes, glucose levels typically increase with time, shifting from the normal range to the range of impaired glucose tolerance and finally to clinical diabetes. The HbA1c test, which correlates with the average plasma glucose concentration over the previous 60 to 90 days, is a useful indicator of long-term glycemic control (Inzucchi, 2006; American Diabetes Association, 2009).

Along with oral antidiabetic medications, the cornerstones of type 2 diabetes treatment are dietary adjustments, exercise therapy, and weight loss. Reduced adipose tissue improves postreceptor insulin action, increases hepatic and peripheral tissue insulin sensitivity, and may even increase insulin secretion (Wood & Trayhurn, 2003).

Strict management of type 2 diabetes offers important advantages in terms of preventing and delaying the development of micro and macrovascular complications of diabetes. Metformin is the first treatment of choice for patients with newly diagnosed type 2 diabetes who are asymptomatic. The medication decreases hepatic gluconeogenesis while increasing glucose transport across cell membranes and glucose utilization by skeletal muscle and adipose tissue. Lactic acidosis is a rare but serious side effect of metformin. Sulfonylureas work by stimulating pancreatic cells to secrete more insulin. They can also boost the consumption of glucose in insulin-stimulated peripheral tissue. Glyburide, glipizide, and glimepiride are second-generation medications that are more potent and have fewer side effects than their predecessors. Unfortunately, due to the nature of type 2 diabetes, which is characterized by reduced β cell function, these drugs are not effective indefinitely. Sulfonylureas can increase the risk of cardiovascular events and prevent protective ischemic cardiac preconditioning after myocardial infarction (De Weille et al., 1988). Gliptins, SGLT-2 inhibitors and thiazolidinediones are the other diabetes medications (Wood & Trayhurn, 2003; Saltiel & Kahn, 2001).

All cases of type 1 diabetes and many cases of type 2 diabetes should be treated with insulin. Insulin is used to treat 30% of patients with type 2 diabetes. Injections are given twice daily in conventional insulin therapy. A continuous infusion or three or more daily injections is necessary for intensive insulin therapy. Different types of insulin include basal insulins, which are either long-acting (Ultralente, glargine, detemir) or intermediate-acting (NPH, Lente, lispro protamine, aspart protamine) and administered twice daily, as well as short-acting or rapid-acting (lispro aspart, glulisine), which control blood sugar levels during meals. For prandial coverage, rapid-acting insulin is preferred over regular insulin. A later onset of action, a longer duration of action, a less pronounced peak of action, and a lower incidence of hypoglycemia, particularly at night, are all characteristics of insulin glargine. To mimic physiologic insulin release with meals, a long-acting insulin is typically prescribed along with a short-acting insulin. Patients with type 1 diabetes typically need 0.5–1 U/kg/day divided into several doses, with approximately 50% administered as basal insulin (American Diabetes Association, 2009; Taniguchi et al., 2006; Herman & Kahn, 2006).

The most common and harmful side effect of insulin therapy is hypoglycemia. A plasma glucose level of less than 55 mg/dl is considered hypoglycemia. Sweating, tachycardia, palpitations, restlessness, exhaustion, confusion, headache, somnolence, convulsions, and coma are among the symptoms. Alcohol, sulfonylureas, biguanides, thiazolidinediones, angiotensin converting enzyme (ACE) inhibitors, monoamine oxidase inhibitors, and non-selective beta-blockers can be administered at the same time and increase the hypoglycemic effect. If the patient is conscious, treatment includes providing sugar cubes, glucose tablets, or soft drinks to the people. If Glasgow Coma Score is decreased, treatment involves giving people glucagon or 0.5 to 1.0 mg of glucose intravenously, intramuscularly, or subcutaneously (Puskas et al., 2007).

Preoperative Evaluation

Cardiovascular, renal, neurological, and musculoskeletal systems should be reviewed in the preoperative evaluation. Since myocardial ischemia and infarction may develop in diabetes, the cardiovascular system should be questioned in the preoperative evaluation. If autonomic neuropathy is present, silent ischemia may occur and patients with multiple cardiac risk factors should undergo stress tests. It is also crucial to pay close attention to the patient's fluid and electrolyte balance, stay away from nephrotoxins, and maintain renal blood flow. The patient is more likely to have intraoperative hypotension and perioperative dysrhythmias if they have autonomic neuropathy. Additionally, hemodynamic disturbances may result from the loss of compensatory sympathetic responses. Joint mobility should be evaluated before induction of anesthesia. Hard and non-pitting edema of the posterior neck and upper back combined with impaired joint mobility can limit the range of motion of the neck and can cause difficult intubation. Gastroparesis can increase the risk of aspiration regardless of the duration of the fast. Oral hypoglycemic drugs or noninsulin injectable drugs should continue to be used until the morning of surgery. Sulfonylureas may increase the risk of hypoglycemia. Insulin management in the preoperative period depends on the type and dose of insulin the patient receives. Although there are different strategies on how insulin should be used in the preoperative period, there is no consensus on the most appropriate strategy (American Diabetes Association, 2009; Bagry et al., 2008; Lipshutz et al., 2009).

A patient who typically administers subcutaneous insulin at bedtime should administer two thirds of this dose (NPH and regular) the night before surgery and one-half of the typical morning NPH dose on the day of surgery. Regular morning insulin doses should be maintained. The overnight rate should be reduced by 30% if the patient uses an insulin pump. The pump can continue to infuse at the basal rate the morning of surgery or it can be stopped and replaced by a continuous insulin infusion at the same rate. As an alternative, subcutaneous glargine can be administered and the pump can be turned off 60 to 90 minutes later. The patient should take the full dose of intermediate acting insulin and two-thirds of long-acting insulin the night before surgery. Preoperatively, oral hypoglycemics should be stopped 24 to 48 hours in advance. Sulfonylureas are advised to be avoided throughout the surgical period because they block the cardiac potassium adenosine triphosphate channels that cause ischemia (American Diabetes Association, 2009; Lipshutz et al., 2009; Schricker et al., 2004).

Intraoperative Management

Intraoperative glycemic control is important. For long and complex procedures, intravenous insulin is usually required. At least two hours before surgery, an insulin infusion should be started. The recommended range for perioperative serum glucose levels is 120–180 mg/dl. One unit of insulin lowers glucose by about 30 mg/dl. A typical rate is 0.02 units/kg/hour. The requirement for insulin infusion is higher for patients undergoing coronary bypass graft surgery, taking steroids, having serious infections, and receiving hyperalimentation or vasopressor infusion (Lipshutz et al., 2009). Insulin infusion should be accompanied by a 5% infusion of dextrose in seminormal saline with potassium chloride 20 mEq at 100 ml/h. At least once per hour, serum glucose levels should be measured. Shorter intervals may be needed if blood sugar levels are below 100 mg/dl if the drop rate is rapid, for patients undergoing cardiovascular surgery. Identification of hypoglycemia may be delayed by anesthetics, analgesics, beta-blockers, or sympatholytics. Bode et al., 2022).

Insulinoma

Insulinomas are infrequent, benign pancreatic islet cell tumors that secrete insulin. They usually appear alone, but can also be a symptom of multiple endocrine neoplasia syndrome. Patients are typically given diazoxide, a drug that directly inhibits the release of insulin from beta cells, before surgery. Verapamil, phenytoin, propranolol, glucocorticoids, and somatostatin analogs are additional medications. Since enucleation is the ideal procedure and 90% of insulinomas are benign, in some centers laparoscopic resection is used. However, pronounced hyperglycemia may follow tumor removal. Profound hypoglycemia can occur during tumor manipulation. Typically, a standard glucometer is used to take serial blood glucose readings every 15 minutes. Since anesthesia may mask hypoglycemia symptoms, intravenous fluids containing glucose should be taken into account (Singh et al., 2022).

Thyroid Diseases

The thyroid gland has two lobes connected by an isthmus and weighs about 20. Each lobe has two parathyroid glands that are located posteriorly. The entire gland is covered by a complex capillary network. The gland is innervated by the adrenergic and cholinergic nervous systems. The recurrent laryngeal nerve and the external motor branch of the superior laryngeal nerve are located close to the gland. The thyroid gland has parafollicular C cells that produce calcitonin (Malhotra & Bhadada, 2022; Verma & Dwivedi, 2022). Most metabolic processes are stimulated by thyroid hormones. It influences tissue development and maturation, improves tissue performance, and promotes protein synthesis, carbohydrate, and lipid metabolism. Cardiovascular myocytes and smooth muscle cells are directly affected by thyroid hormone. Thyroid hormones increase myocardial contractility, lower systemic vascular resistance, and increase intravascular volume. T3 affects cardiac and vascular smooth muscle, which is what causes the exaggerated hemodynamic effects of hyperthyroidism. Despite the fact that hyperthyroid patients appear to have an increase in the number of -adrenergic receptors, these receptors are surprisingly unresponsive to adrenergic stimulation and these patients have normal or low serum catecholamine concentrations (Yamakawa et al., 2021). The hypothalamus, pituitary, and thyroid glands work together as part of a traditional feedback control system to regulate thyroid function. Thyrotropin-releasing hormone is produced by the hypothalamus and travels through the pituitary stalk before activating the anterior pituitary to release thyrotropin stimulating hormone (TSH). TSH binds to specific receptors on the thyroid cell membrane. It improves all the synthesis and secretion processes of T4 and T3. Reduced TSH reduces the size of follicular cells, the production and secretion of T4 and T3, as well as the vascularity of the gland. Production and release of hormones, as well as cellularity and vascularity of the glands, increase when TSH levels increase. Through a negative feedback loop, plasma levels of T4 and T3 also influence TSH secretion. The thyroid gland has an autoregulation mechanism that maintains a constant level of hormone stores in addition to the feedback system (Shahid et al., 2022).

Hyperthyroidism

Diagnosis and Treatment

Hyperthyroidism refers to the overproduction of active thyroid hormones. The most common causes are Graves' disease, toxic multinodular goiter, or toxic adenoma. Hyperthyroidism causes hypermetabolism. Despite increasing appetite, weight loss and osteoporosis can be seen. T3 acts directly on the myocardium and peripheral vessels, causing cardiac responses (Bartalena et al., 2022; Taylor et al., 2018).

The first treatment of choice for this is methimazole or propylthiouracil. If an adequate dosage is used, an euthyroid condition can almost always be achieved in 6 to 8 weeks with both medications. The most serious side effect is agranulocytosis. High doses of iodine reduce all stages of thyroid synthesis and release, leading to a decrease in the size and vascularity of the gland. The effects appear immediately, but are short-lived. Iodide is frequently used to treat severe hyperthyroidism, regulate thyroid storms, and prepare preoperative patients. In a patient with well-controlled thyrotoxicosis, there is no need to delay surgery to begin iodide. Since injection of iodide alone will increase thyroid hormone reserves and worsen thyrotoxicy, antithyroid medication therapy should be started before iodide. Lithium carbonate can be given to patients with iodide allergy. β-adrenergic antagonists can alleviate anxiety, sweating, heat intolerance, tremors, and tachycardia. Propranolol offers additional properties, such as disrupting the peripheral conversion of T4 to T3. Subtotal thyroidectomy corrects thyrotoxicosis in more than 95% of patients; the mortality rate for the procedure is less than 0.1%. Complications of surgery include hypothyroidism, bleeding, damage to the recurrent laryngeal nerve, superior laryngeal nerve, and accidental removal of the parathyroid glands (Rui et al., 2022; Wang et al., 2022).

Anesthesia Management

Preoperative euthyroidism should be provided in operated hyperthyroidism patients. In elective cases, it may take 6 to 8 weeks for antithyroid medications to take effect. Intravenous beta-blockers, glucocorticoids, and propylthiouracil are frequently required in emergencies. Intravenous propylthiouracil is not available, so the drug should be administered orally or rectally. Glucocorticoids must be administered every 6 hours to reduce hormone release and peripheral conversion of T4 to T3 (Verma & Dwivedi, 2022). Chest radiography and computer tomography are useful for evaluating compression or deviation of the trachea caused by goiter. Depending on the type of operation and the patient, invasive arterial monitoring should be performed (Kapre et al., 2020). Hyperthyroidism has not been shown to increase the minimal alveolar concentration. However, it is important to supply sufficient depth of anesthetic to prevent sympathetic system responses. Drugs that stimulate the sympathetic nervous system (e.g., ketamine, ephedrine) should be avoided. The eyes should be protected, especially in patients with proptosis. For the maintenance of anesthesia, any of the inhalational agents can be used. In hyperthyroid patients, careful titration of depolarizing muscle relaxants is recommended, as there may be concomitant muscle diseasesç. Removal of the thyrotoxic gland does not imply immediate resolution of thyrotoxicosis. The half-life of T4 is about 1 week. Therefore, in the postoperative period, β-blocker treatment may need to be continued for up to 1 week (Tang & Hennessey, 2020).

Thyroid Storm

The thyroid storm is a hyperthyroidism exacerbation that can be fatal and is caused by injury, infection, disease, or surgery. Malignant hyperthermia and thyroid storm can both occur during surgery and have similar symptoms. Therefore, the distinction between the two can be difficult. Surprisingly, thyroid hormone levels in a thyroid storm may not be significantly higher than during uncomplicated hyperthyroidism. Therefore, thyroid function tests may not be useful in making a diagnosis. The thyroid storm most commonly occurs during the postoperative period in hyperthyroid patients who are not treated or are not adequately treated after emergency surgery. Thyrotoxicosis should be treated quickly, as well as general supportive care. Vasopressor infusion should be used if there is a hemodynamic compromise. A blocker or digitalis is recommended for atrial fibrillation accompanied by rapid ventricular response (de Mul et al., 2021).

Hypothyroidism

Diagnosis and Treatment

One percent of adults suffer from the disease known as hypothyroidism. Most hypothyroid cases are caused by primary hypothyroidism, which results in decreased thyroid hormone production despite elevated TSH levels (Chiovato et al., 2019). Adult hypothyroidism progresses slowly but gradually. Patients also experience weight gain, accumulation of hydrophilic mucopolysaccharides, and edema over time. It is also typical to have hyponatremia and impaired excretion of free water due to improper antidiuretic hormone secretion. The ventilation response to hypoxia and hypercarbia is decreased, as well as the maximum respiratory capacity and diffusion capacity. Pleural effusions can cause dyspnea. Patients with TSH levels greater than 10 milliunits/L are at increased risk for coronary artery disease. Decreased free T4, T4, T3 and TSH levels, as well as decreased free T4 and T3 levels, are used to diagnose secondary hypothyroidism (Biondi & Cooper, 2019).

The occurrence of abnormal thyroid function test results in seriously ill patients with significant nonthyroid disease is known as euthyroid patient syndrome. Low T3 and T4 levels, together with normal TSH levels, are distinguishing characteristics. The levels of T3 and T4 fall even further as the disease becomes more severe. The etiology of this response is unclear. The physiological reaction to stress that results in euthyroid patient syndrome can be triggered by surgery. Treatment is not required for thyroid function. It can be very challenging to distinguish between euthyroid patient syndrome and hypothyroidism. The best aid is the serum TSH level. Hypothyroidism is indicated by levels greater than 10 milliunits/L, while euthyroidism is indicated by levels less than 5.0 milliunits/L (Hoermann et al., 2019).

L-thyroxine therapy is generally used to treat hypothyroidism. The reduction of TSH level and sodium and water diuresis are the first signs of a therapeutic response to thyroid hormone. Treatment results in improvements in myocardial function in patients with hypothyroid cardiomyopathy (Hoermann et al., 2019).

Anesthesia Management

For a variety of reasons, hypothyroid patients may be more vulnerable when receiving general or regional anesthesia. Vocal cord edema and challenging airways could be risks associated with enlargement of the thyroid gland. Regurgitation and aspiration risk increase with decreased gastric emptying. Surgical stress and cardiac depressant anesthetics can compromise a hemodinamia characterized by decreased cardiac output, stroke volume, heart rate, baroreceptor reflexes, and intravascular volume. Anesthetic agents decrease ventilatory responsiveness to hypoxia and hypercarbia. D Hypothermia occurs quickly and is difficult to treat. Hyponatremia, hypoglycemia, and dysfunctional platelets and coagulation factors are common hematologic abnormalities that require close intraopcrative monitoring (Tang & Hennessey, 2020). Preoperative sedation should be performed with caution, as these patients may be extremely sensitive to narcotics and sedatives. Patients with hypothyroidism seem to be more sensitive to anesthetic medications. Reduced cardiac output, blood volume, liver metabolism, renal excretion, and abnormal baroreceptor function are likely secondary causes of increased sensitivity. Intravascular volume and cardiac status may need to be monitored in patients with hypodynamic cardiovascular systems using invasive monitoring and/or transesophageal echocardiography. Rapid series induction or awake intubation, if there is a difficult airway, should be followed by the administration of general anesthetics through an endotracheal tube. Strong inhalational agents have the potential to myocardially depress patients with hypothyroidism. Vasodilation can cause severe hypotension when there is a risk of hypovolemia and reduced baroreceptor activity. Ephedrine, dopamine, or epinephrine are used instead of a pure adrenergic agonist (phenylephrine) to treat intraoperative hypotension. Steroid administration may be necessary for nonresponsive hypotension. Due to its chronotropic effects, pancuronium is the preferred muscle relaxant from a cardiovascular standpoint; however, careful dosing is necessary due to the decreased activity of the skeletal muscle of the patients and the decrease in liver metabolism (Verma & Dwivedi, 2022).

Controlled ventilation is recommended in all cases because hypoventilation may occur in these patients if spontaneous breathing is permitted. Dextrose in normal saline is the intravenous fluid recommended to prevent hypoglycemia and minimize hyponatremia secondary to impaired free water clearance (Fernandez-Robles et al., 2021).

If urgent surgery is required, there is a substantial risk of serious intraoperative cardiovascular instability and myxedema coma. As soon as possible, intravenous thyroid replacement therapy should start. Compared to IV L-thyroxine, which takes 10–12 days to reach its peak effect, IV triiodothyronine takes just six hours to take effect and reaches its peak basal metabolic rate in 36–72 hours. An appropriate starting dose is 25–50 g of L-triiodothyronine or 300–500 g of levothyroxine administered intravenously. Due to the fact that hypothyroidism frequently coexists with decreased adrenal cortical function, the treatment with hydrocortisone or dexamethasone is required. Since milrinone's mechanism of action does not depend on receptors, whose number and sensitivity may decrease in hypothyroidism, it may be effective in treating reduced myocardial contractility (Fernandez-Robles et al., 2021).

Myxedema Coma

The rare and severe hypothyroid condition known as myxedema coma is characterized by delirium or loss of consciousness, hypoventilation, hypothermia, bradycardia, hypotension, and severe hyponatremia. Hypothyroid patients are more likely to experience a myxedema coma in the presence of infection, trauma, and CNS depressants. Surprisingly, most patients are not unconscious. The primary symptom is hypothermia, which is caused by poor thermoregulation caused by hypothalamic malfunction. With a high mortality rate, myxedema coma is a medical emergency. The preferred treatment is intravenous L-thyroxine or L-triiodothyronine. Intravenous hydration, temperature control, correction of electrolyte imbalances, and hemodynamic stability are necessary when glucose-containing saline solutions are used. Frequently, mechanical ventilation is required. A relative euthyroid state is reached in about 5 days and heart rate, blood pressure, and temperature generally begin to improve within 24 hours. Potential adrenal insufficiency can be treated with hydrocortisone (Talha et al., 2020).

Thyroid Tumors

Goiter is hypertrophy and hyperplasia of the thyroid follicular epithelium. The cause may be inadequate iodine intake, pharmacologic or a defect in the hormonal pathway. Patients with simple non-toxic goiter are euthyroid. However, hypothyroidism or hyperthyroidism can occur in some cases. Mostly, simple non-toxic goiter are idiopatic and treated with L-thyroxine. Thyroidectomy is considered only if medical treatment is ineffective and the airway is compromised (Chen & Chen, 2022).

Major airway obstruction, cardiac compression, and superior vena cava obstruction could occur if the mass enters the substernal region. Following induction of general anesthesia, airway obstruction and cardiac compression may occur. When a patient's position changes or when muscle paralysis first appears, changes in the mechanics of the lung and chest wall lead to airway obstruction. The larger airways are supported by negative intrathoracic pressure during spontaneous respiration, and only the most severe cases of extrinsic compression may be noticeable. With the cessation of spontaneous respiration, compensatory mechanisms are removed, and airway obstruction occurs. Positive pressure ventilation can also show complete airway obstruction. The likelihood of an airway obstruction during general anesthesia is predicted by a preoperative history of dyspnea in the upright or supine position. Examining a CT scan is necessary to determine the extent of the tumor. The degree of cardiac compression can be determined by echocardiography (Pan et al., 2020).

If appropriate, regional anesthesia should be preferred. If general anesthesia is required, it is recommended to reduce the thyroid tumor prior to surgery with radiation or chemotherapy. Unfortunately, goiters are not susceptible to radiation therapy. CT will show anatomical abnormalities. Before intubation, sedatives and narcotics should be avoided or carefully titrated (Verma & Dwivedi, 2022). The best approach to establish the airway is awake intubation.

Surgical removal of the mass may result in underlying tracheomalacia and collapse of the air passage. Therefore, extubation should be done with the same care as intubation. After surgery, a fiberoptic bronchoscopy examination of the airway should be performed to evaluate whether and when extubation is necessary (Kapre et al., 2020).

Complications of Thyroid Surgery

Morbidity due to thyroid surgery may be high. Recurrent laryngeal nerve injury can be unilateral or bilateral and temporary or permanent. Nerve damage may be caused by excessive trauma, unintentional ligation, or transection. The engaged cord assumes a median or paramedian position when the abductor muscles of the vocal cord paralyze. The patient has hoarseness but no airway obstruction if the trauma is unilateral, and function usually returns in 3 to 6 months. Permanent hoarseness is the result of nerve transection or ligation. Since the patient has breathing and coughing problems, bilateral involvement is more serious. Tracheostomy may be required depending on the severity of the damage. The adductor muscles are paralyzed when the adductor fibers of the recurrent laryngeal nerve are damaged, raising the risk of aspiration. Thyroid dissection can also cause injury to the motor branch of the superior laryngeal nerve, which innervates the inferior pharyngeal constrictor and cricothyroid muscles. This harm weakens the voice and makes it difficult to create high tones (Chahardahmasumi et al., 2019).

Complications of thyroid surgery include hypoparathyroidism. Damage to the bloodstream of the parathyroid glands is typically what causes it. All that is required to prevent hypoparathyroidism is a functioning parathyroid gland. Signs and symptoms of hypocalcemia appear within the first 24 to 48 hours after surgery. Stridor could occur, and laryngospasm may worsen. It is necessary to administer calcium chloride or calcium gluconate intravenously as soon as possible (Pãduraru et al., 2019).

After thyroidectomy surgery, acute respiratory failure can occur due to tracheal compression caused by an enlarged hematoma. The first stage of therapy is the evacuation of the emergency hematoma. The patient should be taken back to the operating room as soon as possible. If the peripheric oxygen levels are low, the stitches should be removed at the bedside, the clots should be drained, and the bleeding veins should be fixed to relieve airway obstruction. The tracheostomy kit and surgical equipment should be stored in a place that is easily accessible in the postoperative period. Thus, stitches or clips can be removed, the wound can be opened urgently, and, if necessary, an emergency surgical airway can be provided (Idrees et al., 2021).

Parathyroid Gland Dysfunction

The parathyroid glands are located behind the thyroid gland and release PTH into the systemic circulation through a negative feedback mechanism linked to plasma calcium levels. The release of PTH release is stimulated by hypocalcemia, whereas it is suppressed by hypercalcemia. PTH stimulates calcium movement, maintaining normal serum calcium concentrations (4.5–5.5 mEq/L) (Uslu et al., 2019).

Hyperparathyroidism

Hyperparathyroidism occurs when PTH secretion is elevated. Calcium levels may increase, decrease, or remain unchanged. Primary, secondary, and ectopic hyperparathyroidism are the three types of hyperparathyroidism (Bilezikian et al., 2022b).

Primary Hyperparathyroidism

Due to benign parathyroid adenoma, parathyroid gland carcinoma, or hyperplasia with an excessive amount of PTH secreted, which leads to primary hyperparathyroidism. In approximately 90% of patients, primary hyperparathyroidism is caused by benign parathyroid adenoma (Marques & Moreira, 2020).

Diagnosis and Treatment

Plasma calcium levels >5.5 mEq/L and ionized calcium level >2.5 mEq/L are the hallmarks of primary hyperparathyroidism. Measurement of serum PTH concentrations is not always reliable enough to confirm diagnosis. Twenty-four hour urine calcium and 25-hydroxyvitamin D serum measurements may also be helpful in diagnosis and treatment. (Alore et al., 2019). Symptoms of hypercalcemia reflect changes in ionized calcium concentration. Early signs and symptoms include sedation, vomiting, loss of skeletal muscle strength and mass. Persistent increases in plasma calcium concentrations can cause urine concentration ability and polyuria. Oliguric renal failure can occur in cases of advanced hypercalcemia. Kidney stones, especially in the presence of polyuria and polydipsia, should raise suspicion of primary hyperparathyroidism. The increased serum chloride concentration (>102 mEq/L) is most likely due to the effect of PTH on renal excretion of bicarbonate, which produces mild metabolic acidosis. Anemia, peptic ulcer disease, and abdominal pain are common. When serum calcium concentration exceeds 8 mEq/L, cardiac conduction disorders are likely (Bilezikian et al., 2022a).

The definitive treatment of primary hyperparathyroidism is parathyroidectomy. Successful surgical treatment is reflected in normalization of serum calcium concentrations within 3 to 4 days. The first potential complication in the postoperative period is hypocalcemic tetany. Postoperative hypomagnesemia exacerbates hypocalcemia and makes it resistant to treatment. Hyperchloremic metabolic acidosis may occur temporarily after parathyroidectomy, with impaired renal function (Bilezikian et al., 2022a; Bilezikian et al., 2022b).

Anesthesia Management

There is no evidence that specific anesthetic drugs or techniques are required in patients with primary hyperparathyroidism who undergo elective surgery. Hydration and maintaining urine output are important in the perioperative management of hypercalcemia. Patients with hyperparathyroidism must be placed carefully due to the potential for osteoporosis and their susceptibility to fractures. Somnolence before induction of anesthesia raises the possibility that intraoperative anesthetic requirements may be reduced. Due to its psychotropic effects, ketamine should not be preferred in patients with personality changes that coexist with chronic hypercalcemia. The possibility of coexisting renal dysfunction is an important consideration when using sevoflurane. Coexisting skeletal muscle weakness suggests the possibility of reduced requirements for muscle relaxants, while hypercalcemia may be expected to antagonize the effects of nondepolarizing muscle relaxants. Given the unpredictable response to muscle relaxants, careful titration is recommended. The ECG should be monitored for signs of adverse cardiac effects of hypercalcemia (Verma & Dwivedi, 2022).

Secondary Hyperparathyroidism

Secondary hyperparathyroidism reflects proper overwork of the parathyroid glands as a result of hypocalcemia. For example, chronic kidney disease disrupts phosphorus elimination and reduces vitamin D hydroxylation, which with increased PTH release causes hypocalcemia and compensatory hyperplasia of the parathyroid glands. Secondary hyperparathyroidism rarely causes hypercalcemia. Treatment of secondary hyperparathyroidism aims to control the underlying disease, as is achieved by normalizing serum phosphate concentrations in patients with kidney disease by administering oral phosphate binders (Mizobuchi et al., 2019).

Hypoparathyroidism

Hypoparathyroidism occurs when PTH secretion is absent or deficient or when peripheral tissues are resistant to the effects of the hormone. The absence or deficiency of PTH occurs almost always as a complication of thyroidectomy. Pseudohypoparathyroidism is a congenital disorder in which PTH secretion is intact, but the kidneys do not respond to the hormone. Affected patients have mental retardation, basal ganglia calcification, obesity, and short stature (Gafni & Collins, 2019).

Diagnosis and Treatment

The diagnosis should be suspected in a patient with persistent hypocalcemia with low or inappropriate normal PTH levels and hyperphosphatemia. A serum calcium concentration of less than 4.5 mEq/L and a concentration of ionized calcium of less than 2.0 mEq/L are indicators of hypoparathyroidism (Pasieka et al., 2022).

Symptoms of hypoparathyroidism depend on the speed of the onset of hypocalcemia. Acute hypocalcemia can occur after accidental removal of the parathyroid glands during thyroidectomy. The inspiratory stridor reflects the neuromuscular irritability of the intrinsic laryngeal musculature. Chronic hypocalcemia is associated with fatigue and cramps of the skeletal muscle, which may be associated with a prolonged QT interval on the ECG. The QRS complex, PR interval, and cardiac rhythm usually remain normal. Ulooping, cataract formation, and calcifications involving subcutaneous tissues and basal ganglia can be seen. Chronic renal failure is the most common cause of chronic hypocalcemia (Yao et al., 2022).

Calcium gluconate or calcium chloride is used to treat acute hypocalcemia. Alkalosis needs to be corrected. The approach to the treatment of hypoparathyroidism without symptomatic hypocalcemia is oral administration of calcium and vitamin D. Thiazide diuretics may be useful because these drugs cause sodium depletion without proportional potassium excretion and therefore tend to increase serum calcium concentrations (Khan et al., 2022).

Anesthesia Management

Anesthetic management in the presence of hypocalcemia aims to prevent further reduction in serum calcium concentration and treat the adverse effects of hypocalcemia. Iatrogenic hyperventilation and bicarbonate administration can reduce serum calcium intraoperatively. Routine administration of citrate containing whole blood usually does not reduce serum calcium concentrations because calcium is rapidly mobilized from body stores. However, ionized calcium concentrations can be reduced when blood infusions are rapid, during massive transfusions, or when citrate metabolism or elimination are altered by hypothermia, liver cirrhosis, or renal dysfunction (Traill & Halpern, 2018b).

Adrenal Gland Dysfunction

Glucocorticoids, mineralocorticoids (aldosterone), and androgens are all produced by the adrenal cortex. The corticotropin-releasing hormone (CRH), which is produced in the hypothalamus and delivered to the anterior pituitary, causes the release of corticotropin (ACTH). The adrenal cortex is stimulated by ACTH to produce cortisol. Role of cortisol in helping adrenal medulla convert norepinephrine to epinephrine (Egalini et al., 2022). In response to the release of cortisol, hyperglycemia develops. Cortisol facilitates sodium retention and potassium excretion. At high serum levels of these hormones, the anti-inflammatory effects of glucocorticoids are especially evident. The renin-angiotensin system and serum potassium concentrations control aldosterone secretion. Aldosterone controls the volume of extracellular fluid by encouraging sodium absorption by renal tubules. Aldosterone also encourages potassium excretion from the renal tubular. The adrenal medulla is a specialized part of the sympathetic nervous system that synthesizes norepinephrine and epinephrine. Pheochromocytoma is the disease of the adrenal gland (Egalini et al., 2022).

One of the best and most well-researched activators of the hypothalamic-pituitary-adrenal (HPA) axis is surgery. Normal HPA axis, CRH, ACTH, and cortisol levels increase significantly during surgery. Regional or deep general anesthesia can reduce but not completely prevent this response. The highest level of ACTH occurs with the reversal of muscle relaxants and extubation. ACTH levels increase with surgical incision and increase during urgery. For several days after surgery, hormone levels are elevated. During major surgery, cortisol release can increase from a preoperative level of 15 to 25 mg/day to 75 to 150 mg/day, resulting in a plasma cortisol level of 30 to 50 mg/dl. Patients in the intensive care unit may have plasma cortisol levels of more than 60 mg/dl (Bauer & Currie, 2020; Fernandez-Robles et al., 2021).

Pheochromocytoma

Pheochromocytomas are sympathoadrenal system chromaffin cell-derived catecholamine-secreting tumors. Although it accounts for less than 0.1% of all cases of hypertension, it must be detected as untreatable pheochromo-cytomas are fatal (Leung et al., 2021; Neumann et al., 2019).

Almost 80% of pheochromocytomas are found in the adrenal medulla. The Zuckerkandl organ near the bifurcation of the aorta is the most common extraadrenal region. Most of them are benign. Malignant pheochromocytomas usually spread to the liver and bone through the venous and lymphatic ducts. secrete norepinephrine, while 15% primarily secrete epinephrine. There are also known pheochromocytomas that secrete dopamine. Most pheochromocytomas are not under neurogenic control and secrete catecholamines autonomously (Amodru et al., 2020; Leung et al., 2021).

Pheochromocytoma attacks may be sporadic or frequent. It can occur spontaneously or be triggered by trauma, stress, or drugs. Orthostatic hypotension is another frequent finding linked to impaired vasoconstrictor reflex responses and hypovolemia (Jain et al., 2020). The hemodynamic manifestations are due to the predominant catecholamine secreted. If norepinephrine's α adrenergic effects dominate, patients frequently experience hypertension and reflex bradycardia. Epinephrine has a predominance of β -adrenergic effects, and patients frequently experience systolic hypertension, diastolic hypotension, and tachycardia. Despite the 10-fold higher levels of circulating catecholamines, patients with pheochromocytomas and those with essential hypertension do not exhibit significantly different hemodynamics. Both groups have an increased systemic vascular resistance, usually a normal cardiac output, and a slightly decreased plasma volume. Long-term exposure to high levels of catecholamines does not appear to produce the hemodynamic responses characteristic of acute administration. Desensitization of the cardiovascular system or down-regulation of adrenergic receptors may explain this finding (Y-Hassan & Falhammar, 2020).

Diagnosis and Treatment

A 24-hour urine collection is a helpful screening test for catecholamine measurement in patients who are less likely to have pheochromocytomas. The measurement of non-plasma metanephrines is the most accurate test for high-risk patients. Non-plasma normanephrine level greater than 400 pg/ml and/or metanephrine level greater than 220 pg/ml confirm the diagnosis of pheochromocytoma (Sbardella & Grossman, 2020). CT detects more than 95% of adrenal masses larger than 1.0 cm. Compared to CT, magnetic resonance imaging is better at identifying small lesions (Ilias & Meristoudis, 2019; Nölting et al., 2022).

Phenoxybenzamine is an α blocker most prescribed for preoperative use. Oral dosing is only allowed twice a day due to the prolonged duration of action. Normal blood pressure, symptomatic relief, elimination of changes in ST segment and T wave on ECG, and arrhythmias are the aims of treatment. Orthostatic hypotension caused by overtreatment can be very severe. Phenoxybenzamine's long-term impact on the receptor has led to the recommendation to stop using it 24 to 48 hours prior to surgery to prevent vascular inactivity immediately after tumor removal. Alternatives to phenoxybenzamine include the pure α1-competitive blockers prazosine and doxazosin. They are less tachycardic.

Calcium is a trigger for the release of catecholamines from the tumor. Therefore, calcium canal blockers can be used to control preoperative hypertension. One α_1 blocker and one calcium channel blocker are an effective combination in treatment resistant cases (Srivastava & Naithani, 2022).

B-adrenergic blockers are recommended if tachycardia or other arrhythmias develop as a result of phenoxybenzamine blockade. Blocking the vasodilatory receptors b2 receptors results in unopposed agonism, leading to vasoconstriction. Therefore, non-selective b blockers should never be administered before a blocker. Propranolol (non selective b blocker) is frequently preffered. Atenolol, metoprolol and labetalol have also been used successfully (García et al., 2019).

Preoperative Evaluation

Preoperative administration of an a-adrenergic blocker with or without b blockers and treatment of hypovolemia are essentials for surgical preparation. Intraoperative strategies include avoiding agents or activities that may cause catecholamine release and, preferably, preserving cardiovascular stability using short-acting drugs. During pneumoperitoneum and tumor manipulation, hypertension is common. Significant hypotension may occur after the closure of the vein that drains the tumor. Intraoperative monitoring should be performed using standard and invasive approaches. An arterial catheter and a central venous pressure catheter are probably preferable for patients who do not have cardiac symptoms or other clinical indicators of cardiac involvement (Araujo-Castro et al., 2021). Patients with active tumors may need transesophageal echocardiography or a pulmonary artery catheter. To manage hypotension and maintain intravascular volumes, a large positive fluid balance is needed. Small, functional tumors can be localized and treated with partial adrenalectomies or procedures that spare the adrenal glands using intraoperative ultrasonography. When it is necessary to remove bilateral adrenal pheochromocytomas, adrenal-sparing procedures are especially beneficial. The preferred procedure for tumors under 8 cm in diameter without radiologically malignant features is laparoscopy (Fagundes & Almeida, 2022).

Intraoperative Management

Fear, stress, pain, hypoxia, and hypercarbia are triggers for catecholamine release during surgery and should be kept to a minimum. Although all anesthetic medications have been used successfully, some medications should be avoided to prevent negative hemodynamic reactions. The release of histamine by morphine and atracurium can lead to the production of catecholamines from the tumor. Examples of vasolytic or sympathomimetic drugs that can stimulate the sympathetic nervous system include atropine, ketamine, pancuronium, and succinylcholine. In almost all patients, intraoperatively, increases in systolic arterial pressure can be observed that exceed 200 mmHg. Antihypertensive medication is not available in the operating room. The preferred agent is sodium nitroprusside, a direct vasodilator because of its strength, rapid onset of action, and brief duration of action. Phentolamine, a direct vasodilator and competitive a-adrenergic blocker, is efficient despite its association with tachyphylaxis and tachycardia.

Although nitroglycerin works well, it often needs to be taken in high doses and can make you tachycardic. For tumors that primarily secrete epinephrine, labetalol is preferred due to its higher b-blocking properties in comparison to a-blocking. Magnesium sulfate is a direct vasodilator, antiarrhythmic, and inhibits the release of catecholamines from the peripheral nerve terminals and the adrenal medulla. It also reduces receptor sensitivity to catecholamines. To control hypertension while manipulating a tumor, it is insufficient, as is all antihypertensive medications. Refractory hypertension has been suggested to be controlled with combinations of antihypertensive medications such as nitroprusside, esmolol, diltiazem, and phentolamine. Increasing the depth of anesthesia is also an option, but this approach can deepen the hypotension that accompany tumor vein ligation (Nölting et al., 2022; Srivastava & Naithani, 2022).

Treatment for arrhythmias, which are typically of ventricular origin, includes lidocaine or beta-blockers. Lidocaine has a negligible inotropic effect and a short half-life. Esmolol, a selective 1 blocker, has several benefits, although propranolol is frequently used. The quick onset and short half-life of Esmolol allow adequate heart rate control. As an alternative to beta blockers, amiodarone lengthens the duration of the action potential of the atrial and ventricular muscle, and has been used to treat supraventricular tachycardia caused by hypercatecholamimia (Srivastava & Naithani, 2022).

Following ligation of the tumor vein, hypotension occurs. A sudden decrease in plasma catecholamine levels, secondary vasodilation to phenoxybenzamine, intraoperative fluid, and blood loss are the cause of hypotension. To prevent hypotension, volume dilation with intravenous fluids should be achieved before tumor vein ligation (Jain et al., 2020). Fast-acting vasopressors may also be needed. Residual α-adrenergic blockade and down-regulation of receptors make patients relatively less sensitive to vasopressors. Blood products can cause hypertension secondary to the catecholamine content of blood. Hypotension can be managed by reducing the level of anesthesia. After resection, plasma catecholamine levels drop, insulin levels rise, and hypoglycemia can occur. If a bilateral adrenalectomy is performed or if hypoadrenalism is a concern, glucocorticoid medication should be started (García et al., 2019).

Cushing's Syndrome

The two types of Cushing's syndrome are ACTH-dependent and ACTH-independent. When plasma ACTH levels are abnormally high, as in ACTH-dependent Cushing's syndrome, the adrenal cortex is stimulated to create an excessive amount of cortisol. The excessive synthesis of cortisol by dysfunctional adrenocortical tissue, which is not controlled by CRH and ACTH secretion, is the cause of the ACTH independent type. CRH and ACTH levels are essentially suppressed in this type of Cushing's disease. Cushing's syndrome, which is caused by excessive ACTH release by pituitary ACTH tumors, is known as Cushing's disease. Another type of ACTH-dependent Cushing's syndrome is acute ectopic ACTH syndrome, which is typically associated with small cell lung cancer. Most commonly, benign or malignant adrenocortical tumors are the source of ACTH-independent Cushing's disease (Balomenaki et al., 2022).

Diagnosis and Treatment

The most common symptom is the relatively sudden onset of weight gain, moon faces, and telangiectasias. Systemic hypertension, glucose intolerance, oligomenorrhea, decreased libido, spontaneous ecchymoses, and weakness are common concomitant findings. The diagnosis of Cushing syndrome is confirmed by demonstrating cortisol hypersecretion based on 24-hour urinary secretion of cortisol. Reliable measurements of plasma ACTH are necessary to determine whether a patient's hypercortisolism is ACTH dependent or ACTH independent. The high-dose dexamethasone suppression test distinguishes Cushing disease from ectopic ACTH syndrome. Imaging procedures provide information about the location of a tumor (Balomenaki et al., 2022).

If a clearly delimited microadenoma can be detected, transsphenoidal microadenomectomy is the preferred treatment for those with Cushing disease. In some patients, pituitary irradiation and bilateral total adrenalectomy are required. Surgical removal of the adrenal gland is the treatment of adrenal adenoma or carcinoma (Ferriere & Tabarin, 2020).

Anesthesia Management

The physiological effects of excessive cortisol secretion should be considered. Systemic blood pressure, electrolyte balance, and blood sugar levels should be evaluated before surgery. Osteoporosis is an aspect to consider when positioning patients for the operative procedure. Preoperative drug therapy, induction of anesthesia, and the choice of maintenance of anesthesia are not affected by hypercortisolism. Etomidate may temporarily reduce the synthesis and release of cortisol from the cortex (Pence et al., 2022). Muscle relaxant doses should be initially reduced due to skeletal muscle weakness, which often accompanies hypercortisolism. In addition, the presence of hypokalemia can affect responses to nondepolarizing muscle relaxants. Mechanical ventilation is recommended during surgery because skeletal muscle weakness, with or without coexisting hypokalemia, can reduce the strength of the respiratory muscles. Regional anesthesia should be considered where appropriate. Cortisol levels decrease immediately after resection, and replacement therapy is advised. In patients, acute adrenal insufficiency may develop, which requires the initiation of additional therapy. Transient diabetes insipidus and meningitis may also occur after microadenomectomy (Yang, 2020).

Conn Syndrome

Conn syndrome occurs when there is excessive aldosterone secretion from a functional tumor that acts independently (Lee & Elaraj, 2019). The clinical manifestations are nonspecific. Systemic hypertension is a consequence of sodium retention due to aldosterone and increased volume of extracellular fluids. Aldosterone promotes kidney excretion of potassium, resulting in hypokalaemic metabolic alkalosis. Increased potassium excretion in urine (>30 mEq/day) indicates primary aldosteronism in the presence of hypokalemia. Hypokalaemic nephropathy can cause polyuria and loss of the ability to concentrate urine. Hypomagnesemia and abnormal glucose tolerance can also occur (El-Asmar et al., 2021).

Diagnosis and Treatment

Hypokalemia in the presence of systemic hypertension indicates aldosteronism. Almost all patients with untreated primary aldosteronism have decreased plasma renin activity. Plasma renin activity is elevated in secondary aldosteronism. Plasma aldosterone concentration less than 9.5 ng/dL at the end of a saline infusion excludes primary aldosteronism (Araujo-Castro, 2020).

The first treatment of hyperaldosteronism is the administration of potassium and spironolactone. Skeletal muscle weakness caused by hypokalemia may require intravenous potassium treatment. Systemic hypertension is treated with antihypertensive drugs. Hypokalemia caused by drug-induced diuresis is reduced by using a potassium-sparing diuretic, such as triamteren. The definitive treatment of an aldosterone-secreting tumor is surgical excision. If multiple tumors secreting aldosterone arc found, bilateral adrenalectomy may be required (Araujo-Castro, 2020).

Anesthesia Management

Management of anesthesia in the surgical treatment of hyperaldosteronism is facilitated by correction of hypopotassemia and treatment of hypertension. Persistent hypopotassemia alters responses to non-depolarizing muscle relaxants. Hyperventilation can reduce plasma potassium concentration and should be avoided. Inhalation agents or intravenous anesthetics can be chosen for the maintenance of anesthesia. Measurement of cardiac filling pressures with a right pulmonary artery catheter or monitoring with transesophageal echocardiography may be useful to assess the volume of intravascular fluid. Indicators of underlying hypovolemia include orthostatic hypotension. Plasma electrolyte concentrations and acid-base status should be measured frequently. Surgery to remove a single adrenal cortex adenoma is likely not necessary in this case, nor is exogenous cortisol replacement. However, exogenous cortisol administration may be necessary for bilateral surgery of the adrenal glands (Peramunage & Nikravan, 2020).

Hypoaldosteronism

Hyperpotassemia with normal renal functions suggests the presence of hypoaldosteronism. Hyperpotassemia might suddenly increase with hyperglycemia. Hyperchloremic metabolic acidosis is a predictable finding in the presence of hypoaldosteronism. Orthostatic hypotension, hyponatremia, and arrhythmias resulting from hyperpotassemia may also be present. Isolated lack of aldosterone secretion may be due to congenital aldosterone synthetase deficiency, hyporeninemia caused by defects of the juxtaglomerular apparatus, or treatment with ACE inhibitors, which prevents the stimulation of angiotensin. Patients with chronic kidney disease and/or diabetes mellitus older than 45 years often develop hyporeninemic hypoaldosteronism. This syndrome can be caused by reversible prostaglandin deficiency caused by indomethacin. Treatment of hypoaldosteronism involves a liberal sodium intake and daily administration of fludrocortisone (Husebye et al., 2021).

Adrenal Insufficiency

Adrenal insufficiency includes two types: primary and secondary. In Addison's disease, the adrenal glands cannot produce a sufficient amount of glucocorticoids, mineralocorticoids, and sex hormones. The destruction of both adrenal glands by an autoimmune disease is the most common cause of this rare endocrinopathy (Husebye et al., 2021). The onset of Addison's disease is insidious. Secondary adrenal insufficiency is caused by a failure in CRH or ACTH production caused by hypothalamic-pituitary disease, or by suppression of the hypothalamic-pituitary axis. Unlike Addison's disease, in secondary disease there is only a lack of glucocorticoids. One of the few hormones required for life is cortisol. It plays an important role in the metabolism of proteins and carbohydrates, the release of fatty acids, the maintenance of electrolyte and water balance, and the anti-inflammatory response. Catecholamine synthesis and action are facilitated; receptor synthesis, regulation, pairing, and sensitivity are modulated; and normal vascular permeability, adrenal gland glucocorticoid activity, corticosterone, and cortisone production are some of the activities influenced. Estimated daily cortisol secretion is equivalent to 15 to 25 mg/day or 5 to 7 mg / day of prednisone (Hahner et al., 2021).

Diagnosis and Treatment

The classic definition of adrenal insufficiency includes a low cortisol level that persists even after ACTH stimulation. (Martin-Grace et al., 2020). The most common cause of adrenal insufficiency is exogenous steroids. Long-term steroid users may exhibit signs and symptoms of adrenal insufficiency during periods of stress, such as surgery (Hahner et al., 2021). Recovery from short courses of steroids may take several days. For example, prednisone 25 mg PO twice daily for 5 days results in a reduced response to exogenous ACTH for 5 days. Preoperative glucocorticoid coverage should be provided for patients with adrenal insufficiency or adrenal suppression.

Patients medicated with > 2 g/day of topical steroids or more than 0.8 mg/day of inhaled steroids should be supplemented. In the event of adrenal insufficiency, patients should continue to receive regular steroid treatment in addition to intraoperative supplementation. Supplementation needs to be tailored according to the procedure. It may be wise to think about switching to methylprednisolone instead of hydrocortisone when dosages greater than 100 mg/day are given; due to its lower mineralocorticoid activity, it is less likely to result in fluid retention, edema, and hypopotassemia (Husebye et al., 2021; Woodcock et al., 2020).

Anesthesia Management

In the differential diagnosis of hemodynamic instability, adrenal insufficiency should be taken into account, particularly in patients who do not respond to conventional therapeutic interventions. Treatment options include addressing the underlying cause, replacing circulating glucocorticoids, and replacing sodium and sodium deficits. When replacing glucocorticoids, intravenous hydrocortisone, methylprednisolone, or dexamethasone may be used. Dexamethasone is preferred if ACTH stimulation testing is necessary to aid in the diagnosis of a primary or secondary disease because it does not affect cortisol levels. A viable treatment option is a 100 mg hydrocortisone bolus every 6 hours. Once the patient's condition has stabilized, the steroid dose is decreased and eventually an oral preparation is switched over. Volume deficits may be very large and vasopressor support for hemodynamic stability may be required (He et al., 2018). In the treatment of patients who have or are at risk of adrenal insufficiency, there is no one particular approach. However, etomidate briefly inhibits cortisol synthesis and should be avoided in this population of patients. When under emergency surgery, patients with untreated adrenal insufficiency should be aggressively managed with invasive monitoring, intravenous corticosteroids, and fluid and electrolyte resuscitation. Minimizing anesthetic and drug doses is advised due to the frequent inclusion in the clinical presentation of myocardial depression and weakness of the skeletal muscle (Traill & Halpern, 2018a).

Pituitary Gland Dysfunction

Vasopressin and oxytocin are synthesized in the hypothalamus and then stored in the posterior pituitary. Hormone release is triggered by plasma osmolarity (Dettmeyer, 2018).

The primary cause of excessive anterior pituitary hormone production is excessive ACTH secretion by anterior pituitary adenomas. Hypersecretion of other tropic hormones occurs rarely. Panhypopituitarism is more frequent than underproduction of a single anterior pituitary hormone. Panhypopituitarism symptoms are extremely varied and are dependent on hormone insufficiency. Amenorrhea and impotence are typically the first sign of global pituitary dysfunction. CT and magnetic resonance imaging are useful for evaluation in the pituitary gland (Dettmeyer, 2018).

Acromegaly

Diagnosis and Treatment

Acromegaly develops as a result of excessive growth hormone synthesis, which is often caused by an adenoma in the anterior pituitary gland. Insulin-like growth factor 1 is elevated in patients with acromegaly (Vilar et al., 2017).

The symptoms of acromegaly reflect both the peripheral effects of excess growth hormone and the parasellar spread of the anterior pituitary adenoma. The presence of headache and papilledema is a reflection of elevated intracranial pressure caused by the growth of the pituitary adenoma. Due to the expansion of the surrounding tissues, the optic chiasm may become compressed, causing visual disturbances. Patients are more likely to experience upper airway obstruction due to enlargement of their tongue and epiglottis. Overgrowth of surrounding cartilaginous structures can cause hoarseness, abnormal vocal cord movement, or recurrent laryngeal nerve paralysis. Involvement of the cricoarytenoid joints can also alter the patient's voice as a result of restricted movement of the vocal cord. Peripheral neuropathy is common. Inadequate collateral blood flow from the ulnar artery is present in hands in about 50% of patients with acromegaly. Diabetes mellitus and glucose intolerance may be present. Systemic hypertension, ischemic heart disease, osteoarthritis, and osteoporosis are more common in these patients. Increased lung volume and possible ventilation/perfusion mismatch. Skin becomes thick and greasy, skeletal muscle weakness can be visible, and fatigue complaints are frequent (Vilar et al., 2017; Zahr & Fleseriu, 2018).

The preferred initial treatment for pituitary adenomas is surgical transsphenoidal excision. Surgery or radiation therapy is no longer an option to treat adenomas that have grown beyond the sella turcica; instead, a long-acting somatostatin analog is recommended (Zahr & Fleseriu, 2018).

Anesthesia Management

Anesthetic management in patients with acromegaly is challenged by changes resulting from an overproduction of growth hormone. Specifically, significant changes are those in the upper airway. The positioning of an anesthetic face mask may be complicated by distorted facial anatomy. The enlarged tongue and epiglottis increase the risk of upper airway obstruction and obstruct the ability of direct laryngoscopy to see the vocal cords. Excess growth of the mandible causes an increase in the space between the lips and vocal cords. The expansion of the vocal cords may cause the glottic opening to close. This could require the use of a tracheal tube with a smaller inner diameter than anticipated for the patient's age and size, in addition to subglottic narrowing. The preoperative history of dyspnea, hoarseness, or stridor suggests involvement of the larynx with acromegaly. In this case, indirect laryngoscopy may be indicated to determine the degree of vocal cord dysfunction. When difficulty in placing a tracheal tube is anticipated, an awake fiberoptic tracheal intubation may be considered. When inserting a catheter into the radial artery, it is critical to consider the risk of insufficient collateral circulation at the wrist. In the case of diabetes mellitus or glucose intolerance, monitoring blood glucose concentrations is beneficial. Peripheral nerve stimulation is used to guide the administration of nondepolarizing muscle relaxants, particularly when there is skeletal muscle weakness (Nanjundaswamy & Sridhara, 2018; Smaily & Matar, 2020).

Diabetes Insipidus

Diabetes insipidus reflects the absence of vasopressin (ADH) due to destruction of the posterior pituitary (neurogenic DI) or failure of the renal tubules to respond to ADH (nephrogenic DI). Diabetes insipidus is characterized by polydipsia and high concentration urine output despite an increase in serum osmolarity. Diabetes insipidus due to pituitary gland surgery is usually transient (Lu, 2017). The initial treatment of diabetes insipidus consists of intravenous infusion of electrolyte solutions. Treatment of neurogenic diabetes insipidus is with desmopressin, which can be administered intranasally, in tablet form, or intravenously. Nephrogenic diabetes insipidus is treated with a low-salt, low-protein diet, diuretics, and NSAIDs (Christ-Crain et al., 2019).

Inappropriate Secretion of Antidiuretic Hormone

Inappropriate secretion of ADH can occur in the presence of various pathologic processes, including intracranial tumors, hypothyroidism, porphyria, and carcinoma of the lung. Inappropriate secretion of ADH is alleged to occur in most patients after major surgery. Increased urine sodium concentrations and urine osmolarity in the presence of hyponatremia, as well as reduced serum osmolarity, point to inadequate ADH production. Hyponatremia is due to dilution, reflecting the expansion of the intravascular fluid volume secondary to hormone-induced resorption of water by the renal tubules. Abrupt decreases in serum sodium concentration, especially to less than 110 mEq/L, can result in cerebral edema and seizures (Verbalis et al., 2016).

Treatment of inappropriate ADH secretion consists of restriction of oral fluid intake, high solute intake, and oral salt tablets. Furosemid, vasopressin receptor antagonists, and demeclocycline can also be used. Often, fluid restriction is sufficient treatment for inappropriate secretion of ADH not associated with symptoms secondary to hyponatremia. However, restriction of oral fluid intake and administration of demeclocycline are not immediately effective in the treatment of patients who manifest acute neurologic symptoms resulting from hyponatremia. In these patients, intravenous infusions of hypertonic saline sufficient to increase serum sodium concentrations are recommended. The optimal rate of correction for chronic hyponatremia should be less than 8 mEq/L in a 24-hour period. Overly rapid correction of chronic hyponatremia has been associated with central pontine myelinolysis, a type of brain cell dysfunction caused by the destruction of the myelin sheath of nerve cells in the brain stem (Verbalis et al., 2016).

Conclusion

In practice, the patient with an endocrine imbalance will present substantial obstacles to the anesthesiologist, but a basic understanding of the pathophysiological complexity will reduce the risks associated with these disorders during surgery and will lead to improved surgerical outcomes with successful anesthesia management. Careful and proactive hemodynamic management and foresight of the effects of surgical manipulation improve the management of pheochromocytoma during surgical resection. Similarly to this, better knowledge and early detection of carcinoid crisis have improved the perioperative management of carcinoid syndrome. The risks of thyroid surgery have decreased significantly thanks to advances in preoperative medical care. Finally, the perioperative risk associated with the new generation of sodium-glucose cotransporter 2 inhibitors must be recognized. Given the lack of evidence-based guidelines for the treatment of patients with endocrine disorders in the recent literature, further research should be considered to develop evidence-based guidelines for the treatment of patients with endocrine disorders.

References

Alore, E. A., Suliburk, J. W., Ramsey, D. J., Massarweh, N. N., Balentine, C. J., Singh, H., Awad, S. S., & Makris, K. I. (2019). Diagnosis and management of primary hyperparathyroidism across the Veterans Affairs health care system. *JAMA internal medicine*, *179*(9), 1220-1227. https://doi.org/10.1001/jamainternmed.2019.1747.

Amodru, V., Taieb, D., Guerin, C., Romanet, P., Paladino, N., Brue, T., Cuny, T., Barlier, A., Sebag, F., & Castinetti, F. (2020). MEN2-related pheochromocytoma: current state of knowledge, specific characteristics in MEN2B, and perspectives. *Endocrine*, *69*(3), 496-503. https://doi.org/10.1007/s12020-020-02332-2.

Araujo-Castro, M. (2020). Treatment of primary hyperaldosteronism. *Medicina Clínica, 155*(7), 302-308. https://doi.org/10.1016/j.medcle.2020.04.022.

Araujo-Castro, M., Pascual-Corrales, E., Nattero Chavez, L., Martínez Lorca, A., Alonso-Gordoa, T., Molina-Cerrillo, J., Lorca Álvaro, J., Mínguez Ojeda, C., Redondo López, S., & Barberá Durbán, R. (2021). Protocol for presurgical and anesthetic management of pheochromocytomas and sympathetic paragangliomas: A multidisciplinary approach. *Journal of Endocrinological Investigation*, *44*(12), 2545-2555. https://doi.org/10.1007/s40618-021-01649-7.

American Diabetes Association (2009). Standards of medical care in diabetes—2009. *Diabetes care*, *32*(Suppl 1), S13. https://doi.org/10.2337/dc09-S013.

Bagry, H. S., Raghavendran, S., Carli, F., Warner, D. S., & Warner, M. A. (2008). Metabolic syndrome and insulin resistance: perioperative considerations. *The Journal of the American Society of Anesthesiologists*, *108*(3), 506-523. https://doi.org/10.1097/ALN.0b013e3181649314.

Balomenaki, M., Margaritopoulos, D., Vassiliadi, D. A., & Tsagarakis, S. (2022). Diagnostic workup of Cushing's syndrome. *Journal of Neuroendocrinology*, *34*(8), e13111. https://doi.org/10.1111/jne.13111.

Bartalena, L., Piantanida, E., Gallo, D., Ippolito, S., & Tanda, M. L. (2022). Management of Graves' hyperthyroidism: present and future. *Expert Review of Endocrinology & Metabolism*, *17*(2), 153-166. https://doi.org/10.1080/17446651.2022.2052044.

Bauer, M. B., & Currie, K. P. (2020). Adrenal Medulla Hormones. In *Hormonal Signaling in Biology and Medicine* (pp. 635-653). Elsevier. https://doi.org/10.1016/B978-0-12-813814-4.00029-8.

Bilezikian, J. P., Khan, A. A., Silverberg, S. J., Fuleihan, G. E. H., Marcocci, C., Minisola, S., Perrier, N., Sitges-Serra, A., Thakker, R. V., & Guyatt, G. (2022a). Evaluation and management of primary hyperparathyroidism: summary statement and guidelines from the Fifth International Workshop. *Journal of Bone and Mineral Research*, *37*(11), 2293-2314. https://doi.org/10.1002/jbmr.4677.

Bilezikian, J. P., Silverberg, S. J., Bandeira, F., Cetani, F., Chandran, M., Cusano, N. E., Ebeling, P. R., Formenti, A. M., Frost, M., & Gosnell, J. (2022b). Management of primary hyperparathyroidism. *Journal of Bone and Mineral Research*, *37*(11), 2391-2403. https://doi.org/10.1002/jbmr.4682.

Biondi, B., & Cooper, D. S. (2019). Thyroid hormone therapy for hypothyroidism. *Endocrine*, *66*(1), 18-26. https://doi.org/10.1007/s12020-019-02023-7.

Bode, J., Stewart, H., Ballenger, A., Boutwell, G., & Zaky, A. (2022). 453 Efficacy of the Insulin Infusion Calculator Protocol in the Optimization of Perioperative Blood Glucose Levels in the Cardiac Surgical Patients at UAB. *Journal of Clinical and Translational Science*, *6*(s1), 90-90. https://doi.org/10.1017/cts.2022.266.

Cely, C. M., Arora, P., Quartin, A. A., Kett, D. H., & Schein, R. M. (2004). Relationship of baseline glucose homeostasis to hyperglycemia during medical critical illness. *Chest*, *126*(3), 879-887. https://doi.org/10.1378/chest.126.3.879.

Chahardahmasumi, E., Salehidoost, R., Amini, M., Aminorroaya, A., Rezvanian, H., Kachooei, A., Iraj, B., Nazem, M., & Kolahdoozan, M. (2019). Assessment of the early and late complication after thyroidectomy. *Advanced biomedical research*, *8*. https://doi.org/10.4103/abr.abr_3_19.

Chen, W. H., & Chen, C. Y. (2022). Clinicopathologic characteristics of incidental thyroid carcinoma in euthyroid patients receiving total thyroidectomy for multinodular goiter: A retrospective cohort study. *Journal of the Chinese Medical Association*, *85*(8), 839-844. https://doi.org/10.1097/JCMA.0000000000000758.

Chiovato, L., Magri, F., & Carlé, A. (2019). Hypothyroidism in context: where we've been and where we're going. *Advances in therapy*, *36*(2), 47-58. https://doi.org/10.1007/s12325-019-01080-8.

Christ-Crain, M., Bichet, D. G., Fenske, W. K., Goldman, M. B., Rittig, S., Verbalis, J. G., & Verkman, A. S. (2019). Diabetes insipidus. *Nature Reviews Disease Primers*, *5*(1), 1-20. https://doi.org/10.1038/s41572-019-0103-2.

de Mul, N., Damstra, J., van Dijkum, E. J. N., Fischli, S., Kalkman, C. J., Schellekens, W. J. M., & Immink, R. V. (2021). Risk of perioperative thyroid storm in hyperthyroid patients: a systematic review. *British Journal of Anaesthesia*, *127*(6), 879-889. https://doi.org/10.1016/j.bja.2021.06.043.

De Weille, J., Schmid-Antomarchi, H., Fosset, M., & Lazdunski, M. (1988). ATP-sensitive K+ channels that are blocked by hypoglycemia-inducing sulfonylureas in insulin-secreting cells are activated by galanin, a hyperglycemia-inducing hormone. *Proceedings of the National Academy of Sciences*, *85*(4), 1312-1316. https://doi.org/10.1073/pnas.85.4.1312.

Dettmeyer, R. B. (2018). Endocrine Organs. In *Forensic Histopathology* (pp. 419-439). Springer. https://doi.org/10.1007/978-3-319-77997-3_16.

Egalini, F., Marinelli, L., Rossi, M., Motta, G., Prencipe, N., Rossetto Giaccherino, R., Pagano, L., Grottoli, S., & Giordano, R. (2022). Endocrine disrupting chemicals: effects on pituitary, thyroid and adrenal glands. *Endocrine*, 1-11. https://doi.org/10.1007/s12020-022-03076-x.

El-Asmar, N., Rajpal, A., & Arafah, B. M. (2021). Primary Hyperaldosteronism: Approach to Diagnosis and Management. *Medical Clinics*, *105*(6), 1065-1080. https://doi.org/10.1016/j.mcna.2021.06.007.

Fagundes, G. F., & Almeida, M. Q. (2022). Perioperative Management of Pheochromocytomas and Sympathetic Paragangliomas. *Journal of the Endocrine Society*, *6*(2), bvac004. https://doi.org/10.1210/jendso/bvac004.

Fernandez-Robles, C., Carr, Z. J., & Oprea, A. D. (2021). Endocrine emergencies in anesthesia. *Current Opinion in Anesthesiology*, *34*(3), 326-334. https://doi.org/10.1097/ACO.0000000000000986.

Ferriere, A., & Tabarin, A. (2020). Cushing's syndrome: treatment and new therapeutic approaches. *Best Practice & Research Clinical Endocrinology & Metabolism*, *34*(2), 101381. https://doi.org/10.1016/j.beem.2020.101381.

Gafni, R. I., & Collins, M. T. (2019). Hypoparathyroidism. *New England journal of medicine*, *380*(18), 1738-1747. https://doi.org/10.1056/NEJMcp1800213.

Galicia-Garcia, U., Benito-Vicente, A., Jebari, S., Larrea-Sebal, A., Siddiqi, H., Uribe, K. B., Ostolaza, H., & Martín, C. (2020). Pathophysiology of type 2 diabetes mellitus. *International journal of molecular sciences*, *21*(17), 6275. https://doi.org/10.3390/ijms21176275.

García, M. I. D. O., Palasí, R., Gómez, R. C., Marco, J. L. P., & Merino-Torres, J. F. (2019). Surgical and pharmacological management of functioning pheochromocytoma and paraganglioma. *Exon Publications*, 63-80. https://doi.org/10.15586/paraganglioma.2019.ch4.

Hahner, S., Ross, R. J., Arlt, W., Bancos, I., Burger-Stritt, S., Torpy, D. J., Husebye, E. S., & Quinkler, M. (2021). Adrenal insufficiency. *Nature Reviews Disease Primers*, *7*(1), 1-24. https://doi.org/10.1038/s41572-021-00252-7.

He, X., Findling, J. W., & Auchus, R. J. (2018). Diagnosis and management of adrenal insufficiency. In *Adrenal Disorders* (pp. 199-215). Springer. https://doi.org/10.1007/978-3-319-62470-9_9.

Herman, M. A., & Kahn, B. B. (2006). Glucose transport and sensing in the maintenance of glucose homeostasis and metabolic harmony. *The Journal of clinical investigation*, *116*(7), 1767-1775. https://doi.org/10.1172/JCI29027.

Hoermann, R., Midgley, J. E., Larisch, R., & Dietrich, J. W. (2019). Individualised requirements for optimum treatment of hypothyroidism: complex needs, limited options. *Drugs in context*, *8*. https://doi.org/10.7573/dic.212597.

Husebye, E. S., Pearce, S. H., Krone, N. P., & Kämpe, O. (2021). Adrenal insufficiency. *The Lancet*, *397*(10274), 613-629. https://doi.org/10.1016/S0140-6736(21)00136-7.

Idrees, S., Ahmed, F., & Mayilvaganan, S. (2021). Post-thyroidectomy Bleeding. *Indian Journal of Endocrine Surgery and Research*, *16*(1), 18. https://doi.org/10.5005/jp-journals-10088-11161.

Ilias, I., & Meristoudis, G. (2019). A Bayesian look at the new 2019 guidelines for imaging of pheochromocytoma/paraganglioma with emphasis on extra-adrenal disease. *Hellenic Journal of Nuclear Medicine*, *22*(2), 142-142. https://doi.org/10.1967/s002449911009.

Inzucchi, S. E. (2006). Management of hyperglycemia in the hospital setting. *New England journal of medicine*, *355*(18), 1903-1911. https://doi.org/10.1056/NEJMcp060094.

Jain, A., Baracco, R., & Kapur, G. (2020). Pheochromocytoma and paraganglioma—an update on diagnosis, evaluation, and management. *Pediatric Nephrology*, *35*(4), 581-594. https://doi.org/10.1007/s00467-018-4181-2.

Kapre, V., Deshmukh, S., Deshmukh, P., Sarode, M., & Chaudhary, R. (2020). Anesthesia for Thyroid Surgery. In *Thyroid Surgery* (pp. 57-66). CRC Press. https://doi.org/10.1201/9780429086076-7.

Khan, A. A., Guyatt, G., Ali, D. S., Bilezikian, J. P., Collins, M. T., Dandurand, K., Mannstadt, M., Murphy, D., M'Hiri, I., & Rubin, M. R. (2022). Management of hypoparathyroidism. *Journal of Bone and Mineral Research*. https://doi.org/10.1002/jbmr.4716.

Lee, F. T., & Elaraj, D. (2019). Evaluation and management of primary hyperaldosteronism. *Surgical Clinics*, *99*(4), 731-745. https://doi.org/10.1016/j.suc.2019.04.010.

Leung, A. A., Pasieka, J. L., Hyrcza, M. D., Pacaud, D., Dong, Y., Boyd, J. M., Sadrzadeh, H., & Kline, G. A. (2021). Epidemiology of pheochromocytoma and paraganglioma: population-based cohort study. *European Journal of Endocrinology*, *184*(1), 19-28. https://doi.org/10.1530/EJE-20-0628.

Lipshutz, A. K., Gropper, M. A., Warner, D. S., & Warner, M. A. (2009). Perioperative glycemic control: an evidence-based review. *The Journal of the American Society of*

Anesthesiologists, *110*(2), 408-421. https://doi.org/10.1097/ALN.0b013e3181948a80.

Lu, H. (2017). Diabetes insipidus. *Aquaporins*, 213-225. https://doi.org/10.1007/978-94-024-1057-0_14.

Malhotra, B., & Bhadada, S. K. (2022). Perioperative Management for Non-Thyroidal Surgery in Thyroid Dysfunction. *Indian Journal of Endocrinology and Metabolism*, *26*(5), 428-434. https://doi.org/10.4103/ijem.ijem_273_22.

Marques, J. V. O., & Moreira, C. A. (2020). Primary hyperparathyroidism. *Best Practice & Research Clinical Rheumatology*, *34*(3), 101514. https://doi.org/10.1016/j.berh.2020.101514.

Martin-Grace, J., Dineen, R., Sherlock, M., & Thompson, C. J. (2020). Adrenal insufficiency: Physiology, clinical presentation and diagnostic challenges. *Clinica chimica acta*, *505*, 78-91. https://doi.org/10.1016/j.cca.2020.01.029.

Mizobuchi, M., Ogata, H., & Koiwa, F. (2019). Secondary hyperparathyroidism: pathogenesis and latest treatment. *Therapeutic Apheresis and Dialysis*, *23*(4), 309-318. https://doi.org/10.1111/1744-9987.12772.

Nanjundaswamy, N. H., & Sridhara, R. B. (2018). Perioperative management of patients with acromegaly-a retrospective analysis. *International Journal of Research in Medical Sciences*, *6*(2), 515-520. https://doi.org/10.18203/2320-6012.ijrms20180290.

Neumann, H. P., Young Jr, W. F., & Eng, C. (2019). Pheochromocytoma and paraganglioma. *New England journal of medicine*, *381*(6), 552-565. https://doi.org/10.1056/NEJMra1806651.

Nölting, S., Bechmann, N., Taieb, D., Beuschlein, F., Fassnacht, M., Kroiss, M., Eisenhofer, G., Grossman, A., & Pacak, K. (2022). Personalized management of pheochromocytoma and paraganglioma. *Endocrine Reviews*, *43*(2), 199-239. https://doi.org/10.1210/endrev/bnab019.

Pãduraru, D. N., Ion, D., Carsote, M., Andronic, O., & Bolocan, A. (2019). Post-thyroidectomy hypocalcemia-risk factors and management. *Chirurgia*, *114*(5), 564-570. https://doi.org/10.21614/chirurgia.114.5.564.

Pan, Y., Chen, C., Yu, L., Zhu, S., & Zheng, Y. (2020). Airway Management of Retrosternal Goiters in 22 Cases in a Tertiary Referral Center. *Therapeutics and Clinical Risk Management*, *16*, 1267. https://doi.org/10.2147/TCRM.S281709.

Pasieka, J. L., Wentworth, K., Yeo, C. T., Cremers, S., Dempster, D., Fukumoto, S., Goswami, R., Houillier, P., Levine, M. A., & Pasternak, J. D. (2022). Etiology and pathophysiology of hypoparathyroidism: a narrative review. *Journal of Bone and Mineral Research*. https://doi.org/10.1002/jbmr.4714.

Pence, A., McGrath, M., Lee, S. L., & Raines, D. E. (2022). Pharmacological management of severe Cushing's syndrome: the role of etomidate. *Therapeutic Advances in Endocrinology and Metabolism*, *13*, 20420188211058583. https://doi.org/10.1177/20420188211058583.

Peramunage, D., & Nikravan, S. (2020). Anesthesia for endocrine emergencies. *Anesthesiology Clinics*, *38*(1), 149-163. https://doi.org/10.1016/j.anclin.2019.10.006.

Puskas, F., Grocott, H. P., White, W. D., Mathew, J. P., Newman, M. F., & Bar-Yosef, S. (2007). Intraoperative hyperglycemia and cognitive decline after CABG. *The Annals of thoracic surgery*, *84*(5), 1467-1473. https://doi.org/10.1016/j.athoracsur.2007.06.023.

Rui, Z. Y., Yin, X., Wang, X., Shen, J., & Zheng, W. (2022). A retrospective study of clinical features and prognosis of patients with Graves' disease and ophthalmopathy. *Nuclear Medicine Communications*, 10.1097. https://doi.org/10.1097/MNM.0000000000001649.

Saltiel, A. R., & Kahn, C. R. (2001). Insulin signalling and the regulation of glucose and lipid metabolism. *Nature*, *414*(6865), 799-806. https://doi.org/10.1038/414799a.

Sbardella, E., & Grossman, A. B. (2020). Pheochromocytoma: an approach to diagnosis. *Best Practice & Research Clinical Endocrinology & Metabolism*, *34*(2), 101346. https://doi.org/10.1016/j.beem.2019.101346.

Schricker, T., Galeone, M., Wykes, L., & Carli, F. (2004). Effect of desflurane/remifentanil anaesthesia on glucose metabolism during surgery: a comparison with desflurane/epidural anaesthesia. *Acta anaesthesiologica scandinavica*, *48*(2), 169-173. https://doi.org/10.1111/j.0001-5172.2004.00297.x.

Shahid, M. A., Ashraf, M. A., & Sharma, S. (2022). Physiology, thyroid hormone. In *StatPearls [Internet]*. StatPearls Publishing.

Singh, M., Kapoor, D., Dalal, A. K., Gupta, D., Kang, A., Kumar, A. A., & Singh, N. P. (2022). Perioperative Management of a Rare Pancreatic Insulinoma Resection: Anaesthetic Challenge! *Archives of Anesthesiology and Critical Care*, *8*(1), 79-82. https://doi.org/10.18502/aacc.v8i1.8249.

Smaily, H., & Matar, N. (2020). Laryngeal manifestations in acromegaly: A systematic review of the literature. *Acta Oto-Laryngologica Case Reports*, *5*(1), 57-63. https://doi.org/10.1080/23772484.2020.1809421.

Srivastava, D., & Naithani, B. (2022). Anesthetic Management for Pheochromocytoma. In *Endocrine Surgery* (pp. 396-402). CRC Press. https://doi.org/10.1201/9780429197338-53.

Talha, A., Houssam, B., & Brahim, H. (2020). Myxedema coma: a review. *European Journal of Medical and Health Sciences*, *2*(3). https://doi.org/10.24018/ejmed.2020.2.3.349.

Tang, C. J., & Hennessey, J. V. (2020). Perioperative Management of Patients with Hyperthyroidism or Hypothyroidism Undergoing Nonthyroidal Surgery. In *Handbook of Inpatient Endocrinology* (pp. 85-99). Springer. https://doi.org/10.1007/978-3-030-38976-5_8.

Taniguchi, C. M., Emanuelli, B., & Kahn, C. R. (2006). Critical nodes in signalling pathways: insights into insulin action. *Nature reviews Molecular cell biology*, *7*(2), 85-96. https://doi.org/10.1038/nrm1837.

Taylor, P. N., Albrecht, D., Scholz, A., Gutierrez-Buey, G., Lazarus, J. H., Dayan, C. M., & Okosieme, O. E. (2018). Global epidemiology of hyperthyroidism and hypothyroidism. *Nature Reviews Endocrinology*, *14*(5), 301-316. https://doi.org/10.1038/nrendo.2018.18.

Traill, C., & Halpern, S. H. (2018a). Adrenal Insufficiency. In *Consults in Obstetric Anesthesiology* (pp. 17-19). Springer. https://doi.org/10.1007/978-3-319-59680-8_5.

Traill, C., & Halpern, S. H. (2018b). Hypoparathyroidism. In *Consults in Obstetric Anesthesiology* (pp. 299-301). Springer. https://doi.org/10.1007/978-3-319-59680-8_85.

Uslu, A., Okut, G., Tercan, I. C., Erkul, Z., Aykas, A., Karatas, M., Simsek, C., & Tatar, E. (2019). Anatomical distribution and number of parathyroid glands, and parathyroid function, after total parathyroidectomy and bilateral cervical thymectomy. *Medicine*, *98*(23). https://doi.org/10.1097/MD.0000000000015926.

Verbalis, J. G., Greenberg, A., Burst, V., Haymann, J. P., Johannsson, G., Peri, A., Poch, E., Chiodo III, J. A., & Dave, J. (2016). Diagnosing and treating the syndrome of inappropriate antidiuretic hormone secretion. *The American journal of medicine*, *129*(5), 537. e539-537. e523. https://doi.org/10.1016/j.amjmed.2015.11.005.

Verma, R., & Dwivedi, Y. (2022). Anesthesia for Thyroid and Parathyroid Surgery. In *Endocrine Surgery* (pp. 315-319). CRC Press. https://doi.org/10.1201/9780429197338-41.

Vilar, L., Vilar, C. F., Lyra, R., Lyra, R., & Naves, L. A. (2017). Acromegaly: clinical features at diagnosis. *Pituitary*, *20*(1), 22-32. https://doi.org/10.1007/s11102-016-0772-8.

Wang, Y., Sun, Y., Yang, B., Wang, Q., & Kuang, H. (2022). The management and metabolic characterization: hyperthyroidism and hypothyroidism. *Neuropeptides*, 102308. https://doi.org/10.1016/j.npep.2022.102308.

Wood, I. S., & Trayhurn, P. (2003). Glucose transporters (GLUT and SGLT): expanded families of sugar transport proteins. *British journal of nutrition*, *89*(1), 3-9. https://doi.org/10.1079/BJN2002763.

Woodcock, T., Barker, P., Daniel, S., Fletcher, S., Wass, J., Tomlinson, J., Misra, U., Dattani, M., Arlt, W., & Vercueil, A. (2020). Guidelines for the management of glucocorticoids during the peri-operative period for patients with adrenal insufficiency: Guidelines from the Association of Anaesthetists, the Royal College of Physicians and the Society for Endocrinology UK. *Anaesthesia*, *75*(5), 654-663. https://doi.org/10.1111/anae.14963.

Y-Hassan, S., & Falhammar, H. (2020). Cardiovascular manifestations and complications of pheochromocytomas and paragangliomas. *Journal of clinical medicine*, *9*(8), 2435. https://doi.org/10.3390/jcm9082435.

Yamakawa, H., Kato, T. S., Noh, J. Y., Yuasa, S., Kawamura, A., Fukuda, K., & Aizawa, Y. (2021). Thyroid hormone plays an important role in cardiac function: from bench to bedside. *Frontiers in physiology*, *12*. https://doi.org/10.3389/fphys.2021.606931.

Yang, H. (2020). Management of Patient with Pituitary Tumor (Cushing's Disease). In *Problem Based Learning Discussions in Neuroanesthesia and Neurocritical Care* (pp. 179-190). Springer. https://doi.org/10.1007/978-981-15-0458-7_15.

Yao, L., Guyatt, G., Ye, Z., Bilezikian, J. P., Brandi, M. L., Clarke, B. L., Mannstadt, M., & Khan, A. A. (2022). Methodology for the guidelines on evaluation and management of hypoparathyroidism and primary hyperparathyroidism. *Journal of Bone and Mineral Research*, *37*(11), 2404-2410. https://doi.org/10.1002/jbmr.4687.

Zahr, R., & Fleseriu, M. (2018). Updates in diagnosis and treatment of acromegaly. *European endocrinology*, *14*(2), 57. https://doi.org/10.17925/EE.2018.14.2.57.

Chapter 9

Neurological Insufficiencies and Anesthesia

Sadık Özmen[1], MD
and Yasin Tire[2,3,*], MD

[1]Department of Anesthesia and Reanimation, Antalya Training and Research Hospital, University of Health Sciences, Antalya, Turkiye
[2]Department of Anesthesiology and Reanimation, Konya City Hospital, University of Health Sciences, Konya, Turkiye
[3]Outcomes Research Consortium, Cleveland Clinic, Cleveland, OH, USA

Abstract

This chapter aims to provide information on the clinical features, etiology, and impact of common neurological disorders and deficiencies for anesthesia in adults, as well as the impact that these disorders have on the management of anesthesia. The topic areas in this chapter are ordered based on a combination of prevalence statistics and typical referral questions in general anesthesia clinics. This is done even though the types of neurological disorders seen in practice vary from many different variables (clinician specialty area, age range of the patients, systemic and regional issues, type, and practice affiliation). Dementia, epilepsy, multiple sclerosis, Parkinson's disease, stroke, and traumatic brain injury are some of the diseases covered in this chapter. Anesthesiologists, despite the fact that each of these disorders is unique, are frequently required to think flexibly about the characteristics of anesthesia management.

Keywords: neurological disorders, neuro-anesthesia, brain damage, intracranial pressure, cerebral perfusion

---

* Corresponding Author's Email: dryasintire@hotmail.com.

In: Organ Failure and Anesthesia Practices
Editors: Ahmet Şen and Basar Erdivanli
ISBN: 979-8-89113-486-7

Introduction

Neurological illnesses have been underestimated for decades in global health (Canna & Seligman, 2020). This study showed that the burden of neurological disorders is significantly underestimated by conventional epidemiological and health statistical approaches, which only take mortality rates and ignore disability rates. In particular in low-income and emerging countries, there were disproportionately few neurological services and resources available. Unpredictable increases in neurological and other chronic conditions, as well as impairment from increased life expectancy and global population aging, are all things that governments and healthcare professionals may not be ready to handle, according to a significant body of evidence (Breslow, 2002; pdf, 1948). This chapter on anesthesia management of neurological illnesses was published in response to their challenges. Its goal is to strengthen professional management and severity and concentrate neurological treatment in operating rooms and intensive care units.

Dementia

Dementia disrupts multiple higher cortical processes, including memory, thinking, orientation, comprehension, computation, learning ability, language, and judgment. The mind is unobscured. Dementia doubles every five years in people 65 to 90 years (Jorm & Jolley, 1998). The prevalence doubles every five years after this.

Preoperative Evaluation and Management

Patients with dementia have more comorbidities such as cardiovascular disease, chronic obstructive lung disease, and renal failure, increasing the risk of postoperative complications. In a large retrospective study, patients with dementia experienced greater postoperative complications (pneumonia, urinary tract infection, stroke, septicemia, and acute renal failure) (Hu et al., 2012). Dementia and frailty are linked; however, most frailty criteria do not involve cognitive impairment (Kulmala et al., 2014). Polypharmacy and medication interactions rise. Thus, preoperative examination should focus on the patient's functional status. A multidisciplinary team should decide on dementia surgery that improves quality of life. After preoperative examination, comorbidities should be optimized, medications reviewed, and the ward should be informed of room allocation.

Drug Interactions

Treatment of dementia involves acetylcholinesterase inhibitors. Alzheimer's sufferers have fewer central cholinergic neurons, which may explain their cognitive decline (Fodale et al., 2006). Tacrine, used in anesthesia to reverse neuromuscular block and extend succinylcholine paralysis, was one of the first dementia treatments. Later-generation anticholinesterases like donepezil and rivastigmine used to treat dementia prolong depolarizing neuromuscular blockers and diminish or reverse nondepolarizing ones (Bhardwaj et al., 2011; Crowe & Collins, 2003). Before proceeding with elective surgery, acetylcholinesterase inhibitors should be stopped being taken (Blood, 2012).

Because their respective half-lives are 7–8 hours and 3–4 hours, galantamine and rivastigmine can be stopped a day before surgery. The 70-hour half-life of donepezil requires a washout period of two to three weeks. Due to the potential for irreparable cognitive decline during this period of time without therapy, it is important that this medication be maintained or discontinued prior to any elective surgery. In emergency surgery, anesthesiologists should avoid neuromuscular blocking medications and be careful of drug combinations. There are two neuromuscular blocking drugs that do not cause depolarization in the body. Neostigmine, which may be ineffective due to preexisting cholinesterase inhibition or may extend neuromuscular block via a Phase II-type interaction with succinylcholine, should be replaced with short-acting, spontaneously inactivated drugs such as atracurium and cisatracurium. Sugammadex reliably reverses rocuronium and vecuronium. The safest quick sequence induction alternative for these patients is rocuronium and sugammadex, which avoids the protracted paralysis caused by succinylcholine. Cholinesterase inhibitors and other dementia drugs that improve cognition and behavioral symptoms can interact with anesthetics and increase perioperative problems (Table 1). These patients do not take herbal therapies such as Ginkgo Biloba. Ginkgo leaf is used to treat memory loss; however, taking it within two weeks before surgery may affect platelet function and hemostasis.

Table 1. Some medicines used to treat dementia and its symptoms, as well as their perioperative interactions

Drug group	Indication	Interaction	Example
NMDA receptor antagonists	Cognitive impairment	Enhances side effects of anticholinergic and dopaminergic agonists	Memantine
Herbal medicines	Cognitive impairment	Increases the risk of bleeding—interferes with platelet function	Ginkgo Biloba
Serotonin reuptake inhibitors (SSRI)	Depressive symptoms	Increased risk of serotonin syndrome and enhances effects of opiates and induction agents	Citalopram
Benzodiazepines	For symptoms of agitation, fear	Potentiates effects of anesthetics	Lorazepam
Atypical antipsychotics	For symptoms of aggression, restlessness, hallucinations	Enhances the risk of vasodilation and hypotension with anesthetics	Risperidone
Antiepileptics	Behavioral symptoms, including aggression	Potentiates effects of anesthetics and opioids	Carbamazepine

The Sensitivity of Anesthetic Agents

Dementia may enhance the slow wave and decrease the quick wave EEG activity. This lowers awake BIS scores relative to normal patients. The researchers found that cognitively challenged individuals should not use the BIS target value for sufficient anesthesia. A recent retrospective case-control investigation did not show variation in volatile anesthetic sensitivity in dementia patients (Perez-Protto et al., 2014). An acute state of disorientation known as delirium is characterized by inattention, altered consciousness, disorganized thought, and changing time. Delirium can also cause involuntary movements. Delirium is seen more frequently in elderly people with dementia who are hospitalized (59 versus 13% in one research) (Margiotta et al., 2006).

Analyzing and Treating Pain

Dementia, visual and hearing problems, and age-related physiology can make pain assessment problematic in patients with dementia. Studies show that cognitively impaired patients receive less analgesia for equivalent operational procedures due to their inability to verbalize discomfort or seek more (Lynn et al., 2009). Studies using functional magnetic resonance imaging to examine brain activity in dementia patients in relation to pain experience have shown that pain perception and processing are unaffected by the condition (Cole et al., 2006). Thus, early identification of pain prevents undertreatment. Dementia is not all-or-nothing. Hence, many techniques are needed to quantify pain in people with different cognitive impairments. A verbal rating scale (e.g., "Is your pain mild, moderate, or severe?") beats a numerical scale for mild to moderate cognitive impairment. Severe cognitive impairment: Online observational methods like the Abbey Pain Scale can score pain as absent, mild, moderate, or severe. If pain evaluation is challenging, an empirical analgesia trial may be needed. Analgesia should be provided regularly to this group of patients. When necessary, opioid analgesia should not be avoided, although the risk of side effects, including delirium, is increased. The low-and-slow approach is advised. Intravenous low-dose fentanyl/alfentanil infusions, transdermal patches, or oral controlled-release preparations with breakthrough dosages are better than patient-controlled analgesia. Regional and local anesthetic, including implantation of a perineural catheter, should always be considered to limit opioid use.

Is There a Correlation between Dementia and the Use of Anesthesia or Surgery?

Although much is unknown, anesthesia and surgery can have long-term neurological effects. Anesthesia medicines, especially volatiles, may cause Alzheimer's disease plaques by polymerizing amyloid (A) peptide monomers into oligomers. Nuclear magnetic resonance spectroscopy has indicated that the molecular size of the anesthetic agent influences oligomerization, with propofol having no effect and desflurane having the least (Silverstein, 2014). Surgical stress and the pro-inflammatory condition caused by major surgery can promote cognitive impairment through cortisol and IL6. Regional anesthesia may minimize exposure to anesthetic medicines in this population, which may promote postoperative cognitive damage. If general anesthesia is necessary, reduce the dose and duration. However, these recommendations have not been proven.

Epilepsy

Epilepsy is a chronic neurological disorder that can affect anyone, anywhere. Epileptic seizures are a category of disorders that share symptoms. Brain trauma—systemic, chemical, or metabolic—can cause these seizures. These provoked or acute symptomatic seizures may not reoccur if the underlying cause is treated or the acute phase ends (Banerjee et al., 2009).

AEDs' (Anti-Epileptic Drugs) Underlying Mechanisms of Action

The imbalance of excitatory and inhibitory neuronal activity in the brain causes a seizure. Thus, many cortical neurons fire hypersynchronously. Traditional AEDs decrease glutamate and aspartate levels, increase GABA, and decrease inward voltage-gated positive currents (Na^{+}, Ca^{+2}). New AEDs often operate in unique ways. Novel drug-binding sites include retigabine, ganaxolone, and levetiracetam (Rogawski et al., 2008).

Anesthetic Impact of Antiepileptic Drugs

AEDs and anesthetic medicines interact pharmacologically and dynamically. These factors affect the efficacy of medications and the risk of seizures related to surgery (Anderson & Moor, 2010). AEDs induce and inhibit hepatic cytochrome P450 isoenzymes, the main mechanism of drug interactions. Older AEDs such as carbamazepine, phenytoin, phenobarbital, and primidone induce enzymes. Amiodarone, b-blockers (propranolol and metoprolol), and calcium channel antagonists (nifedipine, felodipine, nimodipine and verapamil) lower plasma concentrations (Patsalos & Perucca, 2003). Before starting or stopping enzyme-inducing AEDs, warfarin patients must monitor their international normalized ratio. Topiramate dose-dependently stimulates hepatic microsomal enzymes. Valproate inhibits hepatic microsomal enzyme systems, which can reduce the clearance of numerous drugs, including other AEDs. A macrolide antibiotic, erythromycin, strongly inhibits CYP3A4. Inhibition of this enzyme causes carbamazepine toxicity. Valproate serum levels can drop significantly when taken with carbapenem antibiotics (Haroutiunian et al., 2009; Mancl & Gidal, 2009).

Epilepsy and the Use of Anesthetics

Many drugs have pro- and anticonvulsant effects, which may impact the anesthetic choice (Kofke, 2010).

Inhalational Anesthetics

Nitrous oxide (N_2O) has caused seizures in cats, but not in people. Mice briefly exposed to N_2O have had withdrawal seizures (Vaughn & Pruhs, 1995). N2O decreased epileptiform activity during electrocorticographic monitoring for epilepsy surgery, but when removed, it returned (Artru et al., 1990). Hyperbaric (1.5 atm) N_2O, coupled with isoflurane or halothane, caused myoclonus in volunteers (Hornbein et al., 1982). There have been multiple reports of seizures or seizure-like activity being induced by sevoflurane, most notably in children (Constant et al., 2005) and in situations where high concentrations of the drug were used in conjunction with hypocapnia (Mohanram et al., 2007). When present in high concentrations, enflurane causes cats and rats to experience periods of suppression interspersed with paroxysmal epileptiform discharges (Sleigh et al., 2009). After receiving enflurane anesthesia, multiple reports have occurred of humans experiencing seizure activity (Kruczek et al., 1980). Isoflurane has anticonvulsant properties that have been extensively studied. Isoflurane and desflurane are both potential treatments for refractory status epilepticus, which will be covered in more detail in a subsequent section (Mirsattari et al., 2004).

Opioids

Meperidine is the opioid most associated with myoclonus and tonic-clonic seizures (Yıllar et al., 2009). On the other hand, patients who take low to moderate doses of fentanyl, alfentanil, or sufentanil, as well as morphine, have been reported to experience generalized seizure activity (Saboory et al., 2007; Tortella, 1988), particularly after intrathecal administration (Borgeat et al., 1988; Parkinson et al., 1990; Shih et al., 2005). It has not been demonstrated that fentanyl or its analogs possess anticonvulsant properties. Opioid anesthetic agents are used in patients diagnosed with focal epilepsy to increase EEG activity. During epilepsy surgery, both remifentanil and alfentanil have been used to induce increased activity in the localization of epileptogenic zones intraoperatively; however, alfentanil seems to be more potent activator. In patients undergoing electroconvulsive therapy (ECT), the addition of alfentanil to the propofol anesthetic prolongs the duration of their seizures (McGuire et al., 2003).

I.V. Anesthetic Agents

Barbiturates—thiopental, methohexital, and pentobarbital—and propofol treat refractory status epilepticus (Brown & Horton, 1967; Lowenstein et al., 1988). All agents have been shown to produce excitatory activity when inducing anesthesia, including myoclonus, opisthotonus, and very rarely generalized seizures. The use of etomidate appears to have the highest incidence (Hymes & Analgesia, 1985), followed by the use of thiopental, methohexital, and propofol. When electroconvulsive therapy (ECT) is performed with etomidate instead of thiopental, longer durations of seizures have been observed (Trzepacz et al., 1993). At higher doses, each of these substances exhibits anticonvulsant activity (Reddy et al., 1993; Smith et al., 1996). Ketamine blocks N-methyl-D-aspartate receptors noncompetitively. This makes it beneficial for treating status epilepticus, which resists other medicines. Ketamine, like other intravenous medications, can worsen seizures in low doses, but is anticonvulsant in higher doses, which can cause sedation or anesthesia (Myslobodsky et al., 1981).

Benzodiazepines

Clinically, all benzodiazepines are effective anticonvulsants (Modica et al., 1990). Status epilepticus is typically treated with benzodiazepines such as diazepam, midazolam, and lorazepam.

Local Anesthetics

Local anesthetics pass the blood-brain barrier and cause drowsiness, analgesia, and widespread convulsions (Steen et al., 1979; USUBIAGA et al., 1967). Accidental intravenous or rapid systemic absorption from a highly vascular location raises blood levels (Veering, 2003). Several small series involving children have shown that intravenous lidocaine can effectively treat status epilepticus (Hamano et al., 2006; Pascual et al., 1992).

Neuromuscular Blocking Agents

There does not appear to be any pro or anticonvulsant activity associated with any of the neuromuscular blocking agents. The primary metabolite of atracurium is laudanosine, and it has been associated with seizure activity on the electroencephalogram (EEG) and the clinical presentation of animals. Patients with hepatic failure, in whom the half-life of laudanosine is significantly prolonged, may benefit from considering this, despite the fact that it has not been replicated in humans. Succinylcholine causes an increase in afferent muscle spindle activity in the brain, which can be suppressed by pretreatment with nondepolarizing neuromuscular blocking agents. There is no evidence that it increases the risk of seizures (Lanier et al., 1986).

Anticholinergics and Anticholinesterases

Central cholinergic blockade can be induced by the administration of atropine or scopolamine, which increases acetylcholine levels (or central anticholinergic syndrome). This can look like mania with stupor, coma, and apnea, or agitation with seizures, hallucinations, and restlessness. Physostigmine is the best medicine for this condition. Because glycopyrrolate cannot penetrate the brain protective barrier, it has no such effects (Schneck & Rupreht, 1989).

Perioperative Management of AEDs

Patients who have a history of epilepsy that has been successfully controlled with medication must take all precautions to prevent disruption of their antiepileptic medication while undergoing surgery. Patients should take their usual medications on the morning of surgery and continue them as soon as possible after surgery. Presurgery drugs should be taken. After day-case surgery, a missed dose should be given as soon as possible. When possible, give antiepileptic medications (AEDs) parenterally to avoid skippepping doses. Phenytoin, sodium valproate, levetiracetam, and carbamazepine can be given intravenously or as suppositories. The patient's regular AED is not accessible in parenteral form. The pharmacokinetics of AEDs are not affected by anesthetics, so perioperative drug level monitoring is rarely needed. However, prolonged stays in the ICU, changes in serum pH and albumin levels, and AED-interacting medicines can influence these medications' blood concentrations. Due to its unusual pharmacokinetics, phenytoin, one of the most common AEDs, is the hardest (Wichards et al., 2013). Dosing in critical care unit patients requires regular check of serum phenytoin concentration.

Status Epilepticus

Status epilepticus, a seizure that lasts more than 30 minutes without regaining consciousness, is largely useful for determining frequency. A convulsive seizure that lasts more than 5 minutes should be treated with emergency antiepileptic medicines because most cease within 2–3 minutes (Lowenstein et al., 1999). The status epilepticus alters the body. Brain metabolism, blood flow, glucose, and lactate increase in convulsive status epilepticus (CSE). Massive catecholamine release increases cardiac output, blood pressure, heart rate, and central venous pressure. Compensatory systems shield the brain for 30 to 60 minutes (Kelso & Cock, 2005). If seizures are not stopped at this time, the compensatory mechanisms of the body break down and the brain may be injured (Figure 1). Cerebral autoregulation fails, causing low oxygen, blood sugar, intracranial pressure, and brain edema. Low sodium, potassium imbalance, and worsening metabolic acidosis occur. The result of coagulopathy, rhabdomyolysis, and organ failure. These changes happen faster in CSE, but can also happen in NCSE (Kelso & Cock, 2005).

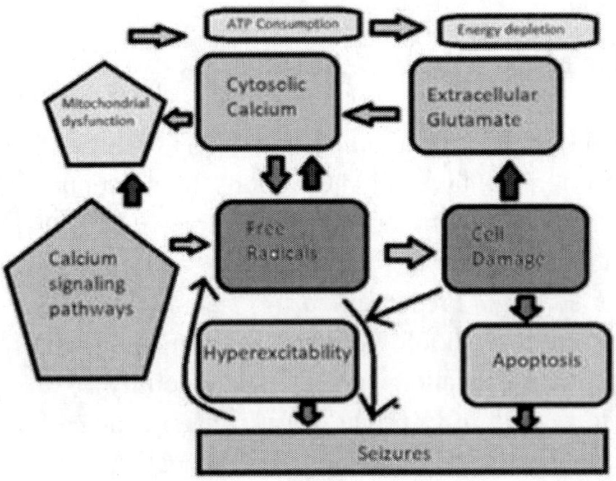

Figure 1. Mechanism of status epilepticus brain damage.

Multiple Sclerosis

The leading cause of disability among young adults worldwide, particularly in Europe and North America, is multiple sclerosis. Despite the low incidence in Asia, there have not been many epidemiological studies there, possibly because there are more neurologists and MRI machines there. Some people have minor handicaps throughout their lives, but by the 20th year following start, as many as 60% are still unable to walk alone, affecting their quality of life and society's expense (Dobson & Giovannoni, 2019).

MS Anesthesia

Anesthetics and MS Drugs

MS medications complicate anesthesia. Baclofen weakens muscles, making them hypersensitive to non-depolarizing muscle relaxants. Avoid agitation, psychosis, and convulsions with a 2-week progressive withdrawal (Handbook, 2011; Møller, 2011). Emergency surgery should give high-dose corticosteroids to patients (Nicholson et al., 1998). IVIG may cause headaches, tachycardia, hypotension, and wheezing. Rare thromboembolic events, severe renal failure, and acute myocardial infarction can worsen anesthesia. Hepatitis and HIV patients can contract viral IVIGs (Orange et al., 2006). Fever, urticaria, hypotension, and citrate-induced hypocalcemia can occur after plasmapheresis. (Shemin et al., 2007) No studies recommend abandoning MS treatment for surgery. Several studies and case reports show MS relapse days or months after stopping treatment (Havla et al., 2012; O'connor, 2011). 20% of 43 patients who stopped interferon-b reported neurological symptoms lasting at least 48 h in 30 days (Siger et al., 2011). All studies suggest that very active diseases cause relapses. Side effects and anesthetic complications should determine the withdrawal of the presurgical medication. Consult a neurologist in tough situations. Restart the medication promptly.

Pre-op Evaluation

Regional procedures involve a complete medical history and physical examination to determine the type of anesthesia based on the patient's type of multiple sclerosis, acute exacerbation, current medications and neurological impairment. Anesthesia involves respiratory failure, which is typical in terminal stages, but can develop sooner (Altintas et al., 2007; Mutluay, 2005). MS patients without impairment exhibited lower FEV1/FVC ratios than healthy controls ($p = 0.06$) and 50% had reduced but normal maximum expiratory pressure (MEP). DLCO impairment, which is common in terminal disease, was also identified (Carvalho et al., 2012). Clinical examination may predict respiratory muscle weakening better than spirometry (Smeltzer et al., 1992). It may also be a side effect of disease management drugs such as baclofen and clonazepam, which relax the pharynx and predispose to OSA (Brass et al., 2010). Perioperative CPAP or bilevel positive airway pressure can minimize hypoxia episodes (De Hert et al., 2011). Patients should undergo an airway blockage examination to reduce hypoxia episodes. Use bilevel or CPAP. The anesthesiologist's main concern is hemodynamic instability, which may be compounded by the drugs' cardiovascular side effects (Makris et al., 2014). Expect severe hypotension and decreased responsiveness to intravenous fluids and vasopressors during induction. 25% of patients had orthostatic dysregulation, bladder or bowel dysfunction, neurocardiogenic syncope, or cardiac dysrhythmias (Lensch & Jost, 2011). Treatment may affect conduction or cardiovascular health, making the cardiac examination crucial. The autonomic nervous system can affect anesthesia administration, thus it must be diagnosed in advance. The anesthesiologist's main concern is hemodynamic instability, which may be compounded by the drugs' cardiovascular side effects (Makris et al., 2014). Expect severe hypotension and decreased responsiveness to intravenous fluids and vasopressors during induction. 25% of patients had orthostatic dysregulation, bladder or bowel dysfunction, neurocardiogenic syncope, or cardiac dysrhythmias (Flachenecker et al., 2001; Lensch & Jost, 2011). Several cardiovascular autonomic system tests have been developed, however, their utility in MS is questionable. Valsalva's maneuver and deep sleep heart rate variability change between active and inactive disease patients (Flachenecker et al., 2001; Merico et al., 2005). Because medication may affect conduction or cardiovascular health, cardiac assessment is crucial.

Intraoperative Care

Anesthesia and surgery worsen the disease. As with any stressful situation, these two treatments can be exacerbated. Therefore, infection, inflammation, fever/hyperpyrexia, delivery, and emotional stress should be effectively treated. The most researched trigger is elevated body temperature. After heat exposure, demyelinated axons exhibit conduction block (Martinez-Rodriguez et al., 2006; Uhthoff, 1890). remains often cited. Multiple sclerosis patients with bilateral hypothalamic involvement might develop difficult-to-treat periodic hyperthermia up to 40 degrees Celsius, which may lead to mortality (Martinez-Rodriguez et al., 2006). In hyperthermia, antibiotics or antipyretics, changes in room temperature, cooling equipment, and cool fluids should be used to monitor and manage temperature. Perioperative pseudorelapses (worsening symptoms of sepsis/fever) should be distinguished from actual exacerbations of the disease. Inhalational and intravenous anesthetic drugs have been used successfully (Sahin et al., 2010; Yamashita et al., 2003) with no clear advantage. Nitrous oxide, sevoflurane, and desflurane have not caused difficulties (Ceyhan et al., 2011; Inoue & Furuya, 2006; Sahin, 2010).

Patients with reduced respiratory function should use midazolam as a premedication with caution. Premedication before surgery helps reduce stress, which can worsen the disease. Induction of general anesthesia with midazolam at 0.2 to 0.3 mg/kg has little effect on thermoregulatory regulation, which is important for patients with MS (Ceyhan et al., 2011). A study found that midazolam inhibits tonic thermoregulatory vasoconstriction, lowering the temperature of the core body. (Honarmand & Safavi, 2008) A bolus dose of 1 lg/kg followed by an infusion of 0.5 lg/kg/h of dexmedetomidine is suitable for monitored anesthesia care. Hypotension and bradycardia were expected, although patient satisfaction was high (Anand et al., 2012). MS patients receive most opioids intraoperatively (Inoue & Furuya, 2006; Sahin et al., 2010). NMBDs require extra caution. MS patients up-regulate skeletal muscle nicotinic acetylcholine receptors. Additionally, constitutional changes in the receptor subunit delay channel opening (Martyn et al., 1992). Succinylcholine can cause hyperkalemia in MS patients, especially during exacerbations (Kyttä & Rosenberg, 1984). Succinylcholine-induced hyperkalemia increases disease progression (Cooperman, 1970). A multiple sclerosis flare caused life-threatening hyperkalemia (Levine & Brown, 2012). Avoid succinylcholine. Resistance to nondepolarizing NMBD has been documented; however, many cases have shown normal responses (Brett et al., 1987; Inoue & Furuya, 2006; Sahin et al., 2010). Muscular weakness and lower muscle mass can increase sensitivity, while a higher number of post-junctional receptors explains resistance (Brett et al., 1987; Briggs & Kirsch, 2003). Neuromuscular monitoring is recommended for the least affected limb. Deep brain stimulation, used to treat tremors and chronic pain, requires additional anesthetic concerns. Intraoperative electrophysiological guiding through microelectrode recording (MER) locates specific nuclei. The most prevalent intravenous anesthetic is propofol, but little is known about its effects on MER (Venkatraghavan & Manninen, 2016).

A supervised anesthetic is used since aware people can locate the target nuclei. Dexmedetomidine is another option for delayed awakening. De-stressing is crucial. Benzodiazepines may work. Sedation causes respiratory depression and intravascular consequences, such as seizures and hemorrhage. High arterial blood pressure increases the risk of bleeding. During surgery, diagnose seizures or extremities weakness differently. Midazolam with propofol cure seizures (Venkatraghavan et al., 2010). Most seizures are brief and do not require treatment. Venous air embolism is a rare procedural complication. ECT is increasingly used to treat severe or medication-resistant depression under general anesthesia (Leiknes et al., 2012). Succinylcholine, a common short-acting agent, should be avoided even in tiny dosages. The reversal of roucuronium, vecuronium and sugammadex is an alternative (Ding et al., 2002). Concerns include worsening autonomic dysfunction. Atropine, glycopyrrolate, b-blockers such as esmolol and labetalol, a2 agonists, Ca blockers, and nitrates (in patients at risk for myocardial ischemia) must be administered to control parasympathetic and sympathetic effects. Studies show a temperature drop (Szuba et al., 1997). We did not find ECT-induced aggravation.

MS Neuraxial Administration

Theoretical concerns about neuraxial procedures are supported by CNS pathophysiological studies. These studies link MS symptoms to neurons binding sodium channel-blocking oligopeptides. MS patients have elevated levels of oligopeptides in their CSF (Weber et al., 2002). QYNAD pentapeptide inhibits excitation in undamaged myelinated rat nerve axons (Weber et al., 2002). Muscle weakness may result from this blockage. Local anaesthetics, especially subarachnoid blocks, may also produce MS symptoms (Brinkmeier et al., 2000). Epidural anesthesia is safe and has no known effect on the progression of the disease (Compston & Coles, 2008; Hebl et al., 2006). Epidural anaesthesia may be beneficial since local anesthetics reach the subarachnoid region at a low concentration (about one-fourth of the concentration administered epidurally) (Warren et al., 1982). Obstetricians have extensively researched epidural blocks. Despite its safety, illness relapse has occurred (Dalmas et al., 2003). Relapse rates increase postpartum (Vukusic & Confavreux, 2006). A pregnant woman received 562.5 mg of bupivacaine over 15 hours, which may have caused labour and caesarean birth (Warren et al., 1982). Fortunately, he recovered fully a few days later. Compared to postpartum relapse rates, three groups of obstetric patients receiving epidural, general, or local anesthesia had similar relapse rates in three months (Bader et al., 1989). Three of five epidural patients who had a postpartum relapse received more than 0.25 percent bupivacaine, and two received 2 percent lidocaine. Despite the danger of inadequate analgesia, central nervous system blockades should use the lowest local anesthetic doses (Bader et al., 1989). They may also not indicate a worsening of the disease. Spinal block no longer causes disease progression (Berger & Ontell, 1987). Despite a transitory exacerbation, nine patients who received 14 spinals for urological surgery had no problems (Bouchard et al., 1984). The rate is comparable to general anesthesia, according to the scientists. Martucci et al. performed a spinal anesthesia for caesarean delivery in a patient with multiple sclerosis, with normal findings for block, intensity, and duration and without exacerbation during the 12 month follow-up (Martucci et al., 2011). Immunologically induced vasculopathy that disrupts the blood–brain barrier in MS patients should be considered, but its clinical importance is unknown (Alvarez et al., 2011; Vercauteren & Heytens, 2007). MS patients have excessively high levels of these oligopeptides in their CSF (Brinkmeier et al., 2000; Weber, 2002). QYNAD pentapeptide inhibits excitation in undamaged myelinated rat nerve axons (Brinkmeier et al., 2000). Muscle weakness may result from this blockage. Local anaesthetics, especially subarachnoid blocks, may also produce MS symptoms (Weber et al., 2002). Despite these methods, epidural anesthesia is safe and does not appear to alter disease progression. Epidural anaesthesia may be beneficial since local anesthetics reach the subarachnoid area at a low concentration (about one-fourth of the concentration delivered epidurally). Obstetricians have extensively researched epidural blocks. Despite being safe, illness relapse has occurred (Dalmas et al., 2003). Relapse rates increase postpartum (Vukusic & Marignier, 2015). A pregnant woman received 562.5 mg of bupivacaine over 15 hours, which may have caused labour and caesarean birth (Warren et al., 1982). Fortunately, he recovered fully a few days later. The relapse rate within three months of three groups of obstetric patients receiving epidural, general, or local anesthesia was comparable to postpartum relapse rates (Bader et al., 1989). Three of five epidural patients who had a postpartum relapse received more than 0.25 percent bupivacaine, and two received 2 percent lidocaine. Despite the danger of inadequate analgesia, central nervous system blockades should use the lowest local anesthetic doses (Dalmas et al., 2003). Neuraxial blockades can cause vasopressor-resistant hypotension. Subarachnoid anesthesia is disputed (Dalmas et al., 2003). Early reports describe illness exposure (Perlas & Chan, 2005). Even if local anesthetics create symptoms such as oculomotor paralysis, they are temporary and reversible. They can also not indicate illness worsening (Perlas & Chan, 2005).

Multiple sclerosis does not exclude spinal anesthesia, and the relapse rate is lower than previously thought (Dobson et al., 2019; Kyttä & Rosenberg, 1984). Actually, spinal anesthesia's first fear has changed. Intravenous lidocaine worsens MS symptoms, especially in the eyes (Sakurai et al., 1992). Intravenous lidocaine and oral mexiletine, which impede conduction, diminish positive symptoms such as spasticity (Sakurai et al., 1992). Ectopic impulses cause good symptoms. Avoid intravenous absorption that could disrupt neural impulses. An epidural blood patch for post-dural puncture headache may increase epidural pressure and disrupt axonal conduction. A recent epidural blood patch went well. To reduce epidural pressure, blood should be injected gently.

MS Peripheral Nerve Plugs

MS is mostly CNS related. Dawson (1916) found that PNS involvement was postmortem. Sensory and motor neuron axonal excitability has changed (Antonini et al., 1995). Postinfectious inflammatory polyneuropathy causes peripheral nerve damage (Poser, 1987). In motor axons, the sluggish potassium current increases, but in sensory axons, the rapid gating of the potassium channel changes. Only 5% of the 60 MS patients who underwent thorough nerve conduction investigations had anomalies suggestive of demyelination (Ng et al., 2013). The clinical importance of PNS involvement is unknown (Vogt et al., 2009). Koff et al., reported severe brachial plexopathy after total shoulder arthroplasty and ultrasound-guided interscalene nerve block. The final diagnosis, inflammatory brachial neuritis, may have been caused by nerve block, showing that preclinical peripheral nerve disease predisposed to autoimmune nerve injury (Koff et al., 2008). Surgery should be considered before diagnosing damage (Koff et al., 2008). Nerve blocks also reduce exacerbations by providing sustained and effective analgesia. Avoid adjuvants causing vasoconstriction such as epinephrine to avoid nerve strain (Ingrosso et al., 2005). Many physicians advocate ultrasound-guided blocks. Ultrasound can reduce mechanical trauma and local anesthetic toxicity, but it cannot remove the risks to the patient and the operation. Ultrasound guidance allows for fewer quantities of local anesthetic, which can reduce neurotoxicity (Ingrosso et al., 2005).

Parkinson's Disease

Parkinson's disease is a chronic progressive neurodegenerative disorder with motor symptoms (bradykinesia, rest tremor, stiffness, and postural problems) that develop gradually. It is also accompanied by a multitude of nonmotor symptoms, which, combined with late-onset motor symptoms such as postural instability and falls, freezing of gait, and speech and swallowing difficulties, constitute one of the greatest obstacles to treating physicians of long-term disease (Davie, 2008).

Preoperative Risk

Parkinson's patients experience more postoperative problems, longer hospital stays, higher hospital costs, and higher mortality rates. Postoperative consequences include pulmonary aspiration, urinary tract infection, wound infection, respiratory insufficiency, hypotension, disorientation, and pressure ulcers. Exacerbation of Parkinson-related motor and non-motor symptoms, bulbar issues, immobility and falls, complex medications, and older age with numerous comorbidities contribute to the higher rate of complication. This condition increases medical and surgical complications and poorer functional outcomes in patients with orthopedic surgery (McClelland III et al., 2017; Newman et al., 2018). Patients with Parkinson's disease are fragile and require intensive anesthetic and perioperative treatment.

Clinical Manifestation

Parkinson's patients have different difficulties. >50% nigrostriatal dopaminergic neuron loss causes motor symptoms. Classic motor symptoms decline as other brainstem and thalamic nuclei degenerate, but nonmotor difficulties arise. Dopaminergic drug dose increases produce variable reactions and dyskinesia. Parkinson's patients may develop abrupt deterioration and increasing motor and nonmotor symptoms during surgery due to concurrent sickness and drug changes. Early-onset, hereditary, and advanced Parkinson's disease increase risk. These consequences include delirium, frequent motor fluctuations, substantial dyskinesia, and akinetic crisis (Simonet et al., 2020). Akinetic crisis, also known as Parkinsonism-hyperpyrexia syndrome, has an incidence of 0.3% (Onofrj & Thomas, 2005) and is difficult to treat due to temporary dopaminergic refractoriness. It can be caused by metoclopramide, haloperidol, or phenothiazines or an abrupt drop in the consumption or enteral absorption of dopamine agonists. Infection, trauma, dehydration, malnutrition, and sympathoadrenal hyperactivity can also occur perioperatively (Onofrj & Thomas, 2005).

Drug Treatment

Pharmacological management prevents acute problems and maintains patient function. Parkinson's disease anesthetists deal with polypharmacy, side effects, drug interactions, decreased drug response, and perioperative medication scheduling. Table 2 lists the frequent antiparkinsonian side effects. Propofol can cause dyskinesia, although Parkinson's disease does not prevent its use. Fentanyl and alfentanil might increase muscular rigidity and produce acute dystonia. Low doses rarely cause this effect. Pethidine or tramadol plus monoamine oxidase inhibitors, antidepressants, or antipsychotics can produce serotonin syndrome.

Table 2. Adverse Effect of Anti-Parkinsonian Medications

•	Orthostatic hypotension
•	Low blood pressure on standing
•	Ankle swelling
•	Nausea (usually mild and transient)
•	Daytime sleepiness
•	Confusion, hallucinations, and delusions

Perioperatively, the patient's antiparkinsonian medication schedule should be maintained if enteral intake is allowed. Adherence to the patient's home schedule, educating healthcare personnel on the timing of medications, and avoiding contraindicated drugs minimize hospital stays (Azmi et al., 2020). Patients with severe conditions who need regular doses or who cannot take oral medication due to fasting or surgery may have trouble. Postoperative fasting, constipation, and enteral feeding must be planned carefully. Levodopa's short half-life necessitates this. Nasogastric tubes can deliver antiparkinsonian drugs intraoperatively and postoperatively. The start and half-life of immediate release levodopa are around 1 and 2 hours, respectively, after normal enteral absorption, so nasogastric delivery can be tailored to guarantee optimal drug action after general anesthesia. Continuous medication delivery and dopaminergic stimulation treatments such as intestinal gel of levodopa-carbidopa, transdermal rotigotine, extended-release levodopa, and subcutaneous apomorphine infusion are being studied to reduce response fluctuation and dyskinesia. Continuous dopaminergic stimulation and medication administration can sustain brain dopamine levels by tonically stimulating dopamine receptors such as normal basal ganglia (Timpka et al., 2016). These innovative perioperative therapies may replace oral dopaminergic therapy. Patients' needs and side effects should guide dose conversion. Sublingual apomorphine (Olanow et al., 2020) is being tested for perioperative use on demand.

Multidisciplinary Perioperative Care

Parkinson's disease patients benefit from multidisciplinary care and an accelerated recovery after surgery (ERAS) protocol due to the complexity of the disease and the high risk of postoperative functional deterioration. Enhanced recovery care packages minimize hospitalization, morbidity, mortality, and expenses for various surgeries (Ljungqvist et al., 2017). ERAS programs can be modified for patients with Parkinson's disease. Anesthetic management goals include medically and functionally optimized and educated patients, reduced Parkinson's disease-related or concomitant problems, early discharge by minimizing unnecessary operations, and a rapid return to premorbid function. Anesthesiologists, surgeons, nurses, neurologists, psychiatrists, other health professionals such as physiotherapists, occupational therapists, speech therapists, and social workers should comprise the multidisciplinary team. Intraoperative anesthesia must avoid hemodynamic, respiratory, and neurological problems. Lenka et al., (2021) provides useful guidance. These patients are at risk of neurocognitive problems after surgery.

Advanced Parkinson's patients who need high-risk surgeries may benefit from integrated care. Unlike traditional multidisciplinary care systems, this involves early active patient decision making in management goals, interdisciplinary consensus building through team meetings and structured referral systems, and specialized care by Parkinson's disease-trained healthcare professionals. This healthcare system is being created (Prizer & Browner, 2012; Rajan et al., 2020), but its adoption will depend on local patient demands and resource availability. These therapies need more testing.

Stroke

Stroke most affects public health. Stroke is the third leading cause of death in most developed countries, after cancer and heart disease. Local cerebral ischemia or hemorrhage causes strokes. Ischemic strokes outnumber hemorrhagic strokes (Warlow, 1998).

Acute ischemic stroke endovascular therapy is an emergency procedure with minimal time for preprocedural patient assessment. Avoid delays by completing the exam quickly (Talke et al., 2014). As mobilization of anesthesia personnel and equipment could delay the move to the interventional radiology suite, the anesthesiologist should be consulted immediately. The presentation of stroke may prevent a patient history. Electronic data, replacement decision makers, and the stroke neurology team often provide additional information. Time and communication constraints make it difficult to clarify the patient's advance directives.

Anticoagulation

The procedural anesthesiologist should know that many patients with acute ischemic stroke start with oral anticoagulants or antiplatelet medications. Depending on their presentation of stroke, many patients underwent intravenous thrombolysis prior to EVT (endovascular treatment). Intravenous heparin helps minimize microcatheter-related thrombotic problems during the procedure; however, dose and monitoring vary by center. If a hemorrhagic problem occurs, reverse the heparin with protamine and investigate alternative pre-existing medicines.

Selecting Anesthesia

Taking into account the needs of the patient and institutional protocols, anesthetic techniques should be chosen individually with aesthetic aims in mind. General anesthesia, sedation, or infiltration of the local groyne puncture are all suitable anesthetic alternatives. EVT is mostly non-stimulating, but manipulating the cerebral arteries during clot extraction can induce discomfort and movement in the patient. The technique requires minimal analgesia. Although each anesthetic method has pros and cons, no data support one over another. Neither general anesthesia nor sedation reduces procedure complications such as artery perforation (Sørensen et al., 2019). Ten years have disputed endovascular stroke anesthesia. In observational studies with hindsight, general anesthesia increased mortality and neurologic outcomes (Abou-Chebl et al., 2010; Davis, 2012; Nichols, 2018). These retrospective investigations have inadequate information on anesthesia technique, intraprocedural physiological measures, and general anesthesia indications. The data may indicate that people with severe strokes need general anesthesia. General anesthesia did not worsen early neurologic recovery, infarct volume, or complication rate in three RCTs (randomised controlled trials) evaluating EVT procedures. The RCTs featured precise inclusion criteria and standardized hemodynamic and ventilatory goals, unlike observational trials.

RCTs avoided hypotension to protect collateral perfusion. Pressure-dependent flow in the ischemic penumbra is sensitive to variations in blood pressure due to loss of autoregulation (Petersen et al., 2019). In 2012, Davis et al., found that the lowest recorded systolic blood pressure of more than 140 mm Hg was related to a better neurologic outcome. In another study, a low mean arterial pressure of more than 70 mm Hg was an independent predictor of a good neurologic outcome (Whalin et al., 2014). Blood pressure affects neurologic outcomes regardless of anesthesia. In sedated patients with EVT, a reduction in mean arterial pressure of more than 10% from baseline strongly indicated a poor prognosis (Whalin et al., 2017). Defining a "safe" level for all patients is difficult. Collateral perfusion may make people more susceptible to blood pressure drops (Petersen et al., 2019). Arterial CO2 concentration affects collateral perfusion. Hypoventilation-related vasodilation in the nonischemic brain can create a steal phenomenon, while hyperventilation can constrict the ischemic area. High and low end-tidal CO2 concentrations have unfavorable effects (Mundiyanapurath et al., 2016). "General anesthesia" refers to several things (Sivasankar et al., 2016). As discussed above, physiological factors change significantly and vary by case. The consequences of the anesthesia agent are unknown. The Society for Neuroscience in Anesthesiology and Critical Care consensus statement and American Heart Association recommendations advocate individualized anesthetic strategy (Powers et al., 2018). Canadian Stroke Best Practise recommends sedation over general anesthesia (Boulanger et al., 2018). General anesthesia is recommended for patients with agitation, vomiting, a poor Glasgow Coma Scale score, or posterior circulation strokes. Patients who can relax flat without respiratory depression or airway impairment may be suitable for sedation. As the stroke worsens, the patient may need general anesthesia. EVT anesthetics are not tested. Patients should choose anesthesias. Due to an unclear fasting status, general anesthesia patients may need rapid sequence induction.

Postoperative Thoughts

Identifying post-procedure consequences such as intracerebral haemorrhage (ICH) requires early neurologic examination. When there are no additional reasons for mechanical breathing, extubation should occur early. Institutional protocols determine the location. After thrombectomy, the stroke neurology and interventional team will discuss blood pressure targets based on reperfusion and intraprocedural problems. Neurological status, extubation capabilities, and local stroke treatment techniques will determine the patient's post-procedure destination.

Brain Trauma

Traumatic brain injury accounts for more than half of trauma-related deaths and disabilities in children and young people around the world. Brain injuries cause years of incapacity and loss of productivity. It also burdens individuals, families, and society economically. Prevention saves lives and prevents years of disability (Tsang et al., 2012).

The Preoperative and Postoperative Periods are Crucial

Due to poor results and secondary insults, the TBI care focuses on preventing the main and secondary injury. Therefore, current TBI care involves in-field resuscitation, rapid triage, emergent surgical evacuation of mass lesions, ICP control, CPP support, multimodal monitoring, and optimization of the physiological environment (Tsang et al., 2012). Perioperative factors can affect TBI treatment. First, despite the vigorous measures of the emergency department to swiftly correct hypoxemia, hypotension, hypo and hypercarbia, and hypo and hyperglycemia, one or more complicating conditions can persist or remain unnoticed when the patient is urgently transferred to the operating room. Thus, preoperative resuscitation and correction of secondary insults are possible. Second, surgery and anesthesia can produce additional secondary ailments, such as intraoperative hypotension from surgical blood loss or anesthetic medications, stress-induced hyperglycemia, etc. which can alter results (Chesnut et al., 1993).

Intracranial/Cerebral Perfusion Pressure Management

The Brain Trauma Foundation published evidence-based guidelines for the treatment of severe traumatic brain injury in 2007. Maintaining cerebral blood flow and oxygenation in the ICU or OR prevents subsequent brain injury. This therapy used to regulate ICP, but now maintains CPP. However, a recent multicenter, randomized trial (BEST: TRIP [Benchmark Evidence from South American Trials: Treatment of Intracranial Pressure]) and a published meta-analysis suggest that rigorous ICP monitoring may not be beneficial (Yuan et al., 2015). Brain Trauma, 2007 recommends keeping the ICP below 20 mm Hg and the cerebral perfusion pressure between 50 and 70 mm Hg. Aggressive therapy to raise CPP above 70 mm Hg has been associated with acute respiratory distress syndrome and other serious effects. With a treatment threshold of less than 15 mm Hg, oxygen tension in brain tissue can be used to monitor resuscitation (Yuan et al., 2015). Elevating the head of the bed by 30 degrees, keeping the neck neutral, and loosening the cervical collar are the first steps to reducing ICP. Reverse Trendelenburg can be used intraoperatively if head-of-bed elevation is not possible (Tankisi et al., 2002).

During Surgery

Traumatic brain damage patients often require additional surgery. Intraoperative anesthetic management avoids brain damage. Quickly securing the airway ensures adequate oxygenation. Trauma patients with reduced GCS or urgent operational intervention should undergo rapid sequence intubation. Assume that all trauma patients have unstable cervical injuries and a full stomach until proven differently. Intubated patients with stabilized cervical spine. For ventilation. Airway protocols may be needed for facial or neck injuries. Nose tubes, endotracheal or gastric, should not be used in patients with skull base fractures or coagulopathy. Etomidate prevents hypotension induction despite concerns about adrenal insufficiency (Cohan et al., 2005). Hypovolemic or hypotensive patients should take propofol and thiopental with caution because they depress the circulatory system. Patients with TBI patients avoid ketamine because it increases intracranial pressure. Chang et al., (2013) question this adage. Intubation requires short-acting paralytics. Avoid hypotonic fluids, which aggravate cerebral edoema. At doses below the minimum alveolar concentration, volatile medications decrease the metabolic rate of brain oxygen. Volatile chemicals can increase ICP and cerebral vasodilation (Engelhard & Werner, 2006). Nitrous oxide increases intracranial pressure. Anesthetics treat TBI. Isoflurane neuroprotected animals by suppressing the apoptotic cytokine cascade (McAuliffe et al., 2007; Segal et al., 2012). Several animal investigations have shown that xenon, an N-methyl-D-aspartate (NMDA) antagonist, protects the body against ischemia and excitotoxic damage, making it a possible general anesthetic (Coburn et al., 2008). Conventional TBI treatments may help. Propofol reduces brain electrical activity and skull pressure to protect the brain. Antioxidants may prevent neurodegeneration.

Conclusion

1. *Dementia:* As older patients with mild cognitive impairment undergo surgery, anesthetists must be aware of the risks of providing safe anesthesia to this population of neurologically susceptible patients. Considerations should include permission, capacity, anesthetic medicines, and the interaction of neuromuscular blocking agents with anti-dementia drugs.
2. *Epilepsy:* Anesthesiologists can help with airway care and general anesthesia for status epilepticus. General anesthesia with midazolam, propofol, or thiopental is the treatment for persistent status epilepticus.
3. *Multiple sclerosis*: Relapses and remissions characterize this chronic demyelinating disease of the neurological system. A complete literature evaluation, including regional approaches, is reassuring despite the long-held idea that anesthesia may cause MS exacerbations or decrease clinical status.
4. *Parkinson's disease:* The complexity of the disease and the drugs make the perioperative period tough. Parkinson's patients may benefit from interdisciplinary perioperative treatment and improved recovery regimens.
5. *Stroke:* Acute ischemic stroke needs immediate treatment. Anesthesiologists must understand all aspects of the procedure, including risks and physiological goals for patients with acute ischemic stroke.
6. *Traumatic brain injury*: TBI comprises many problems of variable severity. Anesthesia teams treating patients with traumatic brain

injury in and out of the operating room should be aware of their special needs and treatments.

References

Abou-Chebl, A., Lin, R., Hussain, M. S., Jovin, T. G., Levy, E. I., Liebeskind, D. S., Yoo, A. J., Hsu, D. P., Rymer, M. M., Tayal, A. H., Zaidat, O. O., Natarajan, S. K., Nogueira, R. G., Nanda, A., Tian, M., Hao, Q., Kalia, J. S., Nguyen, T. N., Chen, M., & Gupta, R. (2010). Conscious sedation versus general anesthesia during endovascular therapy for acute anterior circulation stroke: preliminary results from a retrospective, multicenter study. *Stroke*, *41*(6), 1175-1179. https://doi.org/10.1161/STROKEAHA.109.574129.

Altintas, A., Demir, T., Ikitimur, H. D., & Yildirim, N. (2007). Pulmonary function in multiple sclerosis without any respiratory complaints. *Clinical neurology and neurosurgery*, *109*(3), 242-246. https://doi.org/10.1016/j.clineuro.2006.09.004.

Alvarez, J. I., Cayrol, R., & Prat, A. (2011). Disruption of central nervous system barriers in multiple sclerosis. *Biochimica et Biophysica Acta (BBA)-Molecular Basis of Disease*, *1812*(2), 252-264. https://doi.org/10.1016/j.bbadis.2010.06.017.

Anand, S., Bhatia, A., Sapra, H., Gupta, V., & Mehta, Y. (2012). Dexmedetomidine for monitored anesthesia care in patients undergoing liberation procedure for multiple sclerosis: An observational study. *Saudi Journal of Anaesthesia*, *6*(4), 358. https://doi.org/10.4103/1658-354X.105865.

Anderson, J., & Moor, C. C. (2010). Anti-epileptic drugs: a guide for the non-neurologist. *Clinical medicine*, *10*(1), 54. https://doi.org/10.7861/clinmedicine.10-1-54.

Antonini, G., Millefiorini, E., Borsellino, G., Morino, S., Rasura, M., & Pozzilli, C. (1995). Subclinical peripheral nervous system involvement in multiple sclerosis. *Muscle & nerve*, *18*(10), 1216-1217.

Artru, A. A., Lettich, E., Colley, P. S., & Ojemann, G. A. (1990). Nitrous oxide: suppression of focal epileptiform activity during inhalation, and spreading of seizure activity following withdrawal. *Journal of Neurosurgical Anesthesiology*, *2*(3), 189-193.

Azmi, H., Cocoziello, L., Nyirenda, T., Douglas, C., Jacob, B., Thomas, J., Roth, P., & Thomas, F. P. (2020). Adherence to a strict medication protocol can reduce length of stay in hospitalized patients with Parkinson's Disease. *Clinical Parkinsonism & Related Disorders*, *3*, 100076. https://doi.org/10.1016/j.prdoa.2020.100076.

Bader, A. M., Hunt, C. O., Datta, S., Naulty, J. S., & Ostheimer, G. W. (1988). Anesthesia for the obstetric patient with multiple sclerosis. *Journal of clinical anesthesia*, *1*(1), 21-24. https://doi.org/10.1016/0952-8180(88)90006-2.

Banerjee, P. N., Filippi, D., & Hauser, W. A. (2009). The descriptive epidemiology of epilepsy—a review. *Epilepsy research*, *85*(1), 31-45. https://doi.org/10.1016/j.eplepsyres.2009.03.003.

Berger, J. M., & Ontell, R. (1987). Intrathecal morphine in conjunction with a combined spinal and general anesthetic in a patient with multiple sclerosis. *The Journal of the*

American Society of Anesthesiologists, *66*(3), 400-401. https://doi.org/10.1097/00000542-198703000-00025.

Bhardwaj, A., Dharmavaram, S., Wadhawan, S., Sethi, A., & Bhadoria, P. (2011). Donepezil: A cause of inadequate muscle relaxation and delayed neuromuscular recovery. *Journal of Anaesthesiology, Clinical Pharmacology*, *27*(2), 247.

Blood, S. J. T. P. (2012). *Medication considerations before surgery*. https://doi.org/10.4103/0970-9185.81833.

Borgeat, A., Biollaz, J., Depierraz, B., & Neff, R. (1988). Grand mal seizure after extradural morphine analgesia. *British journal of anaesthesia*, *60*(6), 733-735. https://doi.org/10.1093/bja/60.6.733.

Bouchard, P., Caillet, J. B., Monnet, F., & Banssillon, V. (1984, January). Spinal anesthesia and multiple sclerosis. In *Annales Francaises D'anesthesie et de Reanimation* (Vol. 3, No. 3, pp. 194-198). https://doi.org/10.1016/s0750-7658(84)80053-2.

Boulanger, J. M., Lindsay, M. P., Gubitz, G., Smith, E. E., Stotts, G., Foley, N., Bhogal, S., Boyle, K., Braun, L., Goddard, T., Heran, M., Kanya-Forster, N., Lang, E., Lavoie, P., McClelland, M., O'Kelly, C., Pageau, P., Pettersen, J., Purvis, H., Shamy, M., Tampieri, D., vanAdel, B., Verbeek, R., Blacquiere, D., Casaubon, L., Ferguson, D., Hegedus, Y., Jacquin, G. J., Kelly, M., Kamal, N., Linkewich, B., Lum, C., Mann, B., Milot, G., Newcommon, N., Poirier, P., Simpkin, W., Snieder, E., Trivedi, A., Whelan, R., Eustace, M., Smitko, E., & Butcher, K. (2018). Canadian stroke best practice recommendations for acute stroke management: prehospital, emergency department, and acute inpatient stroke care, update 2018. *International Journal of Stroke*, *13*(9), 949-984. https://doi.org/10.1177/1747493018786616.

Brass, S. D., Duquette, P., Proulx-Therrien, J., & Auerbach, S. (2010). Sleep disorders in patients with multiple sclerosis. *Sleep medicine reviews*, *14*(2), 121-129.

Breslow, L. (Ed.). (2002). *Encyclopedia of Public Health: LR* (Vol. 3). Macmillan reference USA/gale group thomson learning.

Brett, R. S., Schmidt, J. H., Cage, J. S., Schartel, S. A., & Poppers, P. J. (1987). Measurement of acetylcholine receptor concentration in skeletal muscle from a patient with multiple sclerosis and resistance to atracurium. *The Journal of the American Society of Anesthesiologists*, *66*(6), 837-838.

Briggs, E. D., & Kirsch, J. R. (2003). Anesthetic implications of neuromuscular disease. *Journal of anesthesia*, *17*, 177-185. https://doi.org/10.1007/s00540-003-0169-5.

Brinkmeier, H., Aulkemeyer, P., Wollinsky, K. H., & Rüdel, R. (2000). An endogenou s pentapeptide acting as a sodium channel blocker in inflammatory autoimmune disorders of the central nervous system. *Nature Medicine*, *6*(7), 808-811. https://doi.org/10.1038/77543.

Brown, A. S., & Horton, J. M. (1967). Status epilepticus treated by intravenous infusions of thiopentone sodium. *British Medical Journal*, *1*(5531), 27. https://doi.org/10.1136/bmj.1.5531.27.

Carvalho, S. R. S., Alvarenga Filho, H., Papais-Alvarenga, R. M., Chacur, F. H., & Dias, R. M. (2012). Is it useful to perform carbon monoxide diffusion capacity and respiratory muscle function tests in patients with multiple sclerosis without disability?. *Respirology*, *17*(5), 869-875. https://doi.org/10.1111/j.1440-1843.2012.02191.

Ceyhan, A., Uyar, E. T., Gencay, I. Y., & Gunal, S. E. (2011). Anesthesia in multiple sclerosis and obstructive sleep apnea: case report and literature review. *Journal of Research in Medical Sciences: the Official Journal of Isfahan University of Medical Sciences*, *16*(6), 828.

Chang, L. C., Raty, S. R., Ortiz, J., Bailard, N. S., & Mathew, S. J. (2013). The emerging use of ketamine for anesthesia and sedation in traumatic brain injuries. *CNS neuroscience & therapeutics*, *19*(6), 390-395. https://doi.org/10.1111/cns.12077.

Chesnut, R. M., Marshall, L. F., Klauber, M. R., Blunt, B. A., Baldwin, N., Eisenberg, H. M., Jane, J. A., Marmarou, A., & Foulkes, M. A. (2019). The role of secondary brain injury in determining outcome from severe head injury. In *50 Landmark Papers every Trauma Surgeon Should Know* (pp. 63-66). CRC Press.

Coburn, M., Maze, M., & Franks, N. P. (2008). The neuroprotective effects of xenon and helium in an in vitro model of traumatic brain injury. *Critical care medicine*, *36*(2), 588-595. https://doi.org/10.1097/01.CCM.0B013E3181611F8A6.

Cohan, P., Wang, C., McArthur, D. L., Cook, S. W., Dusick, J. R., Armin, B., Swerdloff R, Vespa P, Muizelaar JP, Cryer HG, Christenson PD, & Kelly, D. F. (2005). Acute secondary adrenal insufficiency after traumatic brain injury: a prospective study. *Critical care medicine*, *33*(10), 2358-2366. https://doi.org/0.1097/01.CCM.0000181735.51183.A7.

Cole, L. J., Farrell, M. J., Duff, E. P., Barber, J. B., Egan, G. F., & Gibson, S. J. (2006). Pain sensitivity and fMRI pain-related brain activity in Alzheimer's disease. *Brain*, *129*(11), 2957-2965. https://doi.org/10.1093/brain/awl228.

Constant, I., Seeman, R., & Murat, I. (2005). Sevoflurane and epileptiform EEG changes. *Pediatric Anesthesia*, *15*(4), 266-274. https://doi.org/10.1111/j.1460-9592.2004.01538.x.

Cooperman, L. H. (1970). Succinylcholine-induced hyperkalemia in neuromuscular disease. *Jama*, *213*(11), 1867-1871. https://doi.org/10.1001/jama.1970.03170370051009.

Crowe, S., & Collins, L. (2003). Suxamethonium and donepezil: a cause of prolonged paralysis. *The Journal of the American Society of Anesthesiologists*, *98*(2), 574-575. https://doi.org/10.1097/00000542-200302000-00040.

Dalmas, A. F., Texier, C., Ducloy-Bouthors, A. S., & Krivosic-Horber, R. (2003, December). Obstetrical analgesia and anaesthesia in multiple sclerosis. In *Annales Francaises D'anesthesie et de Reanimation* (Vol. 22, No. 10, pp. 861-864). https://doi.org/10.1016/j.annfar.2003.08.005.

Davie, C. A. (2008). A review of Parkinson's disease. *British medical bulletin*, *86*(1), 109-127.

Davis, M. J., Menon, B. K., Baghirzada, L. B., Campos-Herrera, C. R., Goyal, M., Hill, M. D., & Calgary Stroke Program. (2012). Anesthetic management and outcome in patients during endovascular therapy for acute stroke. *The Journal of the American Society of Anesthesiologists*, *116*(2), 396-405. https://doi.org/10.1097/ALN.0b013e318242a5d2.

Dawson, J. W. (1916). The histology of disseminated sclerosis. *Edinburgh Medical Journal*, *17*(5), 311.

De Hert, S., Imberger, G., Carlisle, J., Diemunsch, P., Fritsch, G., Moppett, I., & Task Force on Preoperative Evaluation of the Adult Noncardiac Surgery Patient of the European Society of Anaesthesiology. (2011). Preoperative evaluation of the adult patient undergoing non-cardiac surgery: guidelines from the European Society of Anaesthesiology. *European Journal of Anaesthesiology| EJA*, *28*(10), 684-722. https://doi.org/10.1097/EJA.0b013e3283499e3b.

Deogaonkar, A., Deogaonkar, M., Lee, J. Y., Ebrahim, Z., & Schubert, A. (2006). Propofol-induced dyskinesias controlled with dexmedetomidine during deep brain stimulation surgery. *The Journal of the American Society of Anesthesiologists*, *104*(6), 1337-1339. https://doi.org/10.1097/00000542-200606000-00029.

Ding, Z., & White, P. F. (2002). Anesthesia for electroconvulsive therapy. *Anesthesia & Analgesia*, *94*(5), 1351-1364. https://doi.org/10.1097/00000539-200205000-00057.

Dobson, R., & Giovannoni, G. (2019). Multiple sclerosis–a review. *European journal of neurology*, *26*(1), 27-40. https://doi.org/10.1111/ene.13819.

Dobson, R., Dassan, P., Roberts, M., Giovannoni, G., Nelson-Piercy, C., & Brex, P. A. (2019). UK consensus on pregnancy in multiple sclerosis:'Association of British Neurologists' guidelines. *Practical neurology*, *19*(2), 106-114. http://dx.doi.org/10.1136/practneurol-2018-002060.

Engelhard, K., & Werner, C. (2006). Inhalational or intravenous anesthetics for craniotomies? Pro inhalational. *Current Opinion in Anesthesiology*, *19*(5), 504-508. https://doi.org/10.1097/01.aco.0000245275.76916.87.

Flachenecker, P., Reiners, K., Krauser, M., Wolf, A., & Toyka, K. V. (2001). Autonomic dysfunction in multiple sclerosis is related to disease activity and progression of disability. *Multiple Sclerosis Journal*, *7*(5), 327-334. https://doi.org/10.1177/1352 45850100700509.

Fodale, V., Quattrone, D., Trecroci, C., Caminiti, V., & Santamaria, L. B. (2006). Alzheimer's disease and anaesthesia: implications for the central cholinergic system. *BJA: British Journal of Anaesthesia*, *97*(4), 445-452. https://doi.org/10.1093/bja/ael233.

Foundation, B. T. (2007). Guidelines for the management of severe traumatic brain injury. *Journal of neurotrauma*, *24*, S1-S106. https://doi.org/10.1089/neu.2007.9999.

Hamano, S. I., Sugiyama, N., Yamashita, S., Tanaka, M., Hayakawa, M., Minamitani, M., Yoshinari, S., & Eto, Y. (2006). Intravenous lidocaine for status epilepticus during childhood. *Developmental medicine and child neurology*, *48*(3), 220-222. https://doi.org/10.1017/S0012162206000466.

Handbook, A. M. (2011). Table B-3 Drugs and CYP enzymes. *Australian Medicines Handbook. Adelaide: AMH Pty Ltd*, 939.

Haroutiunian, S., Ratz, Y., Rabinovich, B., Adam, M., & Hoffman, A. (2009). Valproic acid plasma concentration decreases in a dose-independent manner following administration of meropenem: A retrospective study. *The Journal of Clinical Pharmacology*, *49*(11), 1363-1369. https://doi.org/10.1177/0091270009334377.

Havla, J. B., Pellkofer, H. L., Meinl, I., Gerdes, L. A., Hohlfeld, R., & Kümpfel, T. (2012). Rebound of disease activity after withdrawal of fingolimod (FTY720) treatment. *Archives of Neurology*, *69*(2), 262-264. https://doi.org/10.1001/archneurol.2011.1057.

Hebl, J. R., Horlocker, T. T., & Schroeder, D. R. (2006). Neuraxial anesthesia and analgesia in patients with preexisting central nervous system disorders. *Anesthesia & Analgesia*, *103*(1), 223-228. https://doi.org/10.1213/01.ane.0000220896.56427.53.

Honarmand, A., & Safavi, M. R. (2008). Comparison of prophylactic use of midazolam, ketamine, and ketamine plus midazolam for prevention of shivering during regional anaesthesia: a randomized double-blind placebo controlled trial. *British journal of anaesthesia*, *101*(4), 557-562. https://doi.org/10.1093/bja/aen205.

Hornbein, T. F., Eger, E. I., Winter, P. M., Smith, G., Wetstone, D., & Smith, K. H. (1982). The minimum alveolar concentration of nitrous oxide in man. *Anesthesia & Analgesia*, *61*(7), 553-556.

Hu, C. J., Liao, C. C., Chang, C. C., Wu, C. H., & Chen, T. L. (2012). Postoperative adverse outcomes in surgical patients with dementia: a retrospective cohort study. *World journal of surgery*, *36*, 2051-2058.

Hymes, J. A. (1985). Seizure activity during isoflurane anesthesia. *Anesthesia & Analgesia*, *64*(3), 367-368.

Ingrosso, M., Cirillo, V., Papasso, A., Merolla, V., & Cecere, F. (2005). Femoral and sciatic nerves block (BiBlock) in orthopedic traumatologic lower limbs surgery in patients with multiple sclerosis. *Minerva anestesiologica*, *71*(5), 223 226.

Inoue, S., & Furuya, H. (2006). Sevoflurane is safe for anesthetic management in patients with multiple sclerosis. *Acta Anaesthesiologica Taiwanica: Official Journal of the Taiwan Society of Anesthesiologists*, *44*(3), 187-189.

Jorm, A. F., & Jolley, D. (1998). The incidence of dementia: a meta-analysis. *Neurology*, *51*(3), 728-733.

Kelso, A., & Cock, H. J. P. N. (2005). Status epilepticus. *5*(6), 322-333.

Koff, M. D., Cohen, J. A., McIntyre, J. J., Carr, C. F., & Sites, B. D. (2008). Severe brachial plexopathy after an ultrasound-guided single-injection nerve block for total shoulder arthroplasty in a patient with multiple sclerosis. *The Journal of the American Society of Anesthesiologists*, *108*(2), 325-328. https://doi.org/10.1097/01.anes.0000299833.73804.cd.

Kofke, W. A. (2010). Anesthetic management of the patient with epilepsy or prior seizures. *Current Opinion in Anesthesiology*, *23*(3), 391-399. https://doi.org/10.1097/ACO.0b013e328339250b.

Krauss, J. K., Akeyson, E. W., Giam, P., & Jankovic, J. (1997). Propofol-Induced Dyskinesias in Parkinson's Disease. *Survey of Anesthesiology*, *41*(6), 342-343.

Kruczek, M., Albin, M. S., Wolf, S., & Bertoni, J. M. (1980). Postoperative seizure activity following enflurane anesthesia. *Anesthesiology*, *53*(2), 175-176.

Kruczek, M., Albin, M. S., Wolf, S., & Bertoni, J. M. (1980). Postoperative seizure activity following enflurane anesthesia. *Anesthesiology*, *53*(2), 175-176.

Kyttä, J., & Rosenberg, P. H. (1984, January). Anaesthesia for patients with multiple sclerosis. In *Annales chirurgiae et gynaecologiae,* 73(5), 299-303.

Lanier, W. L., Milde, J. H., & Michenfelder, J. D. (1986). Cerebral stimulation following succinylcholine in dogs. *Anesthesiology*, *64*(5), 551-559.

Leiknes, K. A., Schweder, L. J. V., & Høie, B. (2012). Contemporary use and practice of electroconvulsive therapy worldwide. *Brain and behavior*, *2*(3), 283-344. https://doi.org/10.1002/brb3.37.

Lenka, A., Mittal, S. O., Lamotte, G., & Pagan, F. L. (2021). A pragmatic approach to the perioperative management of Parkinson's disease. *Canadian Journal of Neurological Sciences*, *48*(3), 299-307.

Lensch, E., & Jost, W. H. (2011). Autonomic disorders in multiple sclerosis. *Autoimmune Diseases*, *2011*. https://doi.org/10.4061/2011/803841.

Levine, M., & Brown, D. F. (2012). Succinylcholine-induced hyperkalemia in a patient with multiple sclerosis. *The Journal of Emergency Medicine*, *43*(2), 279-282. https://doi.org/10.1016/j.jemermed.2011.06.062.

Ljungqvist, O., Scott, M., & Fearon, K. C. (2017). Enhanced recovery after surgery: a review. *JAMA surgery*, *152*(3), 292-298. https://doi.org/10.1001/jamasurg.2016.4952.

Lowenstein, D. H., Aminoff, M. J., & Simon, R. P. (1988). Barbiturate anesthesia in the treatment of status epilepticus: clinical experience with 14 patients. *Neurology*, *38*(3), 395-395.

Lowenstein, D. H., Bleck, T., & Macdonald, R. L. (1999). It's time to revise the definition of status epilepticus. *Epilepsia*, 40(1), 120-122.

Löwhagen Hendén, P., Rentzos, A., Karlsson, J. E., Rosengren, L., Leiram, B., Sundeman, H., & Ricksten, S. E. (2017). General anesthesia versus conscious sedation for endovascular treatment of acute ischemic stroke: the AnStroke trial (anesthesia during stroke). *Stroke*, *48*(6), 1601-1607. https://doi.org/10.1161/STROKEAHA.117.016554.

Lynn, C. S., Bloom, K., McDonough, J., & Kalynych, N. M. (2009). Pain management in the elderly: does cognitive function really matter. *AANA J*, *77*(5), 391.

Makris, A., Piperopoulos, A., & Karmaniolou, I. (2014). Multiple sclerosis: basic knowledge and new insights in perioperative management. *Journal of anesthesia*, *28*, 267-278.

Mancl, E. E., & Gidal, B. E. (2009). The effect of carbapenem antibiotics on plasma concentrations of valproic acid. *Annals of Pharmacotherapy*, *43*(12), 2082-2087. https://doi.org/10.1345/aph.1M296.

Margiotta, A., Bianchetti, A., Ranieri, P., & Trabucchi, M. (2006). Clinical characteristics and risk factors of delirium in demented and not demented elderly medical inpatients. *Journal of Nutrition Health and Aging*, *10*(6), 535.

Martinez-Rodriguez, J. E., Munteis, E., & Roquer, J. (2006). Periodic hyperthermia and abnormal circadian temperature rhythm in a patient with multiple sclerosis. *Multiple Sclerosis Journal*, *12*(4), 515-517. https://doi.org/10.1191/135248506ms1321cr.

Martucci, G., Di Lorenzo, A., Polito, F., & Acampa, L. A. (2011). 12-month follow-up for neurological complication after subarachnoid anesthesia in a parturient affected by multiple sclerosis. *Eur Rev Med Pharmacol Sci*, *15*(4), 458-460.

Martyn, J. A., White, D. A., Gronert, G. A., Jaffe, R. S., & Ward, J. M. (1992). Up-and-down regulation of skeletal muscle acetylcholine receptors. Effects on neuromuscular blockers. *Anesthesiology*, *76*(5), 822-843. https://doi.org/10.1097/00000542-199205000-00022.

McAuliffe, J. J., Joseph, B., & Vorhees, C. V. (2007). Isoflurane-delayed preconditioning reduces immediate mortality and improves striatal function in adult mice after neonatal hypoxia–ischemia. *Anesthesia & Analgesia*, *104*(5), 1066-1077. https://doi.org/10.1213/01.ane.0000260321.62377.74.

McClelland III, S., Baker, J. F., Smith, J. S., Line, B. G., Errico, T. J., Ames, C. P., & Bess, R. S. (2017). Impact of Parkinson's disease on perioperative complications and hospital cost in multilevel spine fusion: a population-based analysis. *Journal of Clinical Neuroscience*, *35*, 88-91. https://doi.org/10.1016/j.jocn.2016.10.008.

McGuire, G., El-Beheiry, H., Manninen, P., Lozano, A., & Wennberg, R. (2003). Activation of electrocorticographic activity with remifentanil and alfentanil during neurosurgical excision of epileptogenic focus. *British journal of anaesthesia*, *91*(5), 651-655. https://doi.org/10.1093/bja/aeg241.

Merico, A., Piccione, F., Levedianos, G., Vescovo, G., & Tonin, P. (2005). Autonomic and cardiac testing in multiple sclerosis patients complaining fatigue during rehabilitative treatment. *Basic Appl Myol*, *15*(2), 87-92.

Mirsattari, S. M., Sharpe, M. D., & Young, G. B. (2004). Treatment of refractory status epilepticus with inhalational anesthetic agents isoflurane and desflurane. *Archives of Neurology*, *61*(8), 1254-1259. https://doi.org/10.1001/archneur.61.8.1254.

Modica, P. A., Tempelhoff, R., & White, P. F. (1990). Pro-and anticonvulsant effects of anesthetics (Part I). *Anesthesia & Analgesia*, *70*(3), 303-315.

Mohanram, A., Kumar, V., Iqbal, Z., Markan, S., & Pagel, P. S. (2007). Repetitive generalized seizure-like activity during emergence from sevoflurane anesthesia. *Canadian Journal of Anesthesia*, *54*(8), 657. https://doi.org/10.1007/BF03022961.

Møller, A. R., & Møller, A. R. (2011). Practical aspects of monitoring spinal motor systems. *Intraoperative neurophysiological monitoring*, 207-234.

Mundiyanapurath, S., Stehr, A., Wolf, M., Kieser, M., Möhlenbruch, M., Bendszus, M., Haacke, W., & Bösel, J. (2016). Pulmonary and circulatory parameter guided anesthesia in patients with ischemic stroke undergoing endovascular recanalization. *Journal of neurointerventional surgery*, *8*(4), 335-341. http://dx.doi.org/10.1136/neurintsurg-2014-011523.

Mutluay, F. K., Gürses, H. N., & Saip, S. (2005). Effects of multiple sclerosis on respiratory functions. *Clinical rehabilitation*, *19*(4), 426-432. https://doi.org/10.1191/0269215505cr782oa.

Myslobodsky, M. S., Golovchinsky, V., & Mintz, M. (1981). Ketamine: convulsant or anti-convulsant?. *Pharmacology Biochemistry and Behavior*, *14*(1), 27-33. https://doi.org/10.1016/0091-3057(81)90099-X.

Newman, J. M., Sodhi, N., Dalton, S. E., Khlopas, A., Newman, R. P., Higuera, C. A., & Mont, M. A. (2018). Does Parkinson disease increase the risk of perioperative complications after total hip arthroplasty? A nationwide database study. *The Journal of arthroplasty*, *33*(7), S162-S166. https://doi.org/10.1016/j.arth.2018.01.006.

Ng, K., Howells, J., Pollard, J. D., & Burke, D. (2013). Different mechanisms underlying changes in excitability of peripheral nerve sensory and motor axons in multiple sclerosis. *Muscle & Nerve*, *47*(1), 53-60. https://doi.org/10.1002/mus.23455.

Nichols, C., Carrozzella, J., Yeatts, S., Tomsick, T., Broderick, J., & Khatri, P. (2018). Is periprocedural sedation during acute stroke therapy associated with poorer functional outcomes?. *Journal of neurointerventional surgery*, *10*(Suppl 1), i40-i43. http://dx.doi.org/10.1136/jnis.2009.001768.rep.

Nicholson, G., Burrin, J. M., & Hall, G. M. (1998). Peri-operative steroid supplementation. *Anaesthesia*, *53*(11), 1091-1104.

O'connor, P. W., Goodman, A., Kappos, L., Lublin, F. D., Miller, D. H., Polman, C., Rudick, R. A., Aschenbach, W., & Lucas, N. (2011). Disease activity return during natalizumab treatment interruption in patients with multiple sclerosis. *Neurology*, *76*(22), 1858-1865. https://doi.org/10.1212/WNL.0b013e31821e7c8a.

Olanow, C. W., Factor, S. A., Espay, A. J., Hauser, R. A., Shill, H. A., Isaacson, S., Pahwa, R., Leinonen, M., Bhargava, P., Sciarappa, K., Navia, B., & Blum, D. (2020). Apomorphine sublingual film for off episodes in Parkinson's disease: a randomised, double-blind, placebo-controlled phase 3 study. *The Lancet Neurology*, *19*(2), 135-144. https://doi.org/10.1016/S1474-4422(19)30396-5.

Onofrj, M., & Thomas, A. (2005). Acute akinesia in Parkinson disease. *Neurology,* 64(7), 1162-1169. https://doi.org/10.1212/01.WNL.0000157058.17871.7B.

Orange, J. S., Hossny, E. M., Weiler, C. R., Ballow, M., Berger, M., Bonilla, F. A., Buckley, R., Chinen, J., El-Gamal, Y., Mazer, B. D., Nelson, R. P. Jr, Patel, D. D., Secord, E., Sorensen, R. U., Wasserman, R. L., & Cunningham-Rundles, C. (2006). Use of intravenous immunoglobulin in human disease: a review of evidence by members of the Primary Immunodeficiency Committee of the American Academy of Allergy, Asthma and Immunology. *Journal of Allergy and Clinical Immunology*, *117*(4), S525-S553. https://doi.org/10.1016/j.jaci.2006.01.015.

Parkınson, S. K., Baıley, S. L., Lıttle, W. L., & Mueller, J. B. (1990). Myoclonic seizure activity with chronic high-dose spinal opioid administration. *The Journal of the American Society of Anesthesiologists*, *72*(4), 743-745. https://doi.org/10.1097/00000542-199004000-00025.

Pascual, J., & Berciano, J. (1992). Role of lidocaine (lignocaine) in managing status epilepticus. *Journal of Neurology, Neurosurgery & Psychiatry*, *55*(1), 49-51. http://dx.doi.org/10.1136/jnnp.55.1.49.

Patsalos, P. N., & Perucca, E. (2003). Clinically important drug interactions in epilepsy: interactions between antiepileptic drugs and other drugs. *The Lancet Neurology*, *2*(8), 473-481. https://doi.org/10.1016/S1474-4422(03)00483-6.

Perlas, A., Vincent, W., & Chan, S. (2005). Neuraxial anesthesia and multiple sclerosis. *Canadian Journal of Anesthesia*, *52*(5), 454. https://doi.org/10.1007/BF03016521.

Petersen, N. H., Ortega-Gutierrez, S., Wang, A., Lopez, G. V., Strander, S., Kodali, S., Silverman, A., Zheng-Lin, B., Dandapat, S., Sansing, L. H., Schindler, J. L., Falcone, G. J., Gilmore, E. J., Amin, H., Cord, B., Hebert, R. M., Matouk, C., & Sheth, K. N. (2019). Decreases in blood pressure during thrombectomy are associated with larger infarct volumes and worse functional outcome. *Stroke*, *50*(7), 1797-1804. https://doi.org/10.1161/STROKEAHA.118.024286.

Poser, C. M. (1987). The peripheral nervous system in multiple sclerosis: a review and pathogenetic hypothesis. *Journal of the neurological sciences*, *79*(1-2), 83-90. https://doi.org/10.1016/0022-510X(87)90262-0.

Powers, W. J., Rabinstein, A. A., Ackerson, T., Adeoye, O. M., Bambakidis, N. C., Becker, K., Biller, J., Brown, M., Demaerschalk, B. M., Hoh, B., Jauch, E. C., Kidwell, C. S., Leslie-Mazwi, T. M., Ovbiagele, B., Scott, P. A., Sheth, K. N., Southerland, A. M., Summers, D. V., & Tirschwell, D. L. (2018). 2018 guidelines for the early management of patients with acute ischemic stroke: a guideline for healthcare professionals from the American Heart Association/American Stroke Association. *stroke*, *49*(3), e46-e99. https://doi.org/10.1161/STR.0000000000000158.

Prizer, L. P., & Browner, N. (2012). The integrative care of Parkinson's disease: a systematic review. *Journal of Parkinson's disease*, *2*(2), 79-86.

Rajan, R., Brennan, L., Bloem, B. R., Dahodwala, N., Gardner, J., Goldman, J. G., Grimes, D. A., Iansek, R., Kovács, N., McGinley, J., Parashos, S. A., Piemonte, M. E. P., & Eggers, C. (2020). Integrated care in Parkinson's disease: A systematic review and meta-analysis. *Movement Disorders*, *35*(9), 1509-1531. https://doi.org/10.1002/mds.28097.

Reddy, R. V., Moorthy, S. S., Dierdorf, S. F., Deitch Jr, R. D., & Link, L. (1993). Excitatory effects and electroencephalographic correlation of etomidate, thiopental, methohexital, and propofol. *Anesthesia & Analgesia*, *77*(5), 1008-1011.

Rogawski, M. A., & Bazil, C. W. (2008). New molecular targets for antiepileptic drugs: α2δ, SV2A, and Kv7/KCNQ/M potassium channels. *Current neurology and neuroscience reports*, *8*(4), 345-352.

Saboory, E., Derchansky, M., Ismaili, M., Jahromi, S. S., Brull, R., Carlen, P. L., & El Beheiry, H. (2007). Mechanisms of morphine enhancement of spontaneous seizure activity. *Anesthesia & Analgesia*, *105*(6), 1729-1735. https://doi.org/0.1213/01.ane.0000287675.15225.0b.

Sahin, L., Korkmaz, H. F., Sahin, M., Aydin, T., Toker, S., & Gulcan, E. (2010). Desflurane anaesthesia in a patient with multiple sclerosis in total hip replacement. *Archives of Medical Science*, *6*(6), 984-986. https://doi.org/10.5114/aoms.2010.19314.

Sakurai, M., Mannen, T., Kanazawa, I., & Tanabe, H. (1992). Lidocaine unmasks silent demyelinative lesions in multiple sclerosis. *Neurology*, *42*(11), 2088-2088. https://doi.org/10.1212/WNL.42.11.2088.

Schneck, H. J., & Rupreht, J. (1989). Central anticholinergic syndrome (CAS) in anesthesia and intensive care. *Acta Anaesthesiologica Belgica*, *40*(3), 219-228.

Schönenberger, S., Uhlmann, L., Ungerer, M., Pfaff, J., Nagel, S., Klose, C., Bendszus, M., Wick, W., Ringleb, P. A., Kieser, M., Möhlenbruch, M. A., & Bösel, J. (2018). Association of blood pressure with short-and long-term functional outcome after stroke thrombectomy: post hoc analysis of the SIESTA trial. *Stroke*, *49*(6), 1451-1456. https://doi.org/10.1161/STROKEAHA.117.019709.

Segal, N., Matsuura, T., Caldwell, E., Sarraf, M., McKnite, S., Zviman, M., Aufderheide, T. P., Halperin, H. R., Lurie, K. G., & Yannopoulos, D. (2012). Ischemic postconditioning at the initiation of cardiopulmonary resuscitation facilitates functional cardiac and cerebral recovery after prolonged untreated ventricular fibrillation. *Resuscitation*, *83*(11), 1397-1403. https://doi.org/10.1016/j.resuscitation.2012.04.005.

Shemin, D., Briggs, D., & Greenan, M. (2007). Complications of therapeutic plasma exchange: a prospective study of 1,727 procedures. *Journal of Clinical Apheresis: The Official Journal of the American Society for Apheresis*, *22*(5), 270-276. https://doi.org/10.1002/jca.20143.

Shih, C. J., Doufas, A. G., Chang, H. C., & Lin, C. M. (2005). Recurrent seizure activity after epidural morphine in a post-partum woman. *Canadian Journal of Anesthesia*, *52*(7), 727. https://doi.org/10.1007/BF03016561.

Siger, M., Durko, A., Nicpan, A., Konarska, M., Grudziecka, M., & Selmaj, K. (2011). Discontinuation of interferon beta therapy in multiple sclerosis patients with high pre-treatment disease activity leads to prompt return to previous disease activity. *Journal of the neurological sciences*, *303*(1-2), 50-52. https://doi.org/10.1016/j.jns.2011.01.016.

Silverstein, J. H. (2014). Influence of anesthetics on Alzheimer's disease: biophysical, animal model, and clinical reports. *Journal of Alzheimer's Disease*, *40*(4), 839-848.

Simonet, C., Tolosa, E., Camara, A., & Valldeoriola, F. (2020). Emergencies and critical issues in Parkinson's disease. *Practical neurology*, *20*(1), 15-25. http://dx.doi.org/10.1136/practneurol-2018-002075.

Sivasankar, C., Stiefel, M., Miano, T. A., Kositratna, G., Yandrawatthana, S., Hurst, R., & Kofke, W. A. (2016). Anesthetic variation and potential impact of anesthetics used during endovascular management of acute ischemic stroke. *Journal of neurointerventional surgery*, *8*(11), 1101-1106. http://dx.doi.org/10.1136/neurintsurg-2015-011998.

Sivasankar, C., Stiefel, M., Miano, T. A., Kositratna, G., Yandrawatthana, S., Hurst, R., & Kofke, W. A. (2016). Anesthetic variation and potential impact of anesthetics used during endovascular management of acute ischemic stroke. *Journal of neurointerventional surgery*, *8*(11), 1101-1106. http://dx.doi.org/10.1136/neurintsurg-2015-011998.

Smeltzer, S. C., Skurnick, J. H., Troiano, R., Cook, S. D., Duran, W., & Lavietes, M. H. (1992). Respiratory function in multiple sclerosis: utility of clinical assessment of respiratory muscle function. *Chest*, *101*(2), 479-484. https://doi.org/10.1378/chest.101.2.479.

Smith, M., Smith, S. J., Scott, C. A., & Harkness, W. F. (1996). Activation of the electrocorticogram by propofol during surgery for epilepsy. *British journal of anaesthesia*, *76*(4), 499-502. https://doi.org/10.1093/bja/76.4.499.

Sørensen, L. H., Speiser, L., Karabegovic, S., Yoo, A. J., Rasmussen, M., Sørensen, K. E., & Simonsen, C. Z. (2019). Safety and quality of endovascular therapy under general anesthesia and conscious sedation are comparable: results from the GOLIATH trial. *Journal of neurointerventional surgery*, *11*(11), 1070-1072. http://dx.doi.org/10.1136/neurintsurg-2019-014712.

Steen, P. A., & Michenfelder, J. D. (1979). Neurotoxicity of anesthetics. *The Journal of the American Society of Anesthesiologists*, *50*(5), 437-453. https://doi.org/10.1097/00000542-197905000-00012.

Szuba, M. P., Guze, B. H., & Baxter Jr, L. R. (1997). Electroconvulsive therapy increases circadian amplitude and lowers core body temperature in depressed subjects. *Biological psychiatry*, *42*(12), 1130-1137. https://doi.org/10.1016/S0006-3223(97)00046-2.

Talke, P. O., Sharma, D., Heyer, E. J., Bergese, S. D., Blackham, K. A., & Stevens, R. D. (2014). Society for Neuroscience in Anesthesiology and Critical Care Expert consensus statement: anesthetic management of endovascular treatment for acute ischemic stroke*: endorsed by the Society of NeuroInterventional Surgery and the Neurocritical Care Society. *Journal of neurosurgical anesthesiology*, *26*(2), 95-108. https://doi.org/10.1097/ANA.0000000000000042.

Tankisi, A., Rolighed Larsen, J., Rasmussen, M., Dahl, B., & Cold, G. E. (2002). The effects of 10 reverse Trendelenburg position on ICP and CPP in prone positioned patients subjected to craniotomy for occipital or cerebellar tumours. *Acta neurochirurgica*, *144*, 665-670.

Timpka, J., Mundt-Petersen, U., & Odin, P. (2016). Continuous dopaminergic stimulation therapy for Parkinson's disease–recent advances. *Current opinion in neurology*, *29*(4), 474-479. https://doi.org/10.1097/WCO.0000000000000354.

Tortella, F. C. (1988). Endogenous opioid peptides and epilepsy: quieting the seizing brain?. *Trends in pharmacological sciences*, *9*(10), 366-372. https://doi.org/10.1016/0165-6147(88)90256-8.

Trzepacz, P. T., Weniger, F. C., & Greenhouse, J. (1993). Etomidate anesthesia increases seizure duration during ECT: a retrospective study. *General hospital psychiatry*, *15*(2), 115-120. https://doi.org/10.1016/0163-8343(93)90107-Y.

Tsang, K. K. T., & Whitfield, P. C. (2012). Traumatic brain injury: review of current management strategies. *British Journal of Oral and Maxillofacial Surgery*, *50*(4), 298-308. https://doi.org/10.1016/j.bjoms.2011.03.004.

Uhthoff, W. (1890). Untersuchungen über die bei der multiplen Herdsklerose vorkommenden Angenstörungen. *Archiv für Psychiatrie und Nervenkrankheiten*, *21*(1), 55-116.

Usubiaga, J. E., Moya, F., Wikinski, J. A., Wikinski, R., & Usubiaga, L. E. (1967). Relationship between the passage of local anaesthetics across the blood-brain barrier and their effects on the central nervous system. *British Journal of Anaesthesia*, *39*(12), 943-947. https://doi.org/10.1093/bja/39.12.943.

Vaughn, L. K., & Pruhs, R. J. (1995). Strain-dependent variability in nitrous oxide withdrawal seizure frequency. *Life sciences*, *57*(11), 1125-1130. https://doi.org/10.1016/0024-3205(95)02057-P.

Veering, B. T. (2003). Complications and local anaesthetic toxicity in regional anaesthesia. *Current Opinion in Anesthesiology*, *16*(5), 455-459.

Venkatraghavan, L., & Manninen, P. (2016). Anesthesia for deep brain stimulation. *Current Anesthesiology Reports*, *6*, 233-243.

Venkatraghavan, L., Luciano, M., & Manninen, P. (2010). Anesthetic management of patients undergoing deep brain stimulator insertion. *Anesthesia & Analgesia*, *110*(4), 1138-1145. https://doi.org/10.1213/ANE.0b013e3181d2a782.

Vercauteren, M., & Heytens, L. (2007). Anaesthetic considerations for patients with a pre-existing neurological deficit: are neuraxial techniques safe?. *Acta anaesthesiologica scandinavica*, *51*(7), 831-838. https://doi.org/10.1111/j.1399-6576.2007.01325.x.

Vidal-Jordana, A., & Montalban, X. (2017). Multiple sclerosis: epidemiologic, clinical, and therapeutic aspects. *Neuroimaging Clinics*, *27*(2), 195-204. https://doi.org/10.1016/j.nic.2016.12.001.

Vogt, J., Paul, F., Aktas, O., Müller-Wielsch, K., Dörr, J., Dörr, S., Bharathi, B. S., Glumm, R., Schmitz, C., Steinbusch, H., Raine, C. S., Tsokos, M., Nitsch, R., & Zipp, F. (2009). Lower motor neuron loss in multiple sclerosis and experimental autoimmune encephalomyelitis. *Annals of Neurology: Official Journal of the American Neurological Association and the Child Neurology Society*, *66*(3), 310-322. https://doi.org/10.1002/ana.21719.

Vukusic, S., & Confavreux, C. (2006). Multiple sclerosis and pregnancy. *Revue Neurologique*, *162*(3), 299-309. https://doi.org/10.1016/s0035-3787(06)75016-0.

Vukusic, S., & Marignier, R. (2015). Multiple sclerosis and pregnancy in the'treatment era'. *Nature Reviews Neurology*, *11*(5), 280-289.

Warlow, C. P. (1998). Epidemiology of stroke. *The Lancet*, *352*, S1-S4. https://doi.org/10.1016/S0140-6736(98)90086-1.

Warren, T. M., Datta, S., & Ostheimer, G. W. (1982). Lumbar epidural anesthesia in a patient with multiple sclerosis. *Anesthesia & Analgesia*, *61*(12), 1022-1023.

Weber, F., Rüdel, R., Aulkemeyer, P., & Brinkmeier, H. (2002). The endogenous pentapeptide QYNAD induces acute conduction block in the isolated rat sciatic nerve. *Neuroscience letters*, *317*(1), 33-36. https://doi.org/10.1016/S0304-3940(01)02420-X.

Whalin, M. K., Halenda, K. M., Haussen, D. C., Rebello, L. C., Frankel, M. R., Gershon, R. Y., & Nogueira, R. G. (2017). Even small decreases in blood pressure during conscious sedation affect clinical outcome after stroke thrombectomy: an analysis of hemodynamic thresholds. *American Journal of Neuroradiology*, *38*(2), 294-298. https://doi.org/10.3174/ajnr.A4992.

Whalin, M. K., Lopian, S., Wyatt, K., Sun, C. H. J., Nogueira, R. G., Glenn, B. A., Gershon, R. Y., & Gupta, R. (2014). Dexmedetomidine: a safe alternative to general anesthesia for endovascular stroke treatment. *Journal of neurointerventional surgery*, *6*(4), 270-275. http://dx.doi.org/10.1136/neurintsurg-2013-010773.

Wichards, W. S., Schobben, A. F., & Leijten, F. S. (2013). Perioperative substitution of anti-epileptic drugs. *Journal of neurology*, *260*, 2865-2875.

Yamashita, K., Yokoyama, T., Tokai, H., Imazu, Y., Lee, M., & Manabe, M. (2003). Anesthetic management for a patient with multiple sclerosis at exacerbation stage under general anesthesia. *Masui. The Japanese journal of anesthesiology*, *52*(5), 521-523.

Yıllar, D. O., Akkan, A. G., Akcasu, A., Özüner, Z., Eşkazan, E., & Küçükhüseyin, C. (2009). The effect of oral and subcutaneous meperidine on the maximal electroshock seizure (MES) in mice. *Journal of Basic and Clinical Physiology and Pharmacology*, *20*(2), 159-168. https://doi.org/10.1515/JBCPP.2009.20.2.159.

Yuan, Q., Wu, X., Sun, Y., Yu, J., Li, Z., Du, Z., Mao, Y., Zhou, L., & Hu, J. (2015). Impact of intracranial pressure monitoring on mortality in patients with traumatic brain injury: a systematic review and meta-analysis. *Journal of neurosurgery*, *122*(3), 574-587. https://doi.org/10.3171/2014.10.JNS1460.

Zesiewicz, T. A., Hauser, R. A., Freeman, A., Sullivan, K. L., Miller, A. M., & Halim, T. (2009). Fentanyl-induced bradykinesia and rigidity after deep brain stimulation in a patient with Parkinson disease. *Clinical neuropharmacology*, *32*(1), 48-50. https://doi.org/10.1097/WNF.0b013e31817e23e3.

Chapter 10

Postoperative Critical Care and Organ Failure in Critical Care

Cihangir Doğu*, MD
and Sema Turan, MD
Department of Intensive Care, Ankara Bilkent City Hospital, Ankara, Turkiye

Abstract

More than 300 million patients are admitted to the operation each year. This number has been shown to continue to increase the morality of noncomplication surgery is less than 1%. Postoperative complications result in a five-time increase in mortality. In surgical patients, the risk of death in the first 30 days after surgery is 1000 times higher than the surgery itself. This indicates that postoperative maintenance is as important as the operation itself. Perioperative organ damage can result in neurological complications, myocardial ischemia, acute kidney damage, respiratory failure, intestinal dysfunction, and liver failure. Acute kidney damage (AKI) is a common complication in patients admitted to the intensive care unit (ICU). More than 50% of ICU patients are AKI enhanced and 13.5% will be treated with renal replacement therapy (RRT). Perioperative myocardial injury occurs during surgery or after the administration of anesthesia and/or analgesia. 90% of patients do not show typical symptoms and the clinical diagnosis may be missed. Perioperative pulmonary complication is seen 7.9%, respiratory failure is the most common complication with 3.1%. Delirium is the most common postoperative neurological failure.

* Corresponding Author's Email: cihangirdogu@gmail.com.

In: Organ Failure and Anesthesia Practices
Editors: Ahmet Şen and Basar Erdivanli
ISBN: 979-8-89113-486-7

Keywords: renal insufficiency, heart failure, respiratory insufficiency, intestinal failure, delirium, critical care

Introduction

More than 300 million patients are admitted to the operation each year. This number has been shown to continue to increase (Weiser et al., 2015). The morality of noncomplication surgery is less than 1%. Postoperative complications result in five times the increase in mortality (International Surgical Outcomes Study, 2016). The risk of mortality within 30 days after surgery is greater than the surgery itself (Bartels et al., 2013). This indicates that postoperative maintenance is as important as the operation itself. Treatment of the operation and patient-related risk factors before and after surgery can contribute to improved results. Despite all treatment modalities, acute organ damage is common and is an important cause of morbidity and mortality for surgical patients (Nepogodiev et al., 2019). Perioperative organ damage can lead to neurological complications, myocardial ischemia, acute kidney damage, respiratory failure, intestinal dysfunction, and liver failure (Conrad & Eltzschig, 2020). Perioperative organ failures and their treatments will be presented in this chapter.

Kidney Failure

Acute Kidney Damage (AKI)

AKI is a common complication for patients in the intensive care unit (ICU). The latest epidemiological data shows that more than 50% of ICU patients have enhanced AKI and 13.5% will be treated with renal replacement treatment (RRT) (Hoste et al., 2015). Older patients have a higher incidence of comorbidities such as diabetes, cardiovascular disease, and hypertension, which has led to a significant increase in the proportion of patients treated with RRT over the last decade. The ABH is currently defined by the Kidney Disease Improving Global Outcomes (KDIGO) criteria and is divided into 3 stages depending on the level of serum creatinine and urine output. AKI is an independent risk factor for mortality (Table 1). The mortality rates for AKI that require RRT will vary between 40-55% (Griffin et al., 2020). For this reason, RRT has become an important and widely used treatment option for ICUpatients (Kolhe et al., 2016).

It is manifested by a sudden decrease in glomerular filtration resulting in impaired fluid, electrolyte, and acid-base hemostasis. It is defined by an increase in serum creatinine level or a decrease in urine output (Khwaja, 2012). Kidney Disease Improving Global Outcomes (KDIGO) guidelines require at least one of the following:

- Increase in serum creatinine level of 0.3 mg/dL or more in 48 hours
- Increased serum creatinine level to 1.5 times or more of baseline level within 7 days
- Urine output falling below 0.5 ml/kg/hour for 6 hours

Advanced age, chronic kidney disease, hypertension, heart failure, diabetes among risk factors for AKI, chronic comorbidities such as cirrhosis, and increased severity of the disease during admission to the ICU. Causes that disrupt hemodynamics, such as sepsis and hypovolemia, are the most commonly reported causes of AKI in the intensive care unit (Hoste et al., 2015). AKI is classified anatomically and is named prerenal, intrarenal, or intrinsic, and postrenal.

Table 1. Stages of AKI

Stage	Elevated serum creatinine	Urine output
1	Increase 1.5-1.9 times baseline or 0.3 mg/dl or more	Less than 0.5 ml/kg/hour for 6-12 hours
2	2-2.9 times the baseline value	Less than 0.5 ml/kg/hour for 12 hours or more
3	Increased creatinine 3 times the baseline value or creatinine value of 4 mg/dl or more or initiation of renal replacement therapy	Less than 0.3 ml/kg/hour for 24 hours or more or anuria for 12 hours or more

Prerenal Azothemia

It is associated with renal hypoperfusion and is the most common cause. It accounts for 60 to 70% of causes in the community and 40% of hospital-acquired AKI. Causes of hypoperfusion by reducing effective intravascular volume are excessive diuresis, sepsis, heart failure, or liver failure. Agents that reduce glomerular capillary perfusion, such as non-steroidal anti-inflammatory drugs (NSAIDs), angiotensin receptor blockers, and angiotensin-converting enzyme (ACEI) inhibitors, can cause prerenal ABH. These agents should not be used in patients with renal hypoperfusion.

Intrinsic Acute Kidney Injury

Renal AKI occurs with severe hypoperfusion and cellular damage, with signs of ischemia. Any part of the renal vessels, nephron, or interstitium may be involved. The main causes include ischaemia and septic injury. Furthermore, exposure to radiocontrast and renal toxins, such as aminoglycosides, can damage the tubules both directly and indirectly. The groups of patients most susceptible to toxic kidney injury include hemodynamically unstable patients, geriatric patients with diabetes mellitus, and patients with reduced effective intravascular volume (heart failure, burns, cirrhosis, hypoalbuminaemia). ABH that develops due to interstitial renal damage is called acute interstitial nephritis. The most common causes of interstitial nephritis are penicillins, cephalosporins, sulfonamides, and NSAIDs. Bacterial and viral infections, systemic lupus erythematosus, primary biliary cirrhosis, cryoglobulinaemia, and Sjögren's syndrome are among the causes.

Postrenal Acute Kidney Injury

In the urinary system, it is caused by obstruction from the ureter, bladder, neck of the bladder, or urethra. The most common causes are external compression from benign prostatic hyperplasia, metastatic cancers, neurogenic bladder or retroperitoneal fibrosis, and intrinsic obstruction from stones, crystals, or blood clots.

Management of AKI includes finding the cause and correcting the fluid status. Renal perfusion should be maintained and adequate hemodynamic stabilization should be achieved to prevent further kidney damage. Autoregulation of blood flow should be ensured. Hypotension attacks increase susceptibility to AKI development. If it is only due to dehydration, it is tried to provide renal perfusion by performing fluid replacement. How and with which fluids the replacement will be performed, the patient's age, the presence of hypertension, the accompanying septic picture, heart failure, exposure to contrast material, and pulmonary failure should be evaluated for the patient. For treatment success, urine formation should be observed at 0.5-1 ml/kg/hour per hour. During replacement, fluid load formation should not be allowed by giving too much fluid to the patient and the need for vasopressor support should be taken into consideration. The mean arterial pressure should be at 65 mmHg. In the absence of hemorrhagic shock, preferred fluids are crystalloids (KDIGO, 2012). Hydroxyethylstarch (HES) solutions are not recommended, especially in AKI replacement accompanied by sepsis. HES solutions may disrupt the coagulation cascade by reducing the concentration of von Willebrand factor, factor VIII, and VIIIc. Platelet activity may be altered by blocking the platelet fibrinogen receptor glycoprotein IIb/IIIa. It can also cause a pathological condition known as "osmotic nephrosis," which leads to a potential deterioration in kidney function (Dickenmann et al., 2008). In randomized controlled studies, its use in fluid replacement in septic patients increased mortality (Perner et al., 2012). The sepsis survival campaign also recommends balanced crystalloid solutions as the first choice for fluid replacement in septic patients (Evans et al., 2021). Nephrotoxic agents should be avoided, and treatment of comorbidities that alter nephron perfusion should be organized. If renal failure cannot be cured despite all these efforts, renal replacement therapy can be started.

Indications for RRT include hyperkalemia, persistent pulmonary congestion, uremic symptoms (such as encephalopathy, bleeding, pericarditis), and metabolic acidosis (Tolwani, 2012). Discussions about starting time continue. The authors suggesting early initiation argue that uremic complications can be avoided (Kellum et al., 2012). On the other hand, since spontaneous kidney recovery can be observed even in patients with severe AKI, early initiation of RRT and establishment of vascular access may lead to complications such as risks of the procedure itself (e.g., hypotension, arrhythmia, electrolyte abnormalities, ineffective antibiotic concentrations). The advantages and disadvantages of renal replacement therapies are indicated in Table 2.

Table 2. Advantages and disadvanges of renal replacement therapies

	Intermittent haemodialysis	Sustained low-efficeincy dialysis (SLED)	Continuous renal replacement (CRRT-CVVHD-CVVHDF)
Advantages	Staff used to Widespread Low cost Anticoagulation may not be required	Low cost Haemodynamic tolerability Anticoagulation may not be required	Haemodynamic tolerability Ability to change dosing quickly Probability of improved kidney survival in survivors
Disadvantages	Haemodynamic instability Volüme removal limitations	Limited data on the dosage of antimicrobials Lack of studies comparing efficacy	High cost More complex Need for anticoagulation

Intermittent Haemodialysis (IHD)

IHD is the process of removing solutes from the dialysis membrane by means of a concentration gradient between blood and dialysate. It is typically performed with a catheter placed in the internal jugular, subclavian, or femoral vein. To ensure that a future arteriovenous fistula remains functional, a subclavian venous catheter should be avoided as much as possible to prevent subclavian stenosis. Due to the lower blood flow rates that can be achieved with catheters and the high catabolic rate of critically ill patients, session times of up to 5 hours may be required (Network et al., 2008). Heparin is often neglected due to the bleeding risks often seen in critically ill patients. Blood flow ranges from 200 to 400 ml/min and lower blood flows are used in the first session for patients who may develop a risk of dialysis disequlibrium. In patients with impaired hemodynamics, the use of a hypertonic sodium concentration (e.g., 145 mmol/L) may improve stability by increasing fluid movement from the cell to the extracellular space. Although hyperkalemia is usually an indication for RRT, excessive potassium removal can cause hypokalaemia-mediated arrhythmias. A dialysate potassium concentration of less than 2 mmol/L should be avoided whenever possible. When calculating the ultrafiltration volume in ICU patients with fluid overload, fluid intake from patient infusions and feeding should be taken into account. The main difficulty of IHD is the need to perform relatively large volumes of ultrafiltration in a short time from a patient with unstable hemodynamics. In addition to altering the sodium concentration of the dialysate, intradialytic hypotension can be prevented or alleviated by lowering the temperature of the dialysate or by vasopressor support. However, if hypotension develops during dialysis or if increased doses of vasopressors are needed, switching to slower ultrafiltration modalities should be considered. The duration and frequency of IHD treatment is variable and usually depends on factors such as the patient's planned ultrafiltration and metabolic needs.

Extended-Duration Low-Efficiency Dialysis

Sustained low-efficiency dialysis (SLED), also known as prolonged intermittent renal replacement therapy (PIRRT), is the extension of treatment to 8 to 12 hours to achieve the hemodynamic benefits of SRRT with a conventional hemodialysis device. SLED has gained popularity due to the lack of a survival difference with SRRT compared to IHD, the lack of high costs associated with the administration of SRRT, and the ability to provide safe RRT to hemodynamically unstable patients (Klarenbach et al., 2009). The lack of anticoagulation and intermittent administration are other practical advantages of SLED. However, the fact that it is performed by dialysis nurses and cannot be applied by intensive care specialists limits its use in practice.

Continuous Renal Replacement Therapy

It is a modality in which intermittent dialysis is performed without interruption. Provides slower clearance compared to intermittent treatments. Diffusion (HD), convection (haemofiltration), or a combination of both (haemodiafiltration) are used to remove the solute load. These include continuous venous hemodialysis (CVVHD), continuous venous hemofiltration (CVVHF), and continuous venous hemodiafiltration (CVVHDF). CRRT is believed to cause less hemodynamic stress than IHD in patients with severe ABH. Similar to IHD, diffusion is used for the removal of solutes in CVVHD. In addition to treatment duration, another important difference between CVVHD and IHD is the flow rate of the dialysate. In IHD, the typical dialysate flow rate is 500 to 800 ml/min. In CVVHD, the dialysate flow rate is typically 1 to 2 L/hour and is slow compared to the blood flow rate. Allows low molecular weight solutes to equilibrate between blood and dialysate. Although CRRT provides slower solute clearance, total clearance may be higher as it is typically performed over 24 hours. In CVVHF, the physiological fluid is replaced by the difference in ultrafiltration. Solute removal is equal to the ultrafiltration rate. Dialysate is not used. In continuous hemodiafiltration, the continuous HD dialysate flow is added to the continuous hemofiltration convective ultrafiltration.

The advantages of continuous renal replacement therapies are that it can be administered by an intensive care specialist, the dose and duration can be changed according to the needs of the patient, and it can be administered at lower flows and lower blood pressures without disturbing haemodynamics. The disadvantages include the need for anticoagulation, the inability to predict the plasma level of many treatments, and the need to stop during special procedures and patient transport.

Heart Failure

Perioperative Myocardial Injury

Perioperative myocardial injury (PMI) is defined as acute cardiac muscle cell injury without symptoms, ECG, or imaging findings. Perioperative MI can be detected by preoperative and serial postoperative (e.g., 24 and 48 hours after surgery) cardiac enzyme measurements. Most PMI occurs during surgery or after the administration of anesthesia and/or analgesia. 90% of patients do not show typical symptoms and the clinical diagnosis can be missed (Gualandro et al., 2018). 30-day mortality is 10%. To say that cardiac enzyme elevation is due to myocardial damage, it is necessary to know the preoperative level. To determine the pathophysiology, it is important to differentiate between noncardiac causes (e.g., severe sepsis, pulmonary thromboembolism) and cardiac causes such as tachyarrhythmia and acute heart failure. Myocardial damage can develop due to surgical stress or due to coronary artery disease. In half of PMI patients, the underlying pathophysiology remains unexplained. The prevalence of PMI depends on comorbidities, type of operation, postoperative factors, and the preoperative rate of cardiac enzymes. The incidence of spontaneous MI in the first 30 days after postoperative day 2 is approximately 0.5% (Smilowitz & Berger, 2020). In the early postoperative period (<5 days), bleeding is a major problem and limits the use of antiplatelets and anticoagulants depending on the location and extent of the operation.

Postoperative risk factors include sepsis, hypoxia, continuous tachycardia, hypotension, severe anemia (Abbott et al., 2018). In a study examining patients with postoperative anemia, a hemoglobin of 1 g/dL low increases the risk of PMI by 1.46 times. The optimal hemoglobin value is uncertain and unnecessary transfusions cause both fluid load and immunosuppression (Turan et al., 2021). Antithrombotic therapy appears to be beneficial after PMI. In a post hoc analysis of the POISE trial, aspirin reduced the risk of 30-day mortality (Devereaux et al., 2011). In the POISE study, a reduction in mortality at 30 days was found with statin use, and its benefits for secondary prevention in patients with cardiovascular disease have been proven. Patients taking preoperative angiotensin-converting enzyme (ACE) inhibitors, beta-blockers, or statins should not be interrupted perioperatively. If the drug is discontinued preoperatively in patients using ACE inhibitors, it should be restarted as soon as possible after surgery (Devereaux et al., 2011). If the patient does not use beta blockers, they can be used perioperatively if indicated. However, it is preferable to start 2-7 days before surgery rather than starting on the day of surgery for protection purposes only. Alpha2-adrenergic receptor agonists inhibit central sympathetic discharge, do not alter perioperative hemodynamics, reduce peripheral norepinephrine release, and dilate post-stenotic coronary vessels. For these reasons, they have been proposed as an alternative to perioperative beta-blockers to attenuate the stress response. However, the POISE-2 study showed that it had no beneficial effect on overall stroke, MI or mortality rates (Devereaux & Sessler, 2015). Patients with suspected cardiac ischaemia should be consulted by cardiology. Echocardiography is used to assess cardiac function, left ventricular ejection fraction, wall motion, and valve anomalies. The timing of coronary angiography is uncertain and may depend on clinical findings, the presence of ongoing ischaemia, the elevation of cardiac enzymes, and the risk of bleeding after invasive postoperative angiography.

Heart Failure

Heart failure is a clinical syndrome caused by a structural and/or functional cardiac abnormality. It is characterized by typical symptoms that result in elevated intracardiac pressures and decreased cardiac output with or without stress. Findings such as pulmonary rales, high jugular venous pressure, and peripheral oedema can accompany. Acute heart failure syndromes are a heterogeneous group of diseases. Half of the patients actually have a preserved ejection fraction. End-diastolic volumes and pressures are high. Also, end-systolic volumes may be high. This is transmitted to the pulmonary venous circulation and leads to signs of pulmonary congestion (Michael M. Givertz, 2013). In some patients, it may lead to hepatic congestion and cause liver failure. Decreased contractility can lead to a decrease in stroke volume, which can lead to systemic hypoperfusion.

Eighty per cent of patients with acute heart failure present as an acute exacerbation of chronic heart failure, while 20 per cent are new cases of heart failure (Ponikowski et al., 2016). Increased left ventricular filling pressures, high levels of natriuretic peptides, and echocardiographic findings are helpful in diagnosis.

Table 3. New York Heart Association Functional Classification

Class 1	Patients with heart disease who are not restricted in their usual daily physical activities
Class 2	Patients with mild restriction of physical activity (e.g., shortness of breath with walking)
Class 3	Significant limitation in physical activity, the occurrence of symptoms even with very light activities such as walking around the house
Class 4	Shortness of breath even at rest

Acute Heart Failure

Acute heart failure (AHF) refers to the onset of HF symptoms that are severe enough to require urgent medical intervention and lead to admission to the emergency department. AHF is associated with hospitalization, high mortality, and rehospitalization in people older than 65 years. In-hospital mortality ranges from 4% to 10%. 1-year mortality after discharge can increase by 25-30% (McDonagh et al., 2021). AHF may be the first symptom of new heart failure, but is more often the acute manifestation of chronic HF. New-onset heart failure is associated with higher mortality (Nieminen et al., 2006).

Acute heart failure can present as follows:

1. Acute decompensated heart failure is the most common form (50-70%). It is characterized by progressive fluid retention and systemic congestion. In treatment, triggers are determined, congestion is corrected, and hypoperfusion is tried to prevent.
2. Acute pulmonary oedema is obstruction of the lung. Diagnostic criteria include dyspnea, respiratory failure, tachypnoea, >25 breaths/min, orthopnoea and increased work of breathing. Firstly, continuous positive airway pressure, noninvasive positive pressure ventilation and/or oxygen delivered through a high-flow nasal cannula should be initiated to correct respiratory failure and ensure oxygenation. Subsequently, iv diuretics must be administered and then, in patients with high blood pressure, iv vasodilators may be administered to reduce left ventricular afterload. In patients with advanced heart failure, low cardiac output can be observed with acute pulmonary oedema. Inotropes and vasopressors can be given in these patients to maintain organ perfusion.
3. In isolated right ventricular failure, congestion is observed in the right ventricle, atrium, and systemic circulation. Left ventricular filling may be affected and the flow rate may decrease (Harjola et al., 2016). Noradrenaline and inotropes can be used in cases of decreased cardiac output and in patients with hemodynamic instability. Inotropes that lower cardiac filling pressures may be preferred (e.g., levosimendan, phosphodiesterase type III inhibitors). Since arterial hypotension can increase with inotropes, they can be combined with norepinephrine.
4. Cardiogenic shock is the main cause of cardiac dysfunction due to inadequate cardiac output. Hypoperfusion of tissues can result in multiorgan failure and death. It may develop with MI, myocarditis, or

progression of chronic heart failure. Mental deterioration, cold, sweaty extremities, narrow pulse pressure, oliguria, metabolic acidosis, elevated lactate and creatinine levels are symptoms of hypoperfusion. If compensatory vasoconstriction develops, hypoperfusion is not accompanied by hypotension. Early diagnosis and treatment are crucial in preventing and treating organ dysfunction (Chioncel et al., 2017).

In the evaluation of any patient with cardiac dysfunction, three components are assessed in the history and physical examination: (1) volume status (2) tissue perfusion and (3) the presence of precipitating factors and comorbidities (Table 4, Figure 1).

Oxygen supplementation in patients without hypoxaemia can decrease cardiac output by vasoconstriction (Park et al., 2010). PO_2 target is 60 mmHg, and SO_2 >92%. Impairment in ventilation-perfusion compliance can be observed in patients with COPD who are given high oxygen. This can cause hypercarbia by impairing the respiratory drive. Intermittent non-invasive mechanical ventilation or pressure support can be used. The need for intubation can be reduced (Gray et al., 2008). It should be started when the respiratory rate is >25/min and SO_2<90%. FiO_2 can be increased to 100%. Close blood pressure monitoring should be performed as intrathoracic pressure will increase and venous return will decrease. Caution should be exercised in patients with low preload and intubation should not be delayed in cases of increased respiratory distress.

Diuretics are the cornerstone of the treatment of acute heart failure. They accelerate renal excretion of fluid and salt load. Convolute diuretics are used more frequently due to their rapid onset and high safety index. No significant differences between high initial doses and moderate doses were found in the DOSE study. However, high doses are more effective in reducing dyspnea, weight loss, and moving away from net fluid load (Felker et al., 2011). Furosemide can be started 12 times the daily oral dose of the patient, or equivalent bumetanide, torsemide, can be started intravenously. If the patient does not use furosemide before admission, 20-40 mg of furosemide can be given initially or 10-20 mg of bolus torasemide. Bolus dose of furosemide is an effective way to reach the effective level in serum rapidly. After 2-6 hours, the success of treatment is evaluated by urine sodium and urine volume. Urine sodium 50-70 mEq after 2 hours and urine volume 100-150 ml/h in the 6th hour are indicators of treatment success (Mullens et al., 2019). Thiazide, metazolone, or acetozolamide can be added to the treatment, but close electrolyte monitoring is necessary. After a negative balance is achieved, the dose of convolute diuretic should be reduced.

Table 4. Types of heart failure

Impaired perfusion at rest		Congestion at rest	
		No	Yes
	No	Warm and dry	Warm and wet
	Evet	Cold and dry	Cold and wet

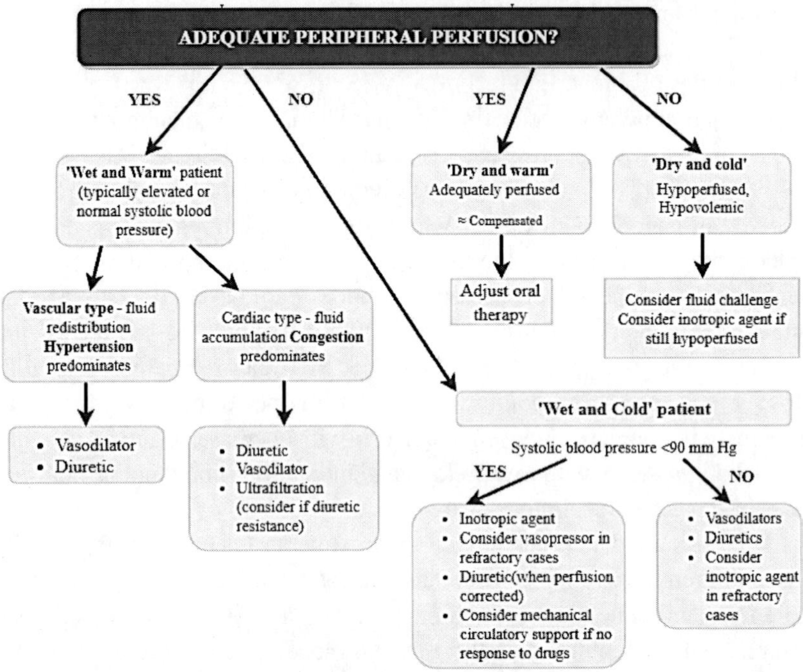

Figure 1. Treatment algorithm for heart failure (Ponikowski et al., 2016).

Vasodilators include nitrates and nitroprusside, which dilate the venous and arterial system, decrease return to the heart, congestion, and afterload, and increase flow rate. Nitrates are effective only in the venous system, whereas nitroprusside is effective in both systems. It is more effective in patients with less fluid accumulation and effective redistubution. In cases where arterial blood pressure exceeds 110 mmHg, a low dose is started and titrated. Treatment can be continued by infusion, or intermittent boluses can be administered. Nitroglycerin may be given in 1-2 mg boluses. Left-ventricular hypertrophic and aortic stenotic patients should use nitroglycerin with caution. Close monitoring is necessary to prevent hypotension attacks.

Inotropes are required in hypotensive patients with low flow. In order to prevent end-organ damage, it is recommended to start and titrate low doses as infusion with close monitoring in patients with left ventricular failure, low flow rate, and hypotensive patients. It may cause sinus tachycardia through adrenergic pathways and increase myocardial ischaemia, arrhythmia, and mortality by increasing the ventricular rate in patients with atrial fibrillation (Maack et al., 2019). Phosphodiesterase inhibitors and levosimendan dobutamine may be preferred in patients using betablockers. Severe hypotension may be observed at bolus or high doses of infusion (Table 5).

Although noradrenaline causes peripheral arterial vasoconstriction, it is the primary choice in severe hypotension. It may increase the left ventricular afterload. For this reason, it would be appropriate to use with inotropes in patients with cardiogenic shock with advanced failure. The use of dopamine as the first choice can increase mortality in patients with cardiogenic shock because it can cause more arrhythmias, but this relationship has not been shown in patients with hypovolaemic and septic shock (De Backer et al., 2010). In a study comparing adrenaline and noradrenaline in patients with cardiogenic shock after acute MI, adrenaline was found to be associated with increased heart rate, higher lactate levels, and refractory shock (Levy et al., 2018).

Table 5. Inotrope dosages for heart failure

Inotropes	Dosage
Dopamin	<5 μg/kg/m; inotropic >5 μg/kg/m: inotropic and vasopressor
Noradrenalin	0.2-1.0 μg/kg/m
Adrenalin	0.05-0.5 μg/kg/m
Levosimendan	0.05-0.2 μg/kg/m
Dobutamin	2-20 μg/kg/m
Milrinon	0.375-0.75 μg/kg/m

Opiates relieve respiratory anxiety and distress. They can be used for sedation during noninvasive positive pressure ventilation. Nausea, hypotension, bradycardia, and respiratory depression can be dose dependent. Retrospective analyzes show that morphine is associated with higher mechanical ventilation, increased length of hospital stay, length of intensive care stay, and mortality (Peacock et al., 2008). Therefore, routine use of opiates is not recommended, although opiates can be used for severe pain, anxiety, and palliation.

Digoxin can be used as a secondary option in patients with AF with a fast ventricular rate (>110 beats/min) despite beta-blockers. 0.25-0.5 mg of iv can be given as boluses. In patients with CKD or on medications that affect digoxin metabolism and/or in the elderly, it is difficult to estimate the maintenance dose; serum concentration measurements should be performed.

Respiratory Failure

Postoperative pulmonary complications (PPCs) are all events that impair respiratory function after surgery. These include infections, respiratory failure, bronchospasm, pleural effusions, pneumothorax, atelectasis, and aspiration pneumonitis. While the PPC rate was 7.9%, respiratory failure was the most common complication with 3.1%. The presence of at least one complication increased hospital mortality by 8.3% (Mazo et al., 2014). The best approach to combating PPC is possible with an appropriate preoperative evaluation and implementation of strategies to prevent the development of complications.

Risk factors for PPC include emergency surgery, advanced age, use of muscle relaxants in abdominal or thoracic surgery, ASA III-IV congestive heart failure, smoking (Merkow et al., 2015). Respiratory failure was defined by the European perioperative clinical outcomes (EPCO) working group as arterial hypoxia in ambient air ($PaO_2 < 60$ mmHg), $PaO_2/FiO_2 < 300$ mmHg or $SO_2 < 90\%$ requiring oxygen support.

Atelectasis plays a major role in the development of respiratory failure. Following the administration of muscle relaxants, the balance between the lung and chest wall elastans is altered by decreased respiratory muscle tone, and functional residual capacity decreases by 0.4-0.5 L (Hedenstierna & Edmark, 2010). The cough reflex is suppressed by pain. Anesthetics and opiates cause respiratory depression. These factors cause a decrease in functional residual capacity and are expected to lead to the development of respiratory failure. Administration of high fraction of oxygen during induction of anesthesia can cause absorption atelectasis. Causes severe hypoxemia as a result of ventilation-perfusion disorder, shunts, impaired gas exchange, and increased pulmonary vascular resistance with a decrease in compliance.

Pulmonary physiotherapy should be started preoperatively to prevent the development of PPC. Postoperative triflov application, deep breathing, and holding exercises are frequently used methods to prevent the formation of atelectasis. Mobilization can be started as early as possible to reduce atelectasis, decrease the use of painkillers, and accelerate recovery. In addition, increased ventilation-perfusion compliance, improved lung capacity, increased airway clearance, and accelerated psychological recovery are also provided (Ambrosino & Gabbrielli, 2010).

The presence of residual muscle relaxants may increase the risk of hypercarbia, hypoxia, pneumonia, atelectasis, and postoperative respiratory failure that may require reintubation. The presence of residual muscle relaxant has been shown in 30-60% of patients admitted to the recovery unit after anaesthesia (Bulka et al., 2016) Upper airway obstruction causing hypoxia, hypercarbia, atelectasis, and hypoventilation is observed in patients. The type of muscle relaxant does not change in terms of the development of complications. However, the age of the patient, the dose of the agent used, the location and duration of the operation affect the development of complications (Murphy et al., 2008) To combat the presence of residual muscle relaxant, at least qualitative Train of four (TOF) monitoring should be performed in all patients to monitor the depth of the block. The TOF ratios should be 0.9 or better before extubation. Various agents can be used to reverse the effects of muscle relaxants. The use of these agents prevents the development of complications.

Pain management is important to prevent respiratory failure by providing airway clearance and preventing muscle weakness. Analgesic regimens should be adjusted considering that opioids can cause respiratory depression. Epidural analgesia is the gold standard for pain control in patients undergoing thoracic and upper abdominal surgery. It is superior to general anesthesia due to the low use of opioids (Amini et al., 2015). Epidural analgesia reduces incisional pain and optimizes lung mechanics by restoring voluntary aspects of spontaneous ventilation. Vital capacity improves after thoracic or upper abdominal surgery. Forced vital capacity does not improve significantly. Premature airway closure is reduced, allowing deeper breathing and more effective coughing (Slinger, 2014) As a result, atelectasis is reduced and mucus clearance is achieved. It has been shown in studies to reduce PPC in patients undergoing hepatic resection, abdominal aortic aneurysm repair, colectomy, and Whipple procedures (Amini et al., 2015; Licker et al., 2013).

Artificial respiratory support should be given to patients who develop respiratory distress in the postoperative period and cannot regress despite previous measures. Application of noninvasive (NIV) methods before invasive respiratory support reduces PPC (Jaber et al., 2010). Noninvasive respiratory support can be applied as continuous positive airway pressure

(CPAP) or bilevel positive airway pressure (BiPAP). With this method, collapse in the airways and alveoli is prevented, functional residual capacity increases, atelectasis development is prevented, interstitial oedema decreases, and gas exchange increases. Furthermore, the heart afterload decreases, diaphragm activity improves, and respiratory workload decreases. Complications of invasive mechanical ventilation are prevented and the need for sedation is reduced. CPAP can be started with a positive pressure of 7-10 cmH_2O, is well tolerated by the patient and no significant haemodynamic effects are observed. In BiPAP mode, it is recommended to start with EPAP, that is, PEEP, and then IPAP should be increased to a maximum of 20-25 cmH_2O, 2 cmH_2O above PEEP, or 6-10 ml/kg expiratory tidal volume, taking into account the number of breaths and comfort. It is recommended to be applied for approximately 60-90 minutes with 2-3 hour intervals, and the total application should be 3-12 hours a day (Pelosi & Jaber, 2010). Absolute contraindications for NIV are severe agitation, cardiac or respiratory arrest, encephalopathy, multiorgan failure, failure to protect the airway. In addition, there is also upper gastrointestinal bleeding or hemoptysis, facial trauma, hemodynamic instability, or unstable cardiac arrhythmias. In case of progression of respiratory failure, invasive mechanical ventilation support should be initiated.

In patients at risk for PPH, high-flow nasal (HFNC) devices reduce reintubation and have been shown to reduce the incidence of respiratory failure requiring mechanical ventilation (Yoo et al., 2016). The HFNC is an oxygen mixer with an active humidifier that allows high oxygen inspiration, bringing the amount of fractionated oxygen close to 100% at maximum flows of 60 L/min. With high flow, the work of breathing is reduced and positive airway pressure can be achieved similar to CPAP (Zhu et al., 2017). It has been shown that airway pressure increases by approximately 5 mm Hg, and when the patient breathes with their mouth closed higher pressures could be achieved (Papazian et al., 2016). Increased pressure also depends on the amount of oxygen administered. Flows of 35 L/min provide a sustained pressure of approximately 2 mm Hg, while flows of approximately 50 L/min provide a positive airway pressure of approximately 5 mm Hg. The dead space in the oropharynx and nasopharynx is reduced (Papazian et al., 2016). Mucociliary activity is maintained with humidified and heated air (Zhu et al., 2017). Functional residual capacity and end-expiratory volumes increase. Oxygenation improves, respiratory work decreases. It has been associated with a lower formation of PPC compared to conventional postoperative oxygen support (Zhu et al., 2017). Patient comfort is also high because there is no mask that limits the patient. The risk of barotrauma is also lower compared to NIV.

Gastrointestinal Failure

Gastrointestinal (GI) problems are common after surgery. Nausea and vomiting, absence of peristalsis, gastroparesis, colonic paresis, dilation, and distention of the colon, diarrhea, and intra-abdominal hypertension are nonspecific symptoms.

Vomiting is known as visible regurgitation of gastric contents, regardless of the amount. It is caused by complex pathways that may be related to the patient, anesthesia, surgery, and inflammation. Antihistamines and anticholinergics, 5-HT(3) antagonists, corticosteroids, dopamine antagonists, and sedatives have been found to be effective in treatment (Griffiths et al., 2012). Preoperative acetominophen has been reported to reduce nausea and vomiting because it reduces pain (Apfel et al., 2013).

Table 6. Aspiration risk factors

Previous documented aspiration
Low level of consciousness (including due to sedation)
Impaired swallowing and cough: - Prolonged intubation - Neuromuscular disease - Age
Gastroesophageal reflux disease
Delayed gastric emptying, ileus
High gastric residues
Vomiting
Naso-enteric tube
Thoracic or abdominal trauma or surgery
Upper respiratory tract intervention/manipulation
Oesophageal surgery or airway surgery
Tracheostomy
Positioning of the spinal (flat head of the bed)
Transport

Gastroparesis is defined as the presence of symptoms of gastric retention and delayed gastric emptying in the absence of mechanical obstruction in the patient (Hasler, 2008). It is defined as gastric residual volume exceeding 200 ml in one measurement and gastric residual volume exceeding 1000 ml in a total of 24 hours. However, if it exceeds 500 ml, it is considered a sign of gastroparesis that requires stoppage of enteral nutrition (Reintam Blaser et al., 2017). It is very important to avoid gastric distention to prevent aspiration after upper GI surgery in patients who spontaneously breathe. Patients receiving noninvasive postoperative ventilation (NIV) may swallow air and gastric distension may be overlooked. It should be noted that there is an increased risk of aspiration in patients taking sedative and opiate analgesics. Aspiration risk factors are presented in Table 6.

Postoperative ileus is a condition characterized by postoperative nausea, vomiting, abdominal distension, and/or delayed stool passage. It may be self-limiting or may result in intestinal distension (Vather et al., 2014). The opioid effect, hormonal modulation, inflammation, electrolyte imbalance and autonomic dysfunction, intestinal hypoperfusion, and oedema are the main mechanisms. Peritonitis is common in sepsis or shock. It can also be a sign of an acute pathology such as ischemia or peritonitis. Fluid management in these patients is difficult, as both hypoperfusion (due to hypovolemia or vasoconstriction) and severe fluid resuscitation can lead to paralytic ileus (Uray et al., 2006). In each case, tissue hypoxia develops in the villi. Oral laxatives and enemas can be administered early to avoid intestinal distension and prevent colonic ileus. In the event of intestinal paralysis (other than mechanical obstruction), neostigmine should be administered as a slow infusion.

Intestinal dilatation is defined as the diameter of the small intestine over 3 cm, the colon over 6 cm, and the cecum over 9 cm (Reintam Blaser et al., 2017). Dilation refers only to enlargement (increase in diameter) and may not cause symptoms. If increased intraluminal pressure develops, distention, bloating, or pain may occur. Bacterial translocation is the most feared complication and may result in perforation. The typical finding is hyper-tympanic percussion. If symptoms are severe and the risk of perforation is thought to be high, imaging should be performed immediately. Severe isolated colon distention is a characteristic condition termed colonic pseudo-obstruction or Ogilvie syndrome. It develops clinically with gross abdominal distention, tenderness, and severe abdominal pain. If the diameter of the cecum exceeds 12 cm, the risk of perforation increases exponentially (Saunders & Kimmey, 2005). Severe distention increases both the risk of aspiration and intra-abdominal hypertension.

Intestinal oedema is defined as the thickness of the small intestine wall greater than 3 mm, the thickness of the colon wall greater than 2 mm if distended and greater than 5 mm if contracted (Fernandes et al., 2014). In critically ill patients, capillary fluid extravasation, decreased lymph flow, increased intra-abdominal pressures, and even right heart failure may develop due to mesenteric venous compression and congestion. Intestinal oedema occurs as a result of fluid overload, increasing the risk of anastomotic leakage (Nessim et al., 2013). Both fluid overload and hypovolaemia should be avoided.

Diarrhea is defined as a stool volume of more than 250 grams or 3 more liquid stools per day (Reintam Blaser et al., 2015). If intestinal ischemia occurs, it can be seen in the early postoperative period and can cause problems in prolonged intensive care hospitalizations. Patients may experience severe loss of fluid, electrolyte and trace elements, and malnutrition may occur due to malabsorption. More importantly, it can be a sign of severe colitis. (e.g., Clostridium difficile or chemotherapy-induced), toxic megacolon or abdominal compartment syndrome (Shaikh et al., 2008).

The condition where intra-abdominal pressure is above 12 mmHg is called intra-abdominal hypertension (IAH). IAH can be seen in up to 30-40% of critically ill patients. Most patients have mild IAH (intra-abdominal pressure (IAP) 12-15 mm Hg). Increased abdominal or intraluminal content, decreased compliance with the abdominal wall, or massive fluid replacement increases the risk of IAH. IAH may alter organ perfusion and cause hypoxia. Hemodynamic instability can be seen by reducing the preload of the heart and increasing its afterload. It can also cause atelectasis, bacterial translocation from the gut, and leading to systemic infection. Risk factors include obesity, abdominal surgery, sepsis, pancreatitis, liver failure/cirrhosis, gastrointestinal bleeding, respiratory failure ($PaO_2/FiO_2<300$), ileus, abdominal distension, hemoperitoneum/
pneumoperitoneum/peritoneal fluid collection, Sequential organ failure score (SOFA) > 4 points, lactate > 1.4 mmol/L, PEEP > 10, use of vasopressor/ inotrope (Holodinsky et al., 2013; Iyer et al., 2014). Pressure measurements are valuable for monitoring the abdominal compartment. Therefore, we recommend the use of intra-abdominal pressure monitoring in all patients after complicated abdominal surgery. Abdominal compartment syndrome is defined as a 25 mmHg elevation of intraabdominal pressure, is a serious consequence of increased IAP and may increase mortality. Enteral nutrition should be reduced in abdominal hypertension; it should be stopped in the compartment. Treatment recommendations are indicated in Table 7.

In addition, perioperative gastrointestinal injury, intraabdominal or retroperitoneal bleeding, anastomotic leakage, and intestinal ischaemia may develop. Short bowel and acute intestinal ischaemia may occur if the size of the resected bowel segment is too large. Short-bowel syndrome can develop when the length of the functional bowel segment is 200 cm short. In this case, intravenous fluid and nutritional support may be required. It is very important that the surgeon and the intensive care specialist communicate closely and decide on manipulations together.

Bleeding or septic complications can occur after liver and biliary tract surgery. Postoperative liver failure can occur due to insufficient liver tissue or dysfunction of the transplanted tissue. Perioperative prolonged hypoperfusion can cause hepatic hypoxia. Bile duct obstruction and portal vein thrombosis are other postoperative complications.

Ischemic hepatitis is a condition that occurs after transient hypotension or ischemia during surgery or shock, characterized by an acute increase in transaminases. Liver enzymes should be monitored in the first postoperative days. Hyperammonemia, which can lead to hepatic encephalopathy and coma, is associated with a bacterial increase that increases ammonia production in the intestine. Lactulose should be applied in the treatment. In the event of inadequate transmission of bile from the intestine, malabsorption of fat digestion and fat-soluble vitamins can develop. The dose of drugs excreted from the liver, such as paracetamol (acetaminophen), should be reevaluated after liver resection and in patients with impaired liver function.

Table 7. Intraabdominal hypertension treatment recommendations

To prevent the development of IAH	If IAH is present and pressure is increasing and/or high compartment risk	If the compartment developed
Avoid fluid overload	Gastric decompression by aspiration of the gastric tube	Deep sedation
Safe and tolerable negative fluid balance	Prokinetics and rectal enemas	Temporary neuromuscular blockade
Adequate analgesia	Decompression of colon distension by colonoscopy	Surgical decompression
	Drainage of intraabdominal or retroperitoneal collections	
	Deep sedation	

Pancreatic insufficiency can occur after pancreatic resection. Postoperative pancreatic fistula, anastomosis leakage, or parenchymal leakage should be expected to be higher than 3 times serum amylase activity if significant fluid drainage develops after 3 days postoperatively. Octreotide and cessation of enteral nutrition are the primary steps in the management of the fistula. Pancreatic secretions can cause severe tissue necrosis, erosive bleeding, and intestinal perforation in extraluminal, intraabdominal, or retroperitoneal areas. Acute severe hemorrhage and permanent fistula are feared complications after infection.

Communication between surgeon, anesthetist, and intensive care specialist is very important. Detailed patient information from the operating room to the intensive care unit, details of the operation, and discussion of future problems are the basic steps in planning and treatment. Description of the surgical procedure, preclosure status of the surgical field, contamination status of the peritoneal cavity, exact location and quality of anastomoses and stoma(s), probability of bleeding, mode of closure of the abdomen, presence of tension during closure, drains should be recorded.

Systemic perfusion must be optimized and euvolemia should be targeted. Ensuring adequate perfusion and oxygenation prevents secondary organ damage. Avoiding electrolyte imbalance is important for maintaining homeostasis and maintaining intestinal motility. Although not proven in studies, high normal potassium and magnesium levels may be beneficial in intestinal paralysis (Reintam Blaser et al., 2018). The analgesic effects of opioids and alpha agonists are frequently used agents in the postoperative period, but caution should be exercised regarding their effects on GI motility. Regular clinical assessment should be followed by monitoring when necessary. If a gastric tube is placed, residual follow-up may be necessary. Drains, stomas, and/or fistulas should be measured daily. In the event of suspicion of ILD, pressure measurements should be started immediately. Monitoring of blood lactate values is a parameter used in monitoring global and splanchnic circulatory disorders and hypoperfusion.

Neurological Failure

Delirium is the most common postoperative neurological problem. Delirium is a cognitive disorder with an acute onset and fluctuating course, characterized by impaired attention and awareness, occurring between the 2nd and 5th postoperative days. The incidence in patients with general surgery can reach 2-3%. It can be as high as 50-70% in high-risk patient groups (Watne et al., 2016). Postoperative delirium is associated with increased morbidity and mortality. It was found to be associated with dementia up to 5 years after postoperative delirium (Lundstrom et al., 2003).

Its incidence increases with age, and in patients over 60 years of age, the incidence is quite high, such as 10%-20% (Drews et al., 2015). Emergency surgery is associated with a 1.5 to three times higher risk of postoperative delirium compared to planned surgery (Chaiwat et al., 2019). Possible pathophysiological mechanisms in the development of delirium include neuroinflammation, decreased acetylcholine levels and alterations in dopamine receptors, and subclinical vascular changes (Picciotto et al., 2012; Plaschke et al., 2010; Yang et al., 2017).

The first step in the fight against postoperative delirium is to identify preoperative risk factors, regulate treatment, apply preventive treatments, and take perioperative precautions. Complicated surgeries, emergency surgery, advanced age, high ASA score, high Charlton comorbidity score, neurological, cardiac, respiratory and metabolic diseases, anticholinergic drug use, hyponatremia, hypernatremia and Parkinson's disease are preoperative risk factors. Perioperative metabolic disorder and pain are risk factors for postoperative delirium (Jin et al., 2020). Scoring systems are being developed to predict the development of postoperative delirium (Kim et al., 2016). Preoperative precautions include avoidance of polypharmacy, prevention of dehydration for more than 6 hours, preoperative pain management, and comprehensive geriatric assessment. Perioperative monitoring by ensuring adequate depth of anesthesia, multimodal opioid-free analgesia, use of paracetamol and nonsteroidal anti-inflammatory drugs, use of dexmethomidine, use of minimally invasive surgery to reduce surgical trauma, avoidance of tricyclic antidepressants, benzodiazepines, gabapentins, and scopolamine in perioperative medications, avoidance of hypothermia, maintenance of intraoperative hemodynamics, and targeted fluid replacement are interventions that can be applied to prevent delirium (Jin et al., 2020).

The patient should be assessed for recognition of delirium in patients who wake up from the operating room or are admitted to intensive care. Richmond Agitation-Sedation Scale (RASS; Table 8) delirium screening tool is used for sedation/agitation (Sessler et al., 2002). High sensitivity can also be obtained with the Confusion Assessment Method (CAM) and the Nursing Delirium Screening Scale (Nu-DESC). However, in a recent study, the sensitivity of both of these tests was lower than expected (Neufeld et al., 2013).

Table 8. Richmond Agitation-Sedation Scale

+4 Irritable
+3 Highly agitated
+2 Agitated
+1 Restless
0 Alert and calm
-1 Sleepy
-2 Light sedation
-3 Moderate sedation
-4 Deep sedation
-5 Cannot be awakened

The first thing to do postoperatively is take nonpharmacological measures. With reorientation of the patient, it can be helped to adapt to the environment and staff. This should minimize staff turnover and patient transfer whenever possible. It can be achieved by introducing employees, accessing natural light and the concept of time, and making reminders. A clinical trial has shown that orientation alone can reduce the incidence of delirium by 40%. Other nonpharmacological interventions include sleep optimization, cognitive exercises, mobilization, vision, and hearing optimization (if using a device), hydration, and nutrition (Colombo et al., 2012). Melatonin is a hormone that is involved in the regulation of sleep and is used to provide circadian rhythm. A meta-analysis reported that perioperative melatonin administration reduced postoperative delirium by 40% (Campbell et al., 2019). Ramelteon is a synthetic melatonin receptor agonist. Similar to melatonin, ramelteon is effective in reducing the risk of postoperative delirium (Wu et al., 2019). However, it is not recommended in the European Society of Anaesthesiology (ASA) postoperative delirium prevention guideline due to insufficient evidence (Aldecoa et al., 2017). Dexamethasone can be used for the prophylaxis of nausea and vomiting. In septic animal models, the administration of dexamethasone has been shown to reduce microglial and astrocyte activation and reduce the expression of inflammatory mediators (Meneses et al., 2017). In the meta-analysis published by Tao et al., high-dose dexamethasone (up to 100 mg) reduced the incidence of postoperative delirium by up to 20%; however, the safety profile without cardiac surgery is unclear (Tao et al., 2018).

Antipsychotic drugs are dopamine antagonists. They have different degrees of affinity for α-adrenergic, muscarinic and serotonergic receptors. The first generation has a higher risk of psychomotor complications and the second generation has a higher risk of metabolic and cardiovascular complications. Olanzapine and risperidone are second-generation antipsychotics. There are studies that report that prophylactic administration reduces the incidence of postoperative delirium. The results of antipsychotic prophylaxis are controversial due to its side effects (Wu et al., 2019). The European Society of Anaesthesiology (ASA) does not recommend routine use (Aldecoa et al., 2017).

Postoperative delirium can be difficult to diagnose, as it can be agitation (hyperactive) or withdrawal (hypoactive). The frequency of hypoactive delirium increases with age. Perioperative hemodynamic fluctuations increase the risk of postoperative delirium in elderly people who are sensitive to hypoxia. Respiratory depression in the recovery room and hypoxia due to analgesia may increase the risk of delirium in the elderly. The elderly need closer monitoring to prevent postoperative delirium. There are studies evaluating spontaneous eye movements, especially blinks, in patients with delirium (van der Kooi et al., 2014). Scales such as Faces Pain Scale and Pain Assessment in Advanced Dementia Scale (Warden et al., 2003) and Non-Communicative Patient Pain Assessment Instrument are available for pain assessment in patients with dementia (Horgas et al., 2007). The European Society of Anaesthesiology (ASA) recommends the application of nonpharmacological measures to reduce delirium. These include maintaining orientation (clock, communication, etc.), audio/visual aids, reducing noise and maintaining day/night rhythm, avoiding unnecessary catheters, early mobilization, and early feeding (Aldecoa et al., 2017).

Management of postoperative delirium requires active multidisciplinary collaboration and implementation of this management in the organization. To achieve this, enthusiastic leadership, active participation, and effective management of stakeholders are required.

Adrenal Failure

Produced in the fasciculata zona of the adrenal cortex, cortisol is the predominant glucocorticoid in humans. It has a circadian rhythm, controlled by adrenocorticotropic hormone (ACTH) and corticotropin releasing hormone (CRH). Up to 20 mg of cortisol is released each day. Following major elective surgery, there is a proportional increase in pro-inflammatory cytokines, CRH, ACTH, and cortisol. Daily oscillations can reach five times the baseline (Prete et al., 2018). During prolonged critical illness, decreased metabolism and clearance contribute to hypercortisolemia (Boonen et al., 2013).

Primary adrenal insufficiency includes adrenal gland diseases such as congenital adrenal hyperplasia and Addison's disease. Cortisol and aldosterone production is insufficient in patients. Patients with secondary adrenal insufficiency due to pituitary or hypothalamic disorders have cortisol deficiency, but aldosterone continues to be secreted in response to renin. Suppression of the hypothalamo-pituitary-adrenal axis can occur with all administration routes (oral; inhaled; topical; intranasal; and intra-articular) (Levin et al., 2014). Although inhaled corticosteroids are claimed to not disrupt the hypothalamo-pituitary-adrenal axis, there are publications against this (Bancos et al., 2015; Chrousos & Harris, 1998). It should also be noted that all patients treated with steroid are at this risk.

Surgical stress can be defined as induced physiological responses that trigger a homeostatic response to counter acute physical or psychological threats before, during, and after surgery. There are three stages of surgical stress:

1. Alarm phase: An immediate response, usually characterized by tachycardia and tachypnoea, mediated by catecholamines produced by the sympathetic nervous system (noradrenaline) and adrenal medulla (adrenaline), is termed the "fight or flight" response.
2. Adaptive phase: Rapid dampening of the alarm phase characterized by neurohormonal release of ADH (vasopressin), glucocorticoid (cortisol) secretion from the adrenal cortex, activation of the renin-angiotensin-aldosterone system. This complex response involves sodium and water retention, reduction of inflammation, and alteration of metabolism.
3. Exhaustion phase: Prolonged exposure to stressor(s) characterized by a persistent adaptive phase and a usually silent alarm phase response.

During the surgical stress response, there is a loss of vasomotor tone with insufficient cortisol production. The responses of the noradrenaline alpha-adrenergic receptor are impaired. Patients may develop orthostatic hypotension, supine hypotension, and severe shock if not corrected. Postoperative water retention and antidiuretic hormone-induced hyponatraemia are common and patients with inadequate aldosterone production are particularly susceptible to hyponatraemia.

Table 9. Recommended doses of steroid replacement for primary and secondary adrenal insufficiency

	Intraoperative	Postoperative
Surgery under anaesthesia (general or regional)	Hydrocortisone 100 mg intravenously at induction, then a continuous infusion of 200 mg/24 h	Hydrocortisone 200 mg/24 h iv vomiting (hydrocortisone 50 mg/6 h im) Enteral – double doses for 48 h or up to a week after major surgery Rapid recoveryenteral-doubledoses for 24 h
Bowel procedures that require laxatives/enema.	Hydrocortisone 100 mg iv/im	Enteral – double hydrocortisone doses for 24 h
Labor and vaginal delivery	Hydrocortisone 100 mg iv at labor, then continuous infusion 200 mg/24 h Alternately, 100 mg im followed by 50 mg/6 h im	Enteral – double hydrocortisone doses for 24 h

Table 10. For adults receiving adrenosuppressive doses of steroids (prednisolone equivalent ≥ 5 mg for 4 weeks or more)

	Intraoperative replacement	Postoperative replacement
Major surgery	Hydrocortisone 100 mg iv on induction, then a continuous infusion 200 mg/24 h Alternatively, dexamethasone 6–8 mg iv for 24 h	Hydrocortisone 200 mg/24 h by iv infusion (alternatively, 50 mg every 6 h by im) Enteral glucocorticoid at double the presurgical therapeutic dose for 48 h Complicated surgery double oral dose for up to a week
Body surface and intermediate surgery	Hydrocortisone 100 mg iv on induction, continuous infusion of 200 mg/24 h Alternatively, dexamethasone 6–8 mg intravenously, if used, will suffice for 24 h	Double regular glucocorticoid dose for 48 h, then continue with the usual treatment dose if not complicated.
Bowel procedures requiring laxatives/enema	Continue normal dose	
Labor and vaginal delivery	Hydrocortisone 100 mg iv in labor, followed by a continuous infusion of hydrocortisone 200 mg/24 h Alternatively, hydrocortisone 100 mg im followed by 50 mg/6 h im	

Half of patients affected by adrenal crisis have a history of adrenal crisis. It can be seen with gastroenteritis and fever and can be triggered by surgery (Hahner et al., 2010). Patients with comorbidities, asthma, and diabetes are more vulnerable to adrenal crisis. Those with mineralocorticoid or vasopressin dependence are also less stable (Bergthorsdottir et al., 2006). Hydrocortisone 100 mg intravenously at the beginning of the operation is recommended followed by 200 mg infusion for 24 hours (Woodcock et al., 2020). If no complications have developed, the oral replacement dose should be doubled in 48 hours. After major surgery, it is recommended to prolong this dose for up to seven days. Subsequently, it should be reduced to the old oral dose. If the patient is in intensive care, continuous intravenous infusion of the stress dose should be continued (Woodcock et al., 2020). The recommended treatment scheme is given in Tables 9 and 10.

Conclusion

Postoperative organ failure may develop depending on the characteristics of the operation and the characteristics of the patient. Mortality and morbidity can be reduced with close follow-up and specialized treatment for failures.

References

Abbott, T. E. F., Pearse, R. M., Archbold, R. A., Ahmad, T., Niebrzegowska, E., Wragg, A., Rodseth, R. N., Devereaux, P. J., Ackland, G. L. (2018). A Prospective International Multicentre Cohort Study of Intraoperative Heart Rate and Systolic Blood Pressure and Myocardial Injury After Noncardiac Surgery: Results of the VISION Study. *Anesth Analg, 126*(6), 1936-1945. https://doi.org/10.1213/ANE.0000000000002560.

Aldam, P., Levy, N., & Hall, G. M. (2014). Perioperative management of diabetic patients: new controversies. *Br J Anaesth, 113*(6), 906-909. https://doi.org/10.1093/bja/aeu259.

Aldecoa, C., Bettelli, G., Bilotta, F, Sanders, R. D., Audisio, R., Borozdina, A., Cherubini, A., Jones, C., Kehlet, H., MacLullich, A., Radtke, F., Riese, F., Slooter, A. J., Veyckemans, F., Kramer, S., Neuner, B., Weiss, B., Spies, C. D. (2017). European Society of Anaesthesiology evidence-based and consensus-based guideline on postoperative delirium. *Eur J Anaesthesiol, 34*(4), 192-214. https://doi.org/10.1097/EJA.0000000000000594.

Ambrosino, N., & Gabbrielli, L. (2010). Physiotherapy in the perioperative period. Best Pract Res Clin *Anaesthesiol, 24*(2), 283-289. https://doi.org/10.1016/j.bpa.2010.02.003.

Amini, N., Kim, Y., Hyder, O., Spolverato, G., Wu, C. L., Page, A. J., & Pawlik, T. M. (2015). A nationwide analysis of the use and outcomes of perioperative epidural analgesia in patients undergoing hepatic and pancreatic surgery. *Am J Surg, 210*(3), 483-491. https://doi.org/10.1016/j.amjsurg.2015.04.009.

Apfel, C. C., Turan, A., Souza, K., Pergolizzi, J., & Hornuss, C. (2013). Intravenous acetaminophen reduces postoperative nausea and vomiting: a systematic review and meta-analysis. *Pain, 154*(5), 677-689. https://doi.org/10.1016/j.pain.2012.12.025.

Bancos, I., Hahner, S., Tomlinson, J., & Arlt, W. (2015). Diagnosis and management of adrenal insufficiency. *Lancet Diabetes Endocrinol*, *3*(3), 216-226. https://doi.org/10.1016/S2213-8587(14)70142-1.

Bartels, K., Karhausen, J., Clambey, E. T., Grenz, A., & Eltzschig, H. K. (2013). Perioperative organ injury. *Anesthesiology*, *119*(6), 1474-1489. https://doi.org/10.1097/ALN.0000000000000022.

Bergthorsdottir, R., Leonsson-Zachrisson, M., Oden, A., & Johannsson, G. (2006). Premature mortality in patients with Addison's disease: a population-based study. *J Clin Endocrinol Metab*, *91*(12), 4849-4853. https://doi.org/10.1210/jc.2006-0076.

Boonen, E., Vervenne, H., Meersseman, P., Andrew, R., Mortier, L., Declercq, P. E., Vanwijngaerden, Y. M., Spriet, I., Wouters, P. J., Vander Perre, S., Langouche, L., Vanhorebeek, I., Walker, B. R., Van den Berghe, G. (2013). Reduced cortisol metabolism during critical illness. *N Engl J Med*, *368*(16), 1477-1488. https://doi.org/10.1056/NEJMoa1214969.

Bulka, C. M., Terekhov, M. A., Martin, B. J., Dmochowski, R. R., Hayes, R. M., & Ehrenfeld, J. M. (2016). Nondepolarizing Neuromuscular Blocking Agents, Reversal, and Risk of Postoperative Pneumonia. *Anesthesiology, 125*(4), 647-655. https://doi.org/10.1097/ALN.0000000000001279.

Campbell, A. M., Axon, D. R., Martin, J. R., Slack, M. K., Mollon, L., & Lee, J. K. (2019). Melatonin for the prevention of postoperative delirium in older adults: a systematic review and meta-analysis. *BMC Geriatr, 19*(1), 272. https://doi.org/10.1186/s12877-019-1297-6.

Chaiwat, O., Chanidnuan, M., Pancharoen, W., Vijitmala, K., Danpornprasert, P., Toadithep, P., & Thanakiattiwibun, C. (2019). Postoperative delirium in critically ill surgical patients: incidence, risk factors, and predictive scores. *BMC Anesthesiol, 19*(1), 39. https://doi.org/10.1186/s12871-019-0694-x.

Chioncel, O., Mebazaa, A., Harjola, V. P., Coats, A. J., Piepoli, M. F., Crespo-Leiro, M. G. Laroche, C., Seferovic, P. M., Anker, S. D., Ferrari, R., Ruschitzka, F., Lopez-Fernandez, S., Miani, D., Filippatos, G., Maggioni, A. P., Investigators, E. S. C. H. F. L. T. R. (2017). Clinical phenotypes and outcome of patients hospitalized for acute heart failure: the ESC Heart Failure Long-Term Registry. *Eur J Heart Fail, 19*(10), 1242-1254. https://doi.org/10.1002/ejhf.890.

Chrousos, G. P., & Harris, A. G. (1998). Hypothalamic-pituitary-adrenal axis suppression and inhaled corticosteroid therapy. 1. General principles. *Neuroimmunomodulation,* 5(6), 277-287. https://doi.org/10.1159/000026348.

Colombo, R., Corona, A., Praga, F., Minari, C., Giannotti, C., Castelli, A., & Raimondi, F. (2012). A reorientation strategy for reducing delirium in the critically ill. Results of an interventional study. *Minerva Anestesiol, 78*(9), 1026-1033. https://www.ncbi.nlm.nih.gov/pubmed/22772860.

Conrad, C., & Eltzschig, H. K. (2020). Disease Mechanisms of Perioperative Organ Injury. *Anesth Analg, 131*(6), 1730-1750. https://doi.org/10.1213/ANE.0000000000005191.

De Backer, D., Biston, P., Devriendt, J., Madl, C., Chochrad, D., Aldecoa, C., Brasseur, A., Defrance, P., Gottignies, P., Vincent, J. L., & Investigators, S. I. (2010). Comparison of dopamine and norepinephrine in the treatment of shock. *N Engl J Med, 362*(9), 779-789. https://doi.org/10.1056/NEJMoa0907118.

Devereaux, P. J., & Sessler, D. I. (2015). Cardiac Complications in Patients Undergoing Major Noncardiac Surgery. *N Engl J Med, 373*(23), 2258-2269. https://doi.org/10.1056/NEJMra1502824.

Devereaux, P. J., Xavier, D., Pogue, J., Guyatt, G., Sigamani, A., Garutti, I., Leslie, K., Rao-Melacini, P., Chrolavicius, S., Yang, H., Macdonald, C., Avezum, A., Lanthier, L., Hu, W., Yusuf, S., Poise Investigators (2011). Characteristics and short-term prognosis of perioperative myocardial infarction in patients undergoing noncardiac surgery: a cohort study. *Ann Intern Med, 154*(8), 523-528. https://doi.org/10.7326/0003-4819-154-8-201104190-00003.

Dickenmann, M., Oettl, T., & Mihatsch, M. J. (2008). Osmotic nephrosis: acute kidney injury with accumulation of proximal tubular lysosomes due to administration of exogenous solutes. *Am J Kidney Dis, 51*(3), 491-503. https://doi.org/10.1053/j.ajkd.2007.10.044.

Drews, T., Franck, M., Radtke, F. M., Weiss, B., Krampe, H., Brockhaus, W. R., Winterer, G., Spies, C. D. (2015). Postoperative delirium is an independent risk factor for posttraumatic stress disorder in the elderly patient: a prospective observational study. *Eur J Anaesthesiol, 32*(3), 147-151. https://doi.org/10.1097/EJA.0000000000000107.

Duncan, A. E. (2012). Hyperglycemia and perioperative glucose management. Curr Pharm Des, *18*(38), 6195-6203. https://doi.org/10.2174/138161212803832236.

Evans, L., Rhodes, A., Alhazzani, W., Antonelli, M., Coopersmith, C. M., French, C., Machado, F. R., McIntyre, L., Ostermann, M., Prescott, H. C., Schorr, C., Simpson, S., Wiersinga, W. J., Alshamsi, F., Angus, D. C., Arabi, Y., Azevedo, L., Beale, R., Beilman, G., Belley-Cote, E., Burry, L., Cecconi, M., Centofanti, J., Coz Yataco, A., De Waele, J., Dellinger, R. P., Doi, K., Du, B., Estenssoro, E., Ferrer, R., Gomersall, C., Hodgson, C., Hylander Moller, M., Iwashyna, T., Jacob, S., Kleinpell, R., Klompas, M., Koh, Y., Kumar, A., Kwizera, A., Lobo, S., Masur, H., McGloughlin, S., Mehta, S., Mehta, Y., Mer, M., Nunnally, M., Oczkowski, S., Osborn, T., Papathanassoglou, E., Perner, A., Puskarich, M., Roberts, J., Schweickert, W., Seckel, M., Sevransky, J., Sprung, C. L., Welte, T., Zimmerman, J., Levy, M. (2021). Surviving Sepsis Campaign: International Guidelines for Management of Sepsis and Septic Shock 2021. *Crit Care Med, 49*(11), e1063-e1143. https://doi.org/10.1097/CCM.0000000000005337.

Felker, G. M., Lee, K. L., Bull, D. A., Redfield, M. M., Stevenson, L. W., Goldsmith, S. R., LeWinter, M. M., Deswal, A., Rouleau, J. L., Ofili, E. O., Anstrom, K. J., Hernandez, A. F., McNulty, S. E., Velazquez, E. J., Kfoury, A. G., Chen, H. H., Givertz, M. M., Semigran, M. J., Bart, B. A., Mascette, A. M., Braunwald, E., O'Connor, C. M., Nhlbi Heart Failure Clinical Research Network (2011). Diuretic strategies in patients with acute decompensated heart failure. *N Engl J Med, 364*(9), 797-805. https://doi.org/10.1056/NEJMoa1005419.

Fernandes, T., Oliveira, M. I., Castro, R., Araujo, B., Viamonte, B., & Cunha, R. (2014). Bowel wall thickening at CT: simplifying the diagnosis. *Insights Imaging, 5*(2), 195-208. https://doi.org/10.1007/s13244-013-0308-y.

Gray, A., Goodacre, S., Newby, D. E., Masson, M., Sampson, F., Nicholl, J., & Trialists, C. P. O. (2008). Noninvasive ventilation in acute cardiogenic pulmonary edema. *N Engl J Med, 359*(2), 142-151. https://doi.org/10.1056/NEJMoa0707992.

Griffin, B. R., Liu, K. D., & Teixeira, J. P. (2020). Critical Care Nephrology: Core Curriculum 2020. *Am J Kidney Dis,* 75*(*3), 435-452. https://doi.org/10.1053/j.ajkd.2019.10.010.

Griffiths, J. D., Gyte, G. M., Paranjothy, S., Brown, H. C., Broughton, H. K., & Thomas, J. (2012). Interventions for preventing nausea and vomiting in women undergoing regional anaesthesia for caesarean section. *Cochrane Database Syst Rev, 2012*(9), CD007579. https://doi.org/10.1002/14651858.CD007579.pub2.

Gualandro, D. M., Puelacher, C., LuratiBuse, G., Lampart, A., Strunz, C., Cardozo, F. A., Yu, P. C., Jaffe, A. S., Barac, S., Bock, L., Badertscher, P., du Fay de Lavallaz, J., Marbot, S., Sazgary, L., Bolliger, D., Rentsch, K., Twerenbold, R., Hammerer-Lercher, A., Melo, E. S., Calderaro, D., Duarte, A. J., de Luccia, N., Caramelli, B., Mueller, C., TropoVasc,, Basel-Pmi Investigators (2018). Comparison of high-sensitivity cardiac troponin I and T for the prediction of cardiac complications after non-cardiac surgery. *Am Heart J, 203*, 67-73. https://doi.org/10.1016/j.ahj.2018.06.012.

Hahner, S., Loeffler, M., Bleicken, B., Drechsler, C., Milovanovic, D., Fassnacht, M., Ventz, M., Quinkler, M., & Allolio, B. (2010). Epidemiology of adrenal crisis in chronic adrenal insufficiency: the need for new prevention strategies. *Eur J Endocrinol*, *162*(3), 597-602. https://doi.org/10.1530/EJE-09-0884.

Harjola, V. P., Mebazaa, A., Celutkiene, J., Bettex, D., Bueno, H., Chioncel, O., Crespo-Leiro, M. G., Falk, V., Filippatos, G., Gibbs, S., Leite-Moreira, A., Lassus, J., Masip, J., Mueller, C., Mullens, W., Naeije, R., Nordegraaf, A. V., Parissis, J., Riley, J. P., Ristic, A., Rosano, G., Rudiger, A., Ruschitzka, F., Seferovic, P., Sztrymf, B., Vieillard-Baron, A., Yilmaz, M. B., & Konstantinides, S. (2016). Contemporary management of acute right ventricular failure: a statement from the Heart Failure Association and the Working Group on Pulmonary Circulation and Right Ventricular Function of the European Society of Cardiology. *Eur J Heart Fail*, *18*(3), 226-241. https://doi.org/10.1002/ejhf.478.

Hasler, W. L. (2008). Gastroparesis--current concepts and considerations. *Medscape J Med*, *10*(1), 16. https://www.ncbi.nlm.nih.gov/pubmed/18324326.

Hedenstierna, G., & Edmark, L. (2010). Mechanisms of atelectasis in the perioperative period. Best Pract Res Clin Anaesthesiol, *24*(2), 157-169. https://doi.org/10.1016/j.bpa.2009.12.002.

Holodinsky, J. K., Roberts, D. J., Ball, C. G., Blaser, A. R., Starkopf, J., Zygun, D. A., Stelfox, H. T., Malbrain, M. L., Jaeschke, R. C, Kirkpatrick, A. W. (2013). Risk factors for intra-abdominal hypertension and abdominal compartment syndrome among adult intensive care unit patients: a systematic review and meta-analysis. *Crit Care*, *17*(5), R249. https://doi.org/10.1186/cc13075.

Horgas, A. L., Nichols, A. L., Schapson, C. A., & Vietes, K. (2007). Assessing pain in persons with dementia: relationships among the non-communicative patient's pain assessment instrument, self-report, and behavioral observations. *Pain Manag Nurs*, *8*(2), 77-85. https://doi.org/10.1016/j.pmn.2007.03.003.

Hoste, E. A., Bagshaw, S. M., Bellomo, R., Cely, C. M., Colman, R., Cruz, D. N., Edipidis, K., Forni, L. G., Gomersall, C. D., Govil, D., Honore, P. M., Joannes-Boyau, O., Joannidis, M., Korhonen, A. M., Lavrentieva, A., Mehta, R. L., Palevsky, P., Roessler, E., Ronco, C., Uchino, S., Vazquez, J. A., Vidal Andrade, E., Webb, S, Kellum, J. A. (2015). Epidemiology of acute kidney injury in critically ill patients: the multinational AKI-EPI study. *Intensive Care Med*, *41*(8), 1411-1423. https://doi.org/10.1007/s00134-015-3934-7.

International Surgical Outcomes Study, g. (2016). Global patient outcomes after elective surgery: prospective cohort study in 27 low-, middle- and high-income countries. *Br J Anaesth*, *117*(5), 601-609. https://doi.org/10.1093/bja/aew316.

Iyer, D., Rastogi, P., Aneman, A., & D'Amours, S. (2014). Early screening to identify patients at risk of developing intra-abdominal hypertension and abdominal compartment syndrome. *Acta Anaesthesiol Scand*, *58*(10), 1267-1275. https://doi.org/10.1111/aas.12409.

Jaber, S., Michelet, P., & Chanques, G. (2010). Role of non-invasive ventilation (NIV) in the perioperative period. *Best Pract Res Clin Anaesthesiol*, *24*(2), 253-265. https://doi.org/10.1016/j.bpa.2010.02.007.

Jin, Z., Hu, J., & Ma, D. (2020). Postoperative delirium: perioperative assessment, risk reduction, and management. *Br J Anaesth*, *125*(4), 492-504. https://doi.org/10.1016/j.bja.2020.06.063.

KDIGO. (2012). Clinical Practice Guidelines for Acute Kidney Injury 2012. Retrieved from https://kdigo.org/guidelines/acute-kidney-injury/.

Kellum, J. A., Bellomo, R., & Ronco, C. (2012). Kidney attack. *Jama, 307*(21), 2265-2266. https://doi.org/10.1001/jama.2012.4315.

Kelly, K. N., & Domajnko, B. (2013). Perioperative stress-dose steroids. *Clin Colon Rectal Surg*, *26*(3), 163-167. https://doi.org/10.1055/s-0033-1351132.

Khwaja, A. (2012). KDIGO clinical practice guidelines for acute kidney injury. *Nephron Clin Pract*, *120*(4), c179-184. https://doi.org/10.1159/000339789.

Kim, M. Y., Park, U. J., Kim, H. T., & Cho, W. H. (2016). DELirium Prediction Based on Hospital Information (Delphi) in General Surgery Patients. *Medicine (Baltimore), 95*(12), e3072. https://doi.org/10.1097/MD.0000000000003072.

Klarenbach, S., Manns, B., Pannu, N., Clement, F. M., Wiebe, N., Tonelli, M., & Alberta Kidney Disease, N. (2009). Economic evaluation of continuous renal replacement therapy in acute renal failure. *Int J Technol Assess Health Care*, *25*(3), 331-338. https://doi.org/10.1017/S0266462309990134.

Kolhe, N. V., Muirhead, A. W., Wilkes, S. R., Fluck, R. J., & Taal, M. W. (2016). The epidemiology of hospitalised acute kidney injury not requiring dialysis in England from 1998 to 2013: retrospective analysis of hospital episode statistics. *Int J Clin Pract*, *70*(4), 330-339. https://doi.org/10.1111/ijcp.12774.

Levin, O. S., Polunina, A. G., Demyanova, M. A., & Isaev, F. V. (2014). Steroid myopathy in patients with chronic respiratory diseases. *J Neurol Sci*, *338*(1-2), 96-101. https://doi.org/10.1016/j.jns.2013.12.023.

Levy, B., Clere-Jehl, R., Legras, A., Morichau-Beauchant, T., Leone, M., Frederique, G., Quenot, J. P., Kimmoun, A., Cariou, A., Lassus, J., Harjola, V. P., Meziani, F., Louis, G., Rossignol, P., Duarte, K., Girerd, N., Mebazaa, A., Vignon, P., Collaborators. (2018). Epinephrine Versus Norepinephrine for Cardiogenic Shock After Acute Myocardial Infarction. *J Am Coll Cardiol*, *72*(2), 173-182. https://doi.org/10.1016/j.jacc.2018.04.051.

Licker, M., Christoph, E., Cartier, V., Mugnai, D., Murith, N., Kalangos, A., Aldenkortt, M., Cassina, T., Diaper, J. (2013). Impact of anesthesia technique on the incidence of major complications after open aortic abdominal surgery: a cohort study. *J Clin Anesth*, *25*(4), 296-308. https://doi.org/10.1016/j.jclinane.2013.01.009.

Lundstrom, M., Edlund, A., Bucht, G., Karlsson, S., & Gustafson, Y. (2003). Dementia after delirium in patients with femoral neck fractures. *J Am Geriatr Soc*, *51*(7), 1002-1006. https://doi.org/10.1046/j.1365-2389.2003.51315.x.

Maack, C., Eschenhagen, T., Hamdani, N., Heinzel, F. R., Lyon, A. R., Manstein, D. J., Metzger, J., Papp, Z., Tocchetti, C. G., Yilmaz, M. B., Anker, S. D., Balligand, J. L., Bauersachs, J., Brutsaert, D., Carrier, L., Chlopicki, S., Cleland, J. G., de Boer, R. A., Dietl, A., Fischmeister, R., Harjola, V. P., Heymans, S., Hilfiker-Kleiner, D., Holzmeister, J., de Keulenaer, G., Limongelli, G., Linke, W. A., Lund, L. H., Masip, J., Metra, M., Mueller, C., Pieske, B., Ponikowski, P., Ristic, A., Ruschitzka, F., Seferovic, P. M., Skouri, H., Zimmermann, W. H,. Mebazaa, A. (2019). Treatments targeting inotropy. *Eur Heart J*, *40*(44), 3626-3644. https://doi.org/10.1093/eurheartj/ehy600.

Mazo, V., Sabate, S., Canet, J., Gallart, L., de Abreu, M. G., Belda, J., Langeron, O., Hoeft, A., Pelosi, P. (2014). Prospective external validation of a predictive score for postoperative pulmonary complications. *Anesthesiology, 121*(2), 219-231. https://doi.org/10.1097/ALN.0000000000000334.

McDonagh, T. A., Metra, M., Adamo, M., Gardner, R. S., Baumbach, A., Bohm, M., Burri, H., Butler, J., Celutkiene, J., Chioncel, O., Cleland, J. G. F., Coats, A. J. S., Crespo-Leiro, M. G., Farmakis, D., Gilard, M., Heymans, S., Hoes, A. W., Jaarsma, T., Jankowska, E. A., Lainscak, M., Lam, C. S. P., Lyon, A. R., McMurray, J. J. V., Mebazaa, A., Mindham, R., Muneretto, C., Francesco Piepoli, M., Price, S., Rosano, G. M. C., Ruschitzka, F., Kathrine Skibelund, A., E. S. C. Scientific Document Group. (2021). 2021 ESC Guidelines for the diagnosis and treatment of acute and chronic heart failure. *Eur Heart J*, *42*(36), 3599-3726. https://doi.org/10.1093/eurheartj/ehab368.

Meneses, G., Gevorkian, G., Florentino, A., Bautista, M. A., Espinosa, A., Acero, G., Diaz, G., Fleury, A., Perez Osorio, I. N., Del Rey, A., Fragoso, G., Sciutto, E, Besedovsky, H. (2017). Intranasal delivery of dexamethasone efficiently controls LPS-induced murine neuroinflammation. *Clin Exp Immunol*, *190*(3), 304-314. https://doi.org/10.1111/cei.13018.

Merkow, R. P., Ju, M. H., Chung, J. W., Hall, B. L., Cohen, M. E., Williams, M. V., Tsai, T. C., Ko, C. Y, Bilimoria, K. Y. (2015). Underlying reasons associated with hospital readmission following surgery in the United States. *Jama, 313*(5), 483-495. https://doi.org/10.1001/jama.2014.18614.

Michael M., & Givertz, W. S. C. (2013). Cardiovascular Therapeutics: *A Companion to Braunwald's Heart Disease* (Fourth Edition). https://doi.org/10.1016/B978-1-4557-0101-8.00014-X.

Mullens, W., Damman, K., Harjola, V. P., Mebazaa, A., Brunner-La Rocca, H. P., Martens, P., Testani, J. M., Tang, W. H. W., Orso, F., Rossignol, P., Metra, M., Filippatos, G., Seferovic, P. M., Ruschitzka, F, Coats, A. J. (2019). The use of diuretics in heart failure with congestion-a position statement from the Heart Failure Association of the European Society of Cardiology. *Eur J Heart Fail, 21*(2), 137-155. https://doi.org/10.1002/ejhf.1369.

Murphy, G. S., Szokol, J. W., Marymont, J. H., Greenberg, S. B., Avram, M. J., & Vender, J. S. (2008). Residual neuromuscular blockade and critical respiratory events in the postanesthesia care unit. *Anesth Analg, 107*(1), 130-137. https://doi.org/10.1213/ane.0b013e31816d1268.

Nepogodiev, D., Martin, J., Biccard, B., Makupe, A., Bhangu, A., & National Institute for Health Research Global Health Research Unit on Global, S. (2019). Global burden of postoperative death. *Lancet, 393*(10170), 401. https://doi.org/10.1016/S0140-6736(18)33139-8.

Nessim, C., Sideris, L., Turcotte, S., Vafiadis, P., Lapostole, A. C., Simard, S., Koch, P., Fortier, L. P., Dube, P. (2013). The effect of fluid overload in the presence of an epidural on the strength of colonic anastomoses. *J Surg Res, 183*(2), 567-573. https://doi.org/10.1016/j.jss.2013.03.030.

Network, V. N. A. R. F. T., Palevsky, P. M., Zhang, J. H., O'Connor, T. Z., Chertow, G. M., Crowley, S. T., Choudhury, D., Finkel, K., Kellum, J. A., Paganini, E., Schein, R. M., Smith, M. W., Swanson, K. M., Thompson, B. T., Vijayan, A., Watnick, S., Star, R. A, & Peduzzi, P. (2008). Intensity of renal support in critically ill patients with acute kidney injury. *N Engl J Med, 359*(1), 7-20. https://doi.org/10.1056/NEJMoa0802639.

Neufeld, K. J., Leoutsakos, J. S., Sieber, F. E., Joshi, D., Wanamaker, B. L., Rios-Robles, J., & Needham, D. M. (2013). Evaluation of two delirium screening tools for detecting post-operative delirium in the elderly. *Br J Anaesth, 111*(4), 612-618. https://doi.org/10.1093/bja/aet167.

Nieminen, M. S., Brutsaert, D., Dickstein, K., Drexler, H., Follath, F., Harjola, V. P., Hochadel, M., Komajda, M., Lassus, J., Lopez-Sendon, J. L., Ponikowski, P., Tavazzi, L, Heart Failure Association, E. S. o. C. (2006). EuroHeart Failure Survey II (EHFS II): a survey on hospitalized acute heart failure patients: description of population. *Eur Heart J*, *27*(22), 2725-2736. https://doi.org/10.1093/eurheartj/ehl193.

Papazian, L., Corley, A., Hess, D., Fraser, J. F., Frat, J. P., Guitton, C., Jaber, S., Maggiore, S. M., Nava, S., Rello, J., Ricard, J. D., Stephan, F., Trisolini, R., & Azoulay, E. (2016). Use of high-flow nasal cannula oxygenation in ICU adults: a narrative review. *Intensive Care Med*, *42*(9), 1336-1349. https://doi.org/10.1007/s00134-016-4277-8.

Park, J. H., Balmain, S., Berry, C., Morton, J. J., & McMurray, J. J. (2010). Potentially detrimental cardiovascular effects of oxygen in patients with chronic left ventricular systolic dysfunction. *Heart*, *96*(7), 533-538. https://doi.org/10.1136/hrt.2009.175257.

Peacock, W. F., Hollander, J. E., Diercks, D. B., Lopatin, M., Fonarow, G., & Emerman, C. L. (2008). Morphine and outcomes in acute decompensated heart failure: an ADHERE analysis. *Emerg Med J*, *25*(4), 205-209. https://doi.org/10.1136/emj.2007.050419.

Pelosi, P., & Jaber, S. (2010). Noninvasive respiratory support in the perioperative period. Curr Opin *Anaesthesiol*, *23*(2), 233-238. https://doi.org/10.1097/ACO.0b013e328335daec.

Perner, A., Haase, N., Guttormsen, A. B., Tenhunen, J., Klemenzson, G., Aneman, A., Madsen, K. R., Moller, M. H., Elkjaer, J. M., Poulsen, L. M., Bendtsen, A., Winding, R., Steensen, M., Berezowicz, P., Soe-Jensen, P., Bestle, M., Strand, K., Wiis, J., White, J. O., Thornberg, K. J., Quist, L., Nielsen, J., Andersen, L. H., Holst, L. B., Thormar, K., Kjaeldgaard, A. L., Fabritius, M. L., Mondrup, F., Pott, F. C., Moller, T. P., Winkel, P., Wetterslev, J., & Scandinavian Critical Care Trials, G. (2012). Hydroxyethyl starch 130/0.42 versus Ringer's acetate in severe sepsis. *N Engl J Med*, *367*(2), 124-134. https://doi.org/10.1056/NEJMoa1204242.

Picciotto, M. R., Higley, M. J., & Mineur, Y. S. (2012). Acetylcholine as a neuromodulator: cholinergic signaling shapes nervous system function and behavior. *Neuron*, *76*(1), 116-129. https://doi.org/10.1016/j.neuron.2012.08.036.

Plaschke, K., Fichtenkamm, P., Schramm, C., Hauth, S., Martin, E., Verch, M., Karck, M., & Kopitz, J. (2010). Early postoperative delirium after open-heart cardiac surgery is associated with decreased bispectral EEG and increased cortisol and interleukin-6. *Intensive Care Med*, *36*(12), 2081-2089. https://doi.org/10.1007/s00134-010-2004-4.

Ponikowski, P., Voors, A. A., Anker, S. D., Bueno, H., Cleland, J. G. F., Coats, A. J. S., Falk, V., Gonzalez-Juanatey, J. R., Harjola, V. P., Jankowska, E. A., Jessup, M., Linde, C., Nihoyannopoulos, P., Parissis, J. T., Pieske, B., Riley, J. P., Rosano, G. M. C., Ruilope, L. M., Ruschitzka, F., Rutten, F. H., van der Meer, P, & Group, E. S. C. S. D. (2016). 2016 ESC Guidelines for the diagnosis and treatment of acute and chronic heart failure: The Task Force for the diagnosis and treatment of acute and chronic heart failure of the European Society of Cardiology (ESC)Developed with the special contribution of the Heart Failure Association (HFA) of the ESC. *Eur Heart J*, *37*(27), 2129-2200. https://doi.org/10.1093/eurheartj/ehw128.

Prete, A., Yan, Q., Al-Tarrah, K., Akturk, H. K., Prokop, L. J., Alahdab, F., Foster, M. A., Lord, J. M., Karavitaki, N., Wass, J. A., Murad, M. H., Arlt, W., & Bancos, I. (2018). The cortisol stress response induced by surgery: A systematic review and meta-analysis. *Clin Endocrinol (Oxf)*, *89*(5), 554-567. https://doi.org/10.1111/cen.13820.

Reintam Blaser, A., Deane, A. M., & Fruhwald, S. (2015). Diarrhoea in the critically ill. *Curr Opin Crit Care*, *21*(2), 142-153. https://doi.org/10.1097/MCC.0000000000000188.

Reintam Blaser, A., Starkopf, J., Alhazzani, W., Berger, M. M., Casaer, M. P., Deane, A. M., Fruhwald, S., Hiesmayr, M., Ichai, C., Jakob, S. M., Loudet, C. I., Malbrain, M. L., Montejo Gonzalez, J. C., Paugam-Burtz, C., Poeze, M., Preiser, J. C., Singer, P., van Zanten, A. R., De Waele, J., Wendon, J., Wernerman, J., Whitehouse, T., Wilmer, A., Oudemans-van Straaten, H. M, Function, E. W. G. o. G. (2017). Early enteral nutrition in critically ill patients: ESICM clinical practice guidelines. *Intensive Care Med*, *43*(3), 380-398. https://doi.org/10.1007/s00134-016-4665-0.

Reintam Blaser, A., Starkopf, J., Moonen, P. J., Malbrain, M., & Oudemans-van Straaten, H. M. (2018). Perioperative gastrointestinal problems in the ICU. *Anaesthesiol Intensive Ther*, *50*(1), 59-71. https://doi.org/10.5603/AIT.a2017.0064.

Saunders, M. D., & Kimmey, M. B. (2005). Systematic review: acute colonic pseudo-obstruction. Aliment Pharmacol Ther, *22*(10), 917-925. https://doi.org/10.1111/j.1365-2036.2005.02668.x.

Sessler, C. N., Gosnell, M. S., Grap, M. J., Brophy, G. M., O'Neal, P. V., Keane, K. A., Tesoro, E. P., Elswick, R. K. (2002). The Richmond Agitation-Sedation Scale: validity and reliability in adult intensive care unit patients. *Am J Respir Crit Care Med*, *166*(10), 1338-1344. https://doi.org/10.1164/rccm.2107138.

Sessler, D. I. (2008). Temperature monitoring and perioperative thermoregulation. *Anesthesiology*, *109*(2), 318-338. https://doi.org/10.1097/ALN.0b013e31817f6d76.

Shaikh, N., Kettern, M. A., Hanssens, Y., Elshafie, S. S., & Louon, A. (2008). A rare and unsuspected complication of Clostridium difficile infection. *Intensive Care Med*, *34*(5), 963-966. https://doi.org/10.1007/s00134-007-0922-6.

Slinger, P. (2014). From the Journal archives: Postoperative analgesia: effect on lung volumes. *Can J Anaesth*, *61*(2), 200-202. https://doi.org/10.1007/s12630-013-0085-6.

Smilowitz, N. R., & Berger, J. S. (2020). Perioperative Cardiovascular Risk Assessment and Management for Noncardiac Surgery: A Review. *Jama*, *324*(3), 279-290. https://doi.org/10.1001/jama.2020.7840.

Tao, R., Wang, X. W., Pang, L. J., Cheng, J., Wang, Y. M., Gao, G. Q., Liu, Y., & Wang, C. (2018). Pharmacologic prevention of postoperative delirium after on-pump cardiac surgery: A meta-analysis of randomized trials. *Medicine (Baltimore)*, *97*(43), e12771. https://doi.org/10.1097/MD.0000000000012771.

Tolwani, A. (2012). Continuous renal-replacement therapy for acute kidney injury. *N Engl J Med*, *367*(26), 2505-2514. https://doi.org/10.1056/NEJMct1206045.

Turan, A., Rivas, E., Devereaux, P. J., Bravo, M., Mao, G., Cohen, B., Maheshwari, K., Pu, X., Ruetzler, K., Li, K., & Sessler, D. I. (2021). Association between postoperative haemoglobin concentrations and composite of non-fatal myocardial infarction and all-cause mortality in noncardiac surgical patients: post hoc analysis of the POISE-2 trial. *Br J Anaesth*, *126*(1), 87-93. https://doi.org/10.1016/j.bja.2020.08.054.

Uray, K. S., Laine, G. A., Xue, H., Allen, S. J., & Cox, C. S., Jr. (2006). Intestinal edema decreases intestinal contractile activity via decreased myosin light chain phosphorylation. *Crit Care Med, 34*(10), 2630-2637. https://doi.org/10.1097/01.CCM.0000239195.06781.8C.

van der Kooi, A. W., Rots, M. L., Huiskamp, G., Klijn, F. A., Koek, H. L., Kluin, J., Leijten, F. S., & Slooter, A. J. (2014). Delirium detection based on monitoring of blinks and eye movements. *Am J Geriatr Psychiatry*, *22*(12), 1575-1582. https://doi.org10.1016/j.jagp.2014.01.001.

Vather, R., O'Grady, G., Bissett, I. P., & Dinning, P. G. (2014). Postoperative ileus: mechanisms and future directions for research. *Clin Exp Pharmacol Physiol, 41*(5), 358-370. https://doi.org/10.1111/1440-1681.12220.

Warden, V., Hurley, A. C., & Volicer, L. (2003). Development and psychometric evaluation of the Pain Assessment in Advanced Dementia (PAINAD) scale. *J Am Med Dir Assoc*, *4*(1), 9-15. https://doi.org/10.1097/01.JAM.0000043422.31640.F7.

Watne, L. O., Idland, A. V., Fekkes, D., Raeder, J., Frihagen, F., Ranhoff, A. H., Chaudhry, F. A., Engedal, K., Wyller, T. B., & Hassel, B. (2016). Increased CSF levels of aromatic amino acids in hip fracture patients with delirium suggests higher monoaminergic activity. *BMC Geriatr*, *16*, 149. https://doi.org/10.1186/s12877-016-0324-0.

Weiser, T. G., Haynes, A. B., Molina, G., Lipsitz, S. R., Esquivel, M. M., Uribe-Leitz, T., Fu, R., Azad, T., Chao, T. E., Berry, W. R., & Gawande, A. A. (2015). Estimate of the global volume of surgery in 2012: an assessment supporting improved health outcomes. *Lancet*, *385*(Suppl 2), S11. https://doi.org/10.1016/S0140-6736(15)60806-6.

Woodcock, T., Barker, P., Daniel, S., Fletcher, S., Wass, J. A. H., Tomlinson, J. W., Misra, U., Dattani, M., Arlt, W., & Vercueil, A. (2020). Guidelines for the management of glucocorticoids during the peri-operative period for patients with adrenal insufficiency: Guidelines from the Association of Anaesthetists, the Royal College of Physicians and the Society for Endocrinology UK. *Anaesthesia*, *75*(5), 654-663. https://doi.org/10.1111/anae.14963.

Wu, Y. C., Tseng, P. T., Tu, Y. K., Hsu, C. Y., Liang, C. S., Yeh, T. C., Chen, T. Y., Chu, C. S., Matsuoka, Y. J., Stubbs, B., Carvalho, A. F., Wada, S., Lin, P. Y., Chen, Y. W, & Su, K. P. (2019). Association of Delirium Response and Safety of Pharmacological Interventions for the Management and Prevention of Delirium: A Network Meta-analysis. *JAMA Psychiatry*, *76*(5), 526-535. https://doi.org/10.1001/jamapsychiatry.2018.4365.

Yang, Y., Zhao, X., Dong, T., Yang, Z., Zhang, Q., & Zhang, Y. (2017). Risk factors for postoperative delirium following hip fracture repair in elderly patients: a systematic review and meta-analysis. *Aging Clin Exp Res*, *29*(2), 115-126. https://doi.org/10.1007/s40520-016-0541-6.

Yoo, J. W., Synn, A., Huh, J. W., Hong, S. B., Koh, Y., & Lim, C. M. (2016). Clinical efficacy of high-flow nasal cannula compared to noninvasive ventilation in patients with post-extubation respiratory failure. *Korean J Intern Med*, *31*(1), 82-88. https://doi.org/10.3904/kjim.2016.31.1.82.

Zhu, Y., Yin, H., Zhang, R., & Wei, J. (2017). High-flow nasal cannula oxygen therapy vs conventional oxygen therapy in cardiac surgical patients: A meta-analysis. *J Crit Care*, *38*, 123-128. https://doi.org/10.1016/j.jcrc.2016.10.027.

Index

A

acute renal failure (ARF), 5, 13, 21, 169, 171, 181, 226, 292
anaesthetics, 70, 238, 259
aortic stenosis, 56, 58, 59, 62, 63, 66, 68, 99
aortic valve regurgitation, 99

B

blood transfusions, 83, 95, 176
brain damage, 136, 225, 234, 247

C

cancer, viii, 13, 34, 39, 69, 70, 71, 72, 73, 74, 75, 76, 77, 78, 79, 80, 82, 83, 84, 85, 86, 87, 88, 89, 90, 91, 92, 93, 94, 95, 96, 115, 127, 132, 209, 243
cancer treatment, viii, 69, 71, 73, 74, 76, 77, 80, 90, 91
cerebral perfusion, 9, 225, 247
chemotherapy, 29, 70, 71, 73, 74, 77, 78, 79, 80, 82, 84, 90, 91, 92, 93, 95, 199, 279
Child-Turcotte-Pugh (CTP), ix, 147, 150, 151, 157, 158
chronic liver disease (CLD), ix, 6, 10, 31, 38, 45, 48, 67, 147, 148, 154, 155, 161, 165
chronic obstructive pulmonary disease (COPD), 3, 5, 6, 8, 16, 17, 32, 39, 111, 121, 127, 128, 131, 137, 138, 141, 145, 271
chronic renal failure (CRF), 22, 35, 38, 50, 51, 52, 53, 59, 62, 63, 64, 65, 66, 67, 112, 168, 169, 176, 177, 183, 186
cirrhosis, ix, 3, 6, 7, 8, 10, 11, 12, 13, 14, 18, 19, 27, 28, 30, 31, 33, 34, 35, 36, 38, 45, 46, 47, 48, 58, 61, 78, 147, 148, 150, 151, 152, 155, 156, 157, 158, 159, 161, 162, 163, 164, 165, 204, 263, 264, 279
colloids, 2, 25, 26
critical care, vi, 32, 34, 35, 37, 65, 67, 144, 145, 146, 162, 164, 182, 184, 185, 222, 233, 245, 258, 261, 262, 290, 294

D

decreased clearance, 47, 168, 172
deep vein thrombosis (DVT), 114, 115, 116, 117, 157
delirium, xi, 9, 198, 228, 229, 241, 254, 261, 262, 281, 282, 283, 284, 287, 288, 289, 291, 292, 293, 294, 295, 296
diabetes mellitus, x, 81, 111, 187, 188, 189, 212, 215, 219, 264
dilated cardiomyopathy, 99

E

endocrine diseases, v, 81, 187, 188
end-stage liver disease model (MELD), ix, 18, 19, 27, 36, 147, 150, 151, 157, 158, 161, 165

F

fluid overload, x, 24, 103, 138, 167, 168, 171, 174, 180, 266, 279, 280, 293

G

glomerular filtration rate (GFR), x, 5, 13, 22, 50, 167, 168, 170, 173, 174, 178

H

heart failure, viii, 7, 9, 18, 21, 22, 27, 31, 32, 33, 37, 39, 44, 47, 51, 54, 65, 77, 97, 98, 99, 100, 101, 102, 103, 104, 105, 106, 107, 108, 110, 115, 116, 117, 118, 138, 153, 155, 262, 263, 264, 267, 268, 269, 270, 271, 272, 273, 274, 279, 288, 290, 292, 293, 294
hematological disorders, 70
high-pressure hypertrophy, 99
high-volume hypertrophy, 99
hormones, 76, 128, 150, 187, 188, 193, 194, 204, 212, 214, 218
hypercarbia, 120, 155, 180, 196, 197, 207, 246, 271, 275
hyperkalemia, 2, 20, 21, 25, 27, 35, 36, 38, 39, 52, 80, 128, 171, 181, 185, 237, 251, 254, 265, 266
hyperthyroidism, 193, 194, 195, 199, 218, 222, 223
hypertrophic obstructive cardiomyopathy, 99
hyponatremia, 2, 18, 19, 23, 32, 34, 79, 128, 152, 155, 156, 158, 180, 196, 197, 198, 212, 216, 282
hypothyroidism, 195, 196, 197, 198, 199, 216, 218, 219, 220, 222, 223
hypoxemia, 3, 51, 120, 128, 130, 131, 132, 136, 137, 142, 143, 153, 246, 274

I

inhalation anesthetics, 2, 3, 4, 86, 88, 90, 93, 108
intestinal failure, 262
intracranial pressure, 9, 214, 225, 234, 247, 260
intravenous anesthetics, 2, 5, 6, 86, 211, 252
IV anesthetics, 5

L

liver failure, v, vii, xi, 1, 14, 18, 20, 28, 32, 45, 46, 47, 61, 147, 148, 150, 151, 157, 160, 261, 262, 263, 269, 279, 280
local anesthetics (LA), 42, 44, 45, 46, 47, 52, 54, 56, 58, 65, 67, 87, 135, 232, 238, 293
low ejection fraction (HFrEF), viii, 97, 98, 99, 100, 102

M

maintenance of normovolemia, 168
major adverse cardiovascular events (MACEs), 98
myocardial stunning, 99

N

neuraxial blocks, 41, 42
neuro-anesthesia, 225
neurological disorders, x, 81, 124, 225, 226
nitrous oxide (N_2O), 3, 68, 88, 89, 179, 186, 231, 253, 259

O

organ failure, v, vi, vii, viii, 1, 2, 18, 26, 30, 41, 42, 57, 58, 80, 81, 141, 142, 234, 261, 262, 279, 287

P

pericardial diseases, 99
perioperative management, 39, 59, 63, 109, 148, 164, 187, 188, 202, 217, 219, 221, 222, 233, 254
peripheral arterial diseases, 97, 110, 111
peripheral nerve blocks (PNB), viii, 41, 42, 44, 45, 48, 50, 52, 53, 55, 56, 57, 59, 63
peripheral vein diseases, 97, 114
positive pressure ventilation (PPV), 25, 120, 121, 122, 123, 124, 126, 136, 137, 143, 181, 270, 273

post-infarct ventricular remodeling, 99
postoperative analgesia, 56, 57, 83, 108, 112, 115, 184
pre-anesthesia evaluation, 80
pulmonary embolism, 53, 114, 131

R

radiotherapy, 70, 71, 72, 73, 77, 78, 84, 90, 92
regional anesthesia, viii, 41, 42, 43, 45, 46, 48, 49, 52, 54, 57, 58, 60, 62, 63, 64, 67, 78, 85, 90, 112, 113, 115, 117, 134, 143, 155, 177, 197, 199
renal insufficiency, 32, 168, 183, 262
respiratory failure, ix, xi, 22, 119, 120, 124, 125, 126, 129, 130, 131, 132, 135, 136, 137, 138, 141, 142, 143, 154, 171, 200, 235, 261, 262, 270, 274, 275, 276, 279, 296
respiratory insufficiency, ix, 119, 133, 135, 241, 262
restrictive cardiomyopathy, 99

S

stem cells, 72
surgical treatment, 71, 73, 98, 105, 202, 211

T

thyroid diseases, 81, 193
total intravenous anesthesia (TIVA), 3, 95, 96, 161, 173, 179, 182, 184
Type 1 diabetes, 188
Type 2 diabetes, 189